# Register Now for Online Access to Your Book!

SPRINGER PUBLISHING
**C⏻NNECT™**

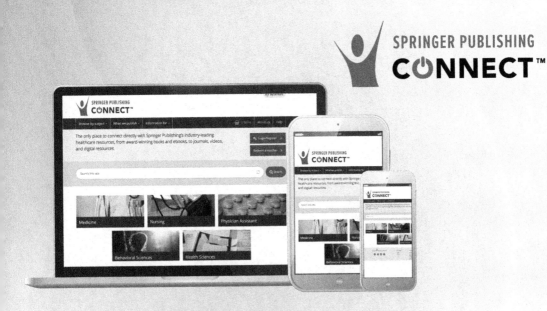

Your print purchase of *Public Health Law* **includes online access to the contents of your book**—increasing accessibility, portability, and searchability!

**Access today at:**
**http://connect.springerpub.com/content/book/978-0-8261-8204-3**
**or scan the QR code at the right with your smartphone**
**and enter the access code below.**

**TYEPB81C**

*Scan here for quick access.*

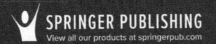
**SPRINGER PUBLISHING**
View all our products at springerpub.com

# PUBLIC HEALTH LAW

**Montrece McNeill Ransom, JD, MPH, ACC,** is a leadership coach, speaker, and professor, with almost 20 years of experience in public health. She has published, presented, and trained on a wide array of topics in public health and public health law and policy, and is an award-winning public health lawyer. She was awarded the Jennifer Robbins Award for the Practice of Public Health Law (American Public Health Association) in 2017 and the American Bar Association Champion for Diversity and Inclusion Award in 2019. She serves as faculty with Walden University's School of Health Sciences, where she teaches the Legal and Ethical Issues in Healthcare, serves as a dissertation mentor, and an instructor in Walden's Competency-Based Education (TEMPO) program. She is also a professor at California State University East Bay, where she teaches health regulation.

Professor Ransom earned her Executive Leadership Coaching Certification from Georgetown University, her law degree from the University of Alabama, and her Master of Public Health degree from Emory University's Rollins School of Public Health. Her undergraduate degree in Speech Communications was earned at Columbus State University. She is also a belonging strategist, certified trainer and facilitator, having received certification through the Association for Talent Development. She is the President-Elect of the American Society for Law, Medicine, and Ethics and serves on the Advisory Committee for the Georgia Campaign for Adolescent Power and Potential.

**Laura Magaña Valladares, PhD, MS,** joined the Association of Schools and Programs of Public Health (ASPPH) as President and CEO in August 2017. Under Dr. Magaña's leadership, ASPPH has continued to advance its mission to strengthen the capacity of members by advancing leadership, excellence, and collaboration for academic public health. During her tenure, ASPPH has significantly grown its global engagement, launched the academic public health leadership institute, and enhanced the voice of academic public health through advocacy efforts.

Prior to joining ASPPH, Dr. Magaña dedicated more than 35 years to successfully leading the transformation and advancements of public and private universities in Mexico, educational organizations in the United States, United Nations programs, and NGOs in Central America and Europe. She was most recently the dean of the School of Public Health in Mexico at the ASPPH-member National Institute of Public Health (INSP). Her diverse portfolio features 90 academic publications and educational technological developments, many of which relate to learning environments, the use of technology in education, and public health education. She has also been a faculty member and lecturer in diverse universities around the world.

# PUBLIC HEALTH LAW

## CONCEPTS AND CASE STUDIES

Montrece McNeill Ransom, JD, MPH, ACC

Laura Magaña Valladares, PhD, MS

EDITORS

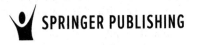
SPRINGER PUBLISHING

Springer Publishing Company, LLC
11 West 42nd Street, New York, NY 10036
www.springerpub.com
connect.springerpub.com/

*Acquisitions Editor*: David D'Addona
*Compositor*: Amnet Systems

*ISBN*: 978-0-8261-8203-6
*ebook ISBN*: 978-0-8261-8204-3
*DOI*: 10.1891/9780826182043

**SUPPLEMENTS:**
**Instructor Materials:**

*Qualified instructors may request supplements by emailing textbook@springerpub.com*
*Instructor's Manual ISBN*: 978-0-8261-8201-2
*Instructor's Test Bank ISBN*: 978-0-8261-8212-8
*Instructor's PowerPoints ISBN*: 978-0-8261-8215-9

21 22 23 24 / 5 4 3 2 1

The author and the publisher of this Work have made every effort to use sources believed to be reliable to provide information that is accurate and compatible with the standards generally accepted at the time of publication. The author and publisher shall not be liable for any special, consequential, or exemplary damages resulting, in whole or in part, from the readers' use of, or reliance on, the information contained in this book. The publisher has no responsibility for the persistence or accuracy of URLs for external or third-party Internet websites referred to in this publication and does not guarantee that any content on such websites is, or will remain, accurate or appropriate.

**Library of Congress Cataloging-in-Publication Data**

Names: Ransom, Montrece McNeill, editor. | Magaña, Laura, editor.
Title: Public health law : concepts and case studies / Montrece McNeill Ransom, Laura Magaña Valladares, editors.
Other titles: Public health law (Ransom)
Description: First Springer Publishing edition. | New York, NY : Springer Publishing Company, LLC 2021. | Includes bibliographical references and index.
Identifiers: LCCN 2020035385 (print) | LCCN 2020035386 (ebook) | ISBN 9780826182036 (paperback) | ISBN 9780826182043 (ebook)
Subjects: MESH: Public Health—legislation & jurisprudence | United States
Classification: LCC RA425 (print) | LCC RA425 (ebook) | NLM WA 33 AA1 | DDC 362.1—dc23
LC record available at https://lccn.loc.gov/2020035385
LC ebook record available at https://lccn.loc.gov/2020035386

Contact us to receive discount rates on bulk purchases.

**Publisher's Note:** New and used products purchased from third-party sellers are not guaranteed for quality, authenticity, or access to any included digital components.

Printed in the United States of America.

# CONTENTS

## Part III    LAW: A TRANSDISCIPLINARY PUBLIC HEALTH TOOL

# CONTRIBUTORS

**Rosa Abraha, MPH**   Public Health Advisor and Founder of Revamped by Rosa, Atlanta Georgia

**Sabrina Adler, JD**   Vice President of Law, ChangeLab Solutions, Oakland, California

**Emily Allender, JD**   University of Kentucky College of Law, Lexington, Kentucky

**Marice Ashe, JD, MPH**   Founder, ChangeLab Solutions, Public Health Law Consultant, Oakland, California

**Ana S. Ayala, JD, LLM**   Global Health Law and Policy Expert, Senior Global Health Officer, U.S. Department of Health and Human Services, Washington, DC

**Georges C. Benjamin, MD**   Executive Director, American Public Health Association, Washington, DC

**Molly Berkery, JD, MPH**   Senior Healthcare Regulatory Consultant, San Diego, California

**Alexandra Bhatti, JD, MPH**   Honors Adjunct Faculty, School for the Science of Health Care Delivery, College of Health Sciences, Arizona State University, Tempe, Arizona

**Derek Carr, JD**   Senior Attorney, ChangeLab Solutions, Oakland, California

**Michelle Castagne, JD**   California Tribal Families Coalition (Sault Ste. Marie Tribe of Chippewa Indians)

**Denise Chrysler, JD**   Director, Mid-States Region, Network for Public Health Law, Edina, Minnesota

**Lindsay K. Cloud, JD**   Director, Policy Surveillance Program, Center for Public Health Law Research, Temple University Beasley School of Law, Philadelphia, Pennsylvania

**Corey Davis, JD, MSPH**   Director, Harm Reduction Legal Project, Deputy Director, Southeast Region, Network for Public Health Law, Edina, Minnesota

**Kelly K. Dineen, PhD, JD, RN**   Associate Professor of Law, Director, Health Law Program, Creighton University, Omaha, Nebraska

**Jessika Douglas, BSHP, MPA, CHES** Department of Social Sciences, Katherine Reese Pamplin College of Arts, Humanities, and Social Sciences, Augusta University, Augusta, Georgia

**Lance Gable, JD, MPH** Associate Professor of Law, Wayne State University Law School, Detroit, Michigan

**Maxim Gakh, JD, MPH** Associate Professor, School of Public Health, Associate Director, University of Nevada, Las Vegas (UNLV) Health Law Program, UNLV, Las Vegas, Nevada

**Siobhan Gilchrist, JD, MPH** Public Health Policy Analyst, IHRC, Inc., in service of Division for Heart Disease and Stroke Prevention, Centers for Disease Control and Prevention, Atlanta, Georgia

**Roojin Habibi, JD, MSc** Fellow, Osgoode Hall Law School and Global Strategy, York University, Toronto, Canada

**Tina Batra Hershey, JD, MPH** Associate Professor, Department of Health Policy and Management, Graduate School of Public Health, Affiliated Professor of Law, School of Law, University of Pittsburgh, Pittsburgh, Pennsylvania

**James G. Hodge, Jr., JD, LLM** Peter Kiewit Foundation Professor of Law, Sandra Day O'Connor College of Law, Arizona State University, Phoenix, Arizona

**Aila Hoss, JD** Assistant Professor of Law, Native American Law Center, University of Tulsa College of Law, Tulsa, Oklahoma

**Mara Howard-Williams, MPH** JD Candidate, University of North Carolina School of Law, Chapel Hill, North Carolina

**Peter D. Jacobson, JD, MPH** Professor Emeritus of Health Law and Policy, Director, Center for Law, Ethics, and Health, University of Michigan School of Public Health, Ann Arbor, Michigan

**Priscilla Keith, JD, MS** Director, Program Management, RIP Medical Debt, New York, New York

**Stacie P. Kershner, JD** Associate Director, Center for Law, Health & Society, Georgia State University College of Law, Atlanta, Georgia

**Fazal Khan, JD, MD** Associate Professor, University of Georgia School of Law, Atlanta, Georgia

**M. Killian Kinney, PhD, MSW, LSW** Postdoctoral Fellow, Wayne State University School of Social Work, Detroit, Michigan

**Donna E. Levin, JD** National Director, The Network for Public Health Law, Edina, Minnesota

**Laura Magaña Valladares, PhD, MS** President and CEO, Association of Schools and Programs of Public Health, Washington, DC

**Keri McDonald Hill, PhD, MPH, CHES**  Director of School-Based Initiatives, Georgia Campaign for Adolescent Power & Potential, Faculty, Department of Health Promotion and Physical Education, Kennesaw State University, Kennesaw, Georgia

**Angela K. McGowan, JD, MPH**  Senior Director, Alliance for Disease Prevention and Response, American Public Health Association, Washington, DC

**Benjamin Mason Meier, PhD, JD, LLM**  Professor of Global Health Policy, University of North Carolina at Chapel Hill, Chapel Hill, North Carolina, and Senior Scholar, O'Neill Institute for National and Global Health Law, Georgetown University, Washington, DC

**Gabrielle Metoyer, MPH**  Associate, Strategic Initiatives, Emory University School of Medicine and Assistant, The Empowermenteur Coaching and Consulting Group, LLC, Atlanta, Georgia

**Harry Nelson, Esq.**  Founder and Managing Partner, Nelson Hardiman, LLP, Los Angeles, California

**Christopher Ogolla, JD, MA, MPH, LLM, BA**  Assistant Professor of Law, Dwayne O. Andreas School of Law, Barry University, Orlando, Florida

**Shade O. Olowookere, MPH, MHA**  Global Public Health Analyst and Associate Research Scientist, Global Health Institute, University of Georgia, Athens, Georgia

**Hayley Penan, JD, MPH**  Deputy Legislative Counsel, State of California Office of Legislative Counsel, Sacramento, California

**Jennifer L. Piatt, JD**  Research Scholar, Center for Public Health Law and Policy, Arizona State University, Phoenix, Arizona

**Montrece McNeill Ransom, JD, MPH, ACC**  Founder, The Empowermenteur Coaching and Consulting Group, LLC, Director, National Coordinating Center for Public Health Training, National Network of Public Health Institutes, Professor, College of Health Sciences, Walden University, and Department of Health Sciences, California State University East Bay

**Floribella Redondo, CHW, BS**  Executive Director, Arizona Community Health Worker Association, Inc., Tucson, Arizona

**Nathan Roush, JD**  Lawyer, Atlanta, Georgia

**Emely Sanchez, JD, MPH**  Public Health Policy Consultant and Founder, Sanchez Solutions, LLC, Washington, DC

**Sharada Shantharam, MPH**  Health Scientist, IHRC, Inc., in service of Division for Heart Disease and Stroke Prevention, Centers for Disease Control and Prevention, Atlanta, Georgia

**Ross D. Silverman, JD, MPH**  Professor, Departments of Health Policy and Management, Indiana University Richard M. Fairbanks School of Public Health, Indiana University Robert H. McKinney School of Law, Indianapolis, Indiana

**LeKara Simmons, MPH, CHES**  Program Manager, College-Based Initiatives, Georgia Campaign for Adolescent Power & Potential, Atlanta, Georgia

**Jason A. Smith, JD, MTS**   ACE Fellow 2021–2022; Associate Professor, California State University East Bay, Hayward, California

**Daniella Thorne, DrPH, MPH, CHES**   W.I.S.E. Program Manager, Georgia Campaign for Adolescent Power and Potential, Atlanta, Georgia

**Lauren Tonti, JD, MPH**   Doctoral Candidate, Max Planck Institute for Social Law & Social Policy, Munich, Germany

**Troy Viger, JD**   Georgia State College of Law, Atlanta, Georgia

**Heather A. Walter-McCabe, JD, MSW**   Associate Faculty, Wayne State University School of Social Work and School of Law, Detroit, Michigan

**Ashley Wennerstrom, PhD, MPH**   Associate Professor, Department of Behavioral and Community Health Sciences, School of Public Health, Center for Healthcare Value and Equity, Louisiana State University Health Sciences Center, New Orleans, Louisiana

**Sarah Wetter, JD, MPH**   Associate, O'Neill Institute for National and Global Health Law, Georgetown University, Washington, DC

**Benjamin D. Winig, JD, MPA**   Founder, ThinkForward Strategies, Walnut Creek, California

**Dana Reed Wise, MPH**   Bureau Chief, Environmental Health, Marion County Public Health Department, Indianapolis, Indiana

**Brianne Bostian Yassine, PhD, MPH, CHES**   Public Health Workforce Education Specialist, University of Georgia College of Education, Athens, Georgia

**Lena Amanti Yueh, JD, MPH**   Health Lawyer, Atlanta, Georgia

# FOREWORD

In 1990, I moved from being the chairman of a department of ambulatory care and community medicine and a practicing emergency physician at the District of Columbia General Hospital in Washington, D.C., to being the health commissioner for public health of our nation's capital. During my time in clinical and administrative medicine, I had a clear understanding of the law and regulatory environment as it applied to outpatient medical care, my hospital, the emergency department, and the emergency medical services in the city. When I became the health commissioner, I suddenly found myself being the top health regulator and health policymaker for a city of 600,000 residents (and over 1 million people during the day when you include commuters). That position came with an enormous increase in responsibility, a sizable jump in the workforce and budget, and a much more complex organization to run. In this role, I had to not only manage the clinical aspects of an outpatient medical system, but also provide oversight of two nursing homes, the medical examiner office, and a host of traditional public health programs.

Actually, I was ready for the managerial task ahead because of sound training in medicine and well-established experience as a health administrator from my previous jobs. But like many of my colleagues who suddenly find themselves in senior public health positions, I was initially unprepared for the profound public health authorities I now processed. Public health is all about policy, and policy assurance is all about one's public health authorities under the law. Most of the early responsibilities I found myself charged with required a full understanding of existing law, regulation, and practice, and my role as an enforcer of these authorities was a tool to protect the public.

My goal became to understand the legal parameters of my new position and how to best use these authorities in a sound and ethical manner using the best science available to guide my decision-making. Initially, I solely relied on knowledgeable staff to advise me, but my most profound discovery was the Code of the District of Columbia. The DC Code is the bible of legal authorities for the nation's capital. This very dry but essential reading defines the parameters of our legal public health world and the rules under which we all live, often unknowingly, and that I was now entrusted to enforce.

For example, as a clinician I understood the childhood vaccine requirements for Washington, D.C., but until I became the health commissioner, I had no role in assuring children had their shots as required by law. Early in my tenure we worked as a region to increase childhood vaccination rates through both education and regulatory actions. Working with my program and legal staff, we had to set our health goals, develop a program strategy, and do so within the context of existing law as well as the practicalities and limits of enforcement. We had to work with the educational system and ensure what we wanted to do was harmonized with law, school policy, and acceptable public health practice. We were successful, but I did have to spend a lot of time reading Title 7 of the Code of the District of Columbia, "Human Health Care and Safety." Later, I had to become acquainted with Title 8 as well, "Environmental and Animal Control and Protection." You see, we provided oversight to the animal shelter through a contract with the D.C. Humane Society and also oversaw a lead hazard and exposure program.

There was a separate department of the environment, but we in public health were of course consulted when several city sanitary workers presented with health problems among workplace exposures to toxins and possible occupationally related disease. My clinical experience was a plus, but I had to learn a lot very quickly abut occupational health law.

I remember signing my first commitment to quarantine a noncompliant patient with tuberculosis, making a regulatory decision concerning a failed restaurant inspection, and managing the intricacy of a hospital closure.

I left my first public health experience to return to the world of emergency medicine but kept my hand in health policy to later return to public health at the state level. First, I became the deputy health officer for public health services and then secretary of health for the state of Maryland. One of my first activities upon appointment was to meet with my department's lawyers and get a broad overview of the legal framework in Maryland and the legal challenges facing the department. My next step was to read, cover to cover, the 24 titles of Maryland Code Health—General. Another dry but essential read. But it made my passage through this 8-year experience productive and effective.

Along the way I learned a lot about the basics of public health law through both my readings and practice experience. I got better over time, but it was sometimes painful and always challenging.

Public health is indeed challenging, but it does not need to be painful, at least from a legal perspective. This text, *Public Health Law: Concepts and Case Studies*, is an excellent tool for improving upon your knowledge of key public health legal concepts. The book puts these concepts into a practice framework through a case study approach. It covers the essential experience of public health practice through a legal framework to aid in effective decision-making. Individuals who work through the 11 cases in this book and who are early in their careers will be better prepared as they enter the field as public health practitioners. Students at the graduate level will find this text a useful way to enhance their public health legal education. It is also an essential read for those who are mid-career when they suddenly, and without warning, find themselves as the chief health strategist for their communities.

*Georges C. Benjamin, MD*
Executive Director
American Public Health Association
Washington, DC

# PREFACE

This book arises from two core beliefs: (1) law is one of the most significant determinants of health; and, (2) a basic understanding of law—as the foundation for public health practice and as an interventional tool—is vital for the effective practice of public health in the 21st century. There is no public health without the law. From the creation of a health department (which is achieved by statute) to a law requiring a state prescription drug monitoring program, law creates the frameworks to make healthy choices the norm.

In today's complex environment where science, policy, and law significantly impact public health programs and health outcomes, it is important that current and emerging public health practitioners and researchers, across the spectrum of public health practice, understand the role of law in advancing the public health goals of the communities they serve. Yet, understanding and analyzing the relationship between law and health outcomes continues to be one of the primary knowledge gaps among public health students and the public health workforce.

Let's face it, the law can be scary. But whether it is by way of policy development or enforcement of existing laws, public health law touches the work of every public health practitioner. The lessons we are learning about the causes of health inequities and the impact of social determinants on our health highlight how law and the legal system necessarily shape our environments and life circumstances, and consequently, influence our health and well-being.

Our goal was to create a textbook that makes law less scary and that empowers students, public health practitioners, and researchers to see law as simply another tool in their toolbox— just like epidemiology, surveillance, biostatistics, and other traditional public health tools. Simply put, we set about creating this textbook because we believe a public health workforce competent in public health law can lead their communities to better well-being and health outcomes. Our hope is that those who study the pages of this book recognize the vastness of public health law and its myriad applications to public health practice and research. Furthermore, we want readers to understand that public health law is constantly evolving, and that law is not, and cannot be, strictly the domain of lawyers. Public health law couples legal might with scientific insight and provides opportunities for public health practitioners to embed evidenced-based, scientific advances into our legal system to protect and advance public health and well-being. By its very nature, public health law is transdisciplinary.

*Public Health Law: Concepts and Case Studies* addresses major topics in public health law and aims to provide a diversity of learners (from beginners to experienced public health practitioners and researchers) with a practice-based overview of the field. It provides students and public health professionals with context and essential concepts in law across a selection of public health topics. This textbook can help students, practitioners, and researchers develop the vocabulary and savvy necessary to engage in productive conversations with their peers, the public, policymakers, partners, and lawyers about laws impacting individual well-being and public health. Additionally, this book is user friendly and easy to read.

This text is also meant to build upon and pay homage to the work of Rick Goodman et al., in the second edition of *Law in Public Health Practice* (Oxford University Press, 2007). Like that text, each chapter in this book is authored by a team of experts in law and public health.

However, this book can be distinguished from the Goodman book, and other public health law-related texts, in at least three ways. First, although we recognize its utility across health-related disciplines, *Public Health Law: Concepts and Case Studies* is specifically designed to be used primarily by undergraduate- and graduate-level schools and programs in public health and by practicing public health professionals. Second, this book is carefully designed for the adult learner and is competency-based. Each chapter includes competency statements from at least one of the three competency models developed by the Centers for Disease Control and Prevention's (CDC) Public Health Law Program, as well as learning objectives that describe the desired results of reading the chapter. Each chapter also includes key terminology, "spark" questions, chapter review questions, and additional resources to help advance learning. Third, this book can be distinguished from others on public health law because it has a health equity underpinning, in that each chapter features a call-out box with health equity-related principles and theories relevant to that chapter's topic.

*Public Health Law: Concepts and Case Studies* is organized into three parts. Part I offers five chapters that cover key legal concepts undergirding the practice of public health and that discuss the origins and nature of the law as it relates to public health. Part II features chapters focused on topics most prevalent in academic public health program areas and many that are addressed in national public health strategies. At the heart of the 11 chapters in Part II are hypothetical case studies, inspired by the traditional law school exam format. These case studies are designed to illustrate how law impacts public health practice in a variety of settings and are intended to help students and practitioners learn how to spot potential legal issues and identify when law might be a tool for, or perhaps a barrier to, effective public health practice. Part III has five chapters exploring the transdisciplinary and multi-sectoral nature of the practice and implementation of public health law and includes discussions of law and public health decision-making, law as a social determinant of health, health in all policies, and legal epidemiology. For instructors who adopt this text, we have also designed several ancillary materials, including an instructor's guide and accompanying lecture slides.

We are indebted to many people for their encouragement, ideas, and considerable effort in the creation of this book. First, we would like to thank the dedicated, brilliant group of public health and public health law professionals who served as authors and contributed to making this book a reality. They are masters at their craft, and we were privileged to work with them. Colleagues at the CDC's Public Health Law Program, the American Public Health Association, the Network for Public Health Law, and the Association of Schools and Programs of Public Health served as important resources and were incredibly supportive of this effort. We thank you all—those who are listed in this book as chapter authors and those who are too numerous to list but whose contributions and inspiration nevertheless measure large. We are also deeply proud of the diversity of our contributors, and are honored to make this contribution to the field. We acknowledge, with gratitude, the valuable advice we received from Fred Shaw, Matthew Penn, and Marice Ashe during the early planning stages of this book. Special thanks to Gabrielle Metoyer, MPH student at Emory University's Rollins School of Public Health, who was gracious enough to read each chapter and was instrumental in ensuring the quality and usefulness of this book from a student perspective. We are also immensely grateful to Andrea Ciria, Executive Editorial Assistant, who contributed her editorial expertise to ensuring the quality and coherence of each chapter of the text. Finally, but perhaps most importantly, we thank our families who have supported and encouraged us as we worked on this project. Thank you for your inspiration, patience and understanding.

*Montrece McNeill Ransom*
*Laura Magaña Valladares*

# INTRODUCTION

## Getting the Most Out of This Text

*"In the realm of public health…it's the law that really does the work. That's been demonstrated time and time again in areas ranging from mandating vaccinations to requiring automobile seatbelts; improving workplace safety; the inspection of meat products; and fluoridation of water. Public health succeeds by making healthy choices the norm."*

MICHAEL BLOOMBERG, Mayor of New York City, 2002–2013
In an address at the Harvard School of Public Health, October 29, 2007

## INTRODUCTION

### Defining Public Health Law

On March 9, 2020, Governor Mike DeWine of Ohio signed an executive order declaring a public health emergency, and on March 12, the state became the first in the nation to close schools in an effort to stop the spread of SARS-CoV-2, the virus that causes COVID-19 (Executive Order 2020-01D, 2020). States across the country quickly followed suit as the impact of the virus on state health systems became dire. DeWine and other governors used public health legal tools within their authority and at their disposal to balance the needs of students and parents with the urgent need to protect the health of the community—particularly the states' most vulnerable citizens.

Public health law can be defined as the legal powers and duties of the state, defined to include state, Tribal, local, and territorial governments, to ensure the conditions for people to be healthy, and the limitations on the power of the state to constrain the autonomy, privacy, liberty, proprietary, or other legally protected interests of individuals for the protection and promotion of community health (Gostin, 2007). This definition underscores the fact that when practitioners take steps in the name of public health, they must be mindful of balancing both the needs of the community as well as those of the individual. Public health law, whether in an emergency or in routine situations, is a balancing act between keeping the public healthy and protecting individual freedoms. And, in this balancing, individual rights must at times give way to the common good. As stated by Justice Harlan in the seminal case of *Jacobson v. Massachusetts*, "…there are manifold restraints to which we are all necessarily subject for the common good." (*Jacobson v. Massachusetts*, 1905).

Consider this through the lens of the everyday practice of public health. To ensure community immunity against a specific infectious disease, a state may enforce a vaccination requirement for school attendance, and in doing so, might impact individual autonomy, or a person's ability to choose for themselves. Public health might infringe on a person's privacy when a practitioner, complying with mandatory reporting requirements for the protection of children, reports child abuse to the appropriate officials. Enforcing an isolation or quarantine order, to prevent the spread of an infectious disease, may implicate liberty interests by limiting a person's movements. Proprietary interests may be impacted when a public health official suspends the license of a restaurant owner.

## Public Health Law's Two Major Domains: A Sailboat Analogy

Public health law can be further organized into two major categories or domains: (1) foundational and (2) interventional. Foundational public health law concerns itself with the legal authority for public health action, sources of law, and constitutional principles. This domain of public health law has also been called infrastructural law (Moulton et al., 2009). Interventional public health law includes specific laws implemented and enforced by public health practitioners to promote and protect the public's health.

Think about it like a sailboat. The hull forms the foundation of the sailboat. Without it, there is no footing, structure, or base. The sails are used to power the sailboat, and the rudder guides it in the right direction, keeps it on the right course toward the destination or goal. Similarly, foundational public health law—which consists of constitutional frameworks and legal authorities for public health practice—forms the base of the system in which public health practitioners operate. An example of a foundational public health law is a statute that establishes a state or local health department and authorizes its actions. And, just as the sail powers the sailboat

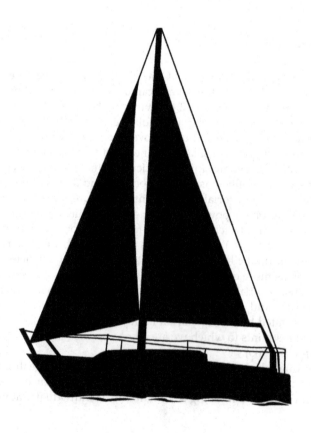

and the rudder steers and changes its direction, interventional public health law can be used to steer society toward better health choices and change the context in which people live, learn, play, worship, work, and age. It has been said that public health law can deliver a public health intervention to hundreds of thousands of individuals with the stroke of a pen (Burris et al., 2016). Examples of interventional public health laws include local clean indoor air ordinances and state prescription drug monitoring or vaccine laws.

## Public Health Law Is Transdisciplinary

A sailboat also needs a captain, officers, sailors, a deck crew, maintenance workers, etc.—a variety of players, with multiple skillsets, to move it forward. As does public health law. This book is intended for graduate and undergraduate students in schools and programs in public health, as well as current public health practitioners, because public health law is not and cannot be strictly the domain of lawyers. It is, by its nature, transdisciplinary. The transdisciplinary model couples legal might with scientific insight and it provides opportunities to embed scientific advances into our legal systems and structures (Burris et al., 2016).

The coupling of law and public health is not new. Law is a tool that has been used to advance public health goals for centuries. Consider the 10 Public Health Achievements of the 20th Century (CDC, 1999). Advancements in vaccinations, healthier mothers and babies, reduction in heart disease and stroke, safer drinking water—just to name a few—all can be attributed to linking scientific and legal elements. A transdisciplinary approach.

## Integrating Public Health and the Law: A Historical Example

One illustrative example of the impact of coupling legal might with public health insight comes from New York City in the late 19th Century. By the mid-19th century, the population in America's urban centers began to explode, and New York City was doubling in population size every decade from the early 1800s to 1880 (Garfield, 2017). Population density and unsanitary human waste disposal, including outdoor privies and cesspools, began to prove both inadequate and unsafe, especially when located near water sources.

There were calls for comprehensive sanitary reform in the city as early as 1832, in response to a cholera outbreak. The New York City Medical Society strongly urged the establishment of emergency hospitals, the disinfection of cesspools and privies, and a clean-up of streets, yards, and vacant lots. But the city government ignored the Medical Society's suggestions. A total of 3,513 persons died during that epidemic, mostly in poorer neighborhoods (Olsen, 2015). In 1848, cholera struck again, this time spreading beyond the slums and infecting the rich and the poor alike (Olsen, 2015). Newspapers reported that several of the cholera victims were members of the "respectable classes, including even ladies" (Miller, 1998). The calls for sanitary reforms could no longer be ignored.

One of the most immediate reforms after the outbreak was the development of a sewer system. However, despite the new sewer system, street cleaning and regular trash collection were not widely available. Only those who could afford those services received them. In the absence of regular garbage collection, pigs were allowed to roam the streets and convert at least a portion of the waste to food (Liboiron, 2013). Garbage, including dead animals, horse urine and manure, food waste, used furniture, and other filth, accumulated on the streets and alleyways in the city's neighborhoods, as shown in Figure I.1 (Liboiron, 2013). The stench was so bad that "travelers six miles away could rely on their noses to tell them when they were approaching the city" (Zeliadt, 2010).

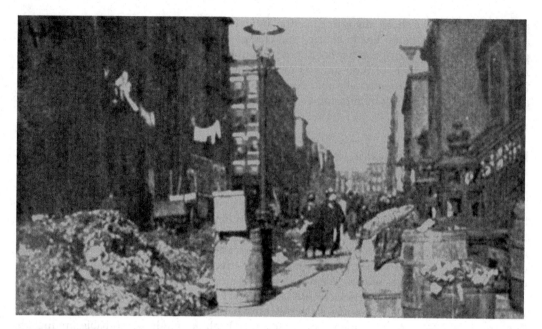

**FIGURE I.1** Varick Street in 1893 New York City.

Comprehensive sanitary reform did not occur until 1895, with the appointed Commissioner of Street Cleaning in New York City (Olsen, 2015). Waring was a Civil War colonel and a sanitary engineer who recognized the need for better drainage and sewer systems that would keep domestic waste away from drinking wells to better protect the population from the infectious disease epidemics common during this period. He was an early designer and advocate of sewer systems that kept domestic sewage separate from storm runoff, and before his appointment in New York City, Waring helped the city of Memphis end its era of epidemics by constructing a separated sewer system (Olsen, 2015).

Waring applied this scientific insight to lead New York City through a massive clean-up effort. As Commissioner of Street Cleaning, Waring used his legal authority (foundational public health law) to establish a Street Cleaning Department, a white-uniformed corps of workers pushing wheeled carts who were tasked with cleaning up city streets (Sante, 1991). Waring created a system for hauling away trash from all neighborhoods, regardless of socioeconomic status, and initiated a law that required horses and carts to be stabled overnight, instead of being left on the street (interventional public health law). Waring's men cleared a shin-deep accumulation of waste across the city. Horse carcasses were removed from the streets and sold for glue; horse manure was sold for fertilizer. Other refuse was sent to dumps along the waterfront. Waring's crew even removed snow, packing it into trucks and dumping it into the rivers (Sante, 1991).

As depicted in Figure I.2, Waring's efforts were successful in that they highlighted the crucial role of sanitation in improving the public's health. Although Waring served as New York's sanitation commissioner for only 3 years, his reforms had a lasting impact. His efforts changed the image of the sanitation department and introduced the fundamentals that would lead to modern systems of recycling, street-cleaning, and waste collection. (White Wings, n.d.). The sanitary reforms of Waring's era led to decreased disease burden and mortality and set the stage for sanitary reforms across the country. Today, New York City's Department of Sanitation is one of the largest in the world (Liboiron, 2013). Not only is the department responsible for trash and snow, but its public health service has been extended to disaster response, providing first responder services after the September 11, 2001, terrorist attacks and Hurricane Sandy (Liboiron, 2013).

Pivotal moments like the story of New York City sanitation reform, and others explored in this text, are important because they show how both foundational and interventional public

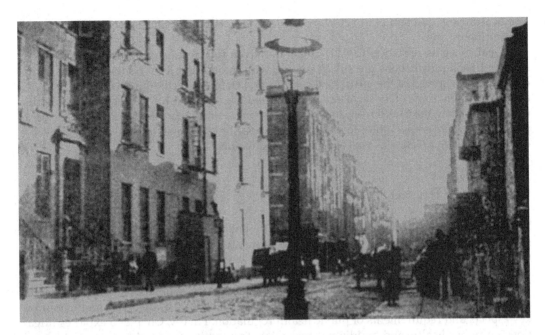

**FIGURE I.2**  Varick Street in 1895 New York City.

health law, when integrated with public health and scientific insight, can lead to improved health outcomes.

## BUILDING THE CAPACITY OF THE MODERN PUBLIC HEALTH PRACTITIONER

Today's public health challenges are daunting, including an increasing aging population; the burden of the social determinants of health leading to increased mortality and morbidity from chronic and other noncommunicable diseases; national disasters; the opioid epidemic; the health impacts of climate change and environmental pollution; and the rapid transfer of infectious pathogens and the potential for global pandemics. As we go to print with this text, public health agencies, healthcare workers, emergency managers, policymakers, and partners across the health spectrum are grappling with core public health legal issues as they work to mitigate the impact of the COVID-19 pandemic in the United States and around the world.

The pandemic has raised a host of foundational public health law-related constitutional questions about the distribution of power among the federal, state, and local governments, and how state and local governments can use their police powers to implement and enforce social distancing policies. Legal issues related to the use of quarantine and isolation, civil liberties and human rights, data sharing, and privacy are just a few of the interventional law-related issues that public health practitioners are dealing with in response to COVID-19.

The COVID-19 pandemic has also served to highlight significant health inequities in the United States and globally. Communities of color, people with low income, immigrants, and other underserved groups are disproportionately impacted by the virus. These groups are particularly vulnerable because of our system of existing laws and policies that impact the fundamental drivers of health inequities (Rojas et al., 2020). "The law, our legal systems and legal structures exert a powerful influence on health by structuring, perpetuating, and mediating the risk factors and underlying conditions known as the social determinants of health: education, food, housing, income, employment, sanitation, and health care" (Gostin et al., 2019, p. 1859). The COVID-19 pandemic provides a vivid illustration of this.

Legal concerns related to COVID-19 are not given full treatment in this text since many state and local jurisdictions are still grappling with the myriad legal issues associated with controlling the spread of the virus. However, several chapters, including Chapters 6, 7, 10, 11, and 14, highlight some of the legal issues at play and their relationship to specific public health topics. Ultimately, the COVID-19 pandemic has served to underscore the need for public health practitioners, across specialties, to increase their capacity to understand and use law in every-day public health practice, as well as emergency situations.

## Components of This Text

Part I is aimed at ensuring that readers from different backgrounds or levels of study share some key concepts and principles related to foundational public health law. To that end, Chapter 1 examines the structure of the U.S. legal system and the sources of authority for public health action. Chapter 2 provides an overview of key constitutional principles, including federalism and police powers. Preemption, which places limitations on public health action, is explored in Chapter 3. Chapter 4 focuses on administrative law and examines key aspects and requirements of public health regulation. Finally, Chapter 5 explores litigation and public health, and highlights cases related to obesity, food poisoning, opioids, and bleach poisoning.

Part II focuses on interventional public health law or law as a public health tool. Through hypothetical case studies, a feature of each chapter in Part II, readers will learn the instrumental role that law plays in 21st-century public health practice. As explored in Chapter 6, vaccination law helps to ensure high community immunity thresholds are maintained by maximizing the number of people who are vaccinated for each of the 18 vaccine-preventable diseases. Chapter 7 discusses how law can be used to prevent and control the spread of infectious diseases. Legal tools can also be used to define the scope of practice for chronic disease prevention and health equity, as addressed in Chapter 8. While approaches may vary, states are also enacting laws like "Erin's Law" to promote adolescent sexual health, as addressed in Chapter 9. Another example of modern applications of law as an intervention in the area of opioid use disorder, which is the subject of Chapter 10. As described in Chapter 11, laws and legal frameworks equip government agencies with the tools and processes necessary to effectively prepare for and appropriately respond to public health emergencies. Modern public health practitioners are also beginning to understand ways in which public health law and global health governance, discussed in Chapter 12, can help foster coordination and build public health capacity across the globe. And, local governments can use law and regulations to address environmental public health issues, such as healthy housing, as outlined in Chapter 13.

Law is also being used to address population-specific public health issues. For example, as discussed in Chapter 14, in the context of public health practice, laws and legal frameworks govern the relationships between Tribes, states, and the federal government. Public health also has a role in understanding how law can be used to promote the health of LGBTQ communities, as addressed in Chapter 15. Further, law can be used as a barrier to or facilitator for a woman's access to reproductive and sexual healthcare, as described in Chapter 16.

Part III offers five chapters that describe public health law as a transdisciplinary tool. Chapter 17 defines and discusses racism as a public health issue. Law-based approaches to health in all policies are discussed in Chapter 18. Legal epidemiology, defined as the scientific study of the impact of law on health, is addressed in Chapter 19. Chapter 20 is focused on public health ethics and the law. Finally, public health decision-making and liability are discussed in Chapter 21.

## GETTING THE MOST OUT OF THIS TEXT

Each chapter was designed with the readers' engagement and active participation in mind. So, getting the most out of this text involves taking advantage of the learning activities featured in each chapter. These learning activities include not only chapter review questions, but also a Spark Question(s) (at the beginning of the chapter) to ignite the reader's thinking, as well as a set of internet activities that have been crafted to allow the reader to assess and apply what they've learned from the reading. These appear at the end of the chapter. Examples of internet activities include online scavenger hunt activities and legal research tasks that allow the reader to explore public health laws in their jurisdiction. Several chapters also feature links to the Public Health Law Academy, an online, on-demand portal of trainings in public health law.

### Reflect on the Law-Related Competencies Covered by Each Chapter

*Public Health Law: Concepts and Case Studies* is a competency-based text. At the beginning of each chapter, the reader will find at least two public health law competencies that the chapter addresses. Competencies are logical building blocks upon which assessments of educational and professional development can be based. The chapters also include chapter objectives that outline the substantive areas covered. The competencies and chapter objectives ensure that readers have a common understanding of the specific knowledge and skills that they should gain as a result of studying the chapter. Readers have the opportunity to apply the knowledge they learned by completing chapter review questions and internet activities.

The competencies relied on for this textbook are derived from one or more of the three competency models developed by CDC's Public Health Law Program:

a. the public health emergency law competency model,
b. the public health law competency model, and
c. the legal epidemiology competency model.

These competency models expand upon and give context to the law and policy-related competencies identified by the Council on Education for Public Health (CEPH) and the Association of Schools and Programs of Public Health. This is important because public health law, as a distinct policy tool, is not specifically contemplated in the foundational competencies for Master of Public Health (MPH) students. Rather, the CEPH competencies include statements that highlight the need, for example, to ensure students can "compare regulatory systems across national and international settings" (CEPH MPH Competency #5; Council on Education for Public Health, 2016) and "discuss multiple dimensions of the policy-making process, including the roles of ethics and evidence" (CEPH MPH Competency #12; Council on Education for Public Health, 2016). If graduating public health students are to have a grounding in these competencies, in particular, it is critical that they understand the basics of public health law.

Because each chapter touches on health equity and calls out specific health equity principles, this text also effectively supports achievement of the CEPH competencies focused on health equity (CEPH MPH Competency #15) and the social determinants (CEPH MPH Competency #6).

This text, and the three law-based competency models upon which it relies, also supports CEPH competencies related to leadership and systems thinking can also be strengthened by a firm understanding of foundational public health law. Through case studies, this text also brings a practical perspective to how policy-related CEPH competencies are implicated and applied in the day-to-day public health practice.

To benefit fully from this text, readers should take note of the competencies that each chapter addresses. As they move through the chapter, readers should reflect on how each section of that chapter has increased their knowledge base in that specific competency and ways that competency might be applied beyond reading the text or the classroom environment. For example, a reader might pause after reading each major chapter section, and ask themselves, "What have I learned about this competency so far?" or "What does this mean in public health practice?" "How might the concepts and principles presented in the chapter be applicable to other public health issues?" This is a form of active learning that can help with comprehension of information, knowledge transfer, and decision-making.

## Look for the Health Equity Discussion in Each Chapter

*Health equity is* the "attainment of the highest level of health for all people" (CDC, 2019). Health disparities are the preventable differences in the health of one group over another as the result of factors such as race, sexual orientation, gender, disability, age, socioeconomic status, or geographic location (CDC, 2019).

While health equity and health disparities are two distinct concepts in public health, they are necessarily linked. Health equity can be achieved **only** by eliminating health disparities. Law is central to this pursuit. In fact, law itself is a determinant of health, as alluded to above and articulated in Chapter 17. As acknowledged in a *Lancet* report on the legal determinants of health, "law can...be a formidable barrier to achieving global health and equity" (Gostin et al., 2019, p. 1859). One obvious example of this is in the "separate but equal" doctrine that allowed racial segregation in housing, healthcare, education, employment, transportation. We see the consequences of this specific use of law today, in seemingly undefeatable health disparities.

As such, rather than limiting this discussion to one chapter on health equity and the law, each chapter in this text features a call-out box with a quote or statistic related to health equity or health disparities or a discussion of health equity principles. This approach to centering health equity demonstrates that **every public health issue is an equity issue**. Readers can use the information to reflect on ways the legal system has served as a facilitator for or a barrier to achieving health equity.

## When Reading the Hypothetical Case Studies, Start With the Questions First

Each of the 11 chapters in Part II features a hypothetical case study. Each of these hypothetical case studies concludes with a number of questions and is followed by text that answers those questions. To get the most out of these hypothetical case studies, the reader should start first with the questions, read the hypothetical case study, and then work through answering the questions in their own words. Lastly, the reader should focus on the explanatory text and compare their thoughts with the author's explanation of the potential legal solutions, frameworks, or approaches.

## CONCLUSION

The field of public health made significant advances in the health outcomes in the 19th and 20th century. Reflecting on the sailboat analogy, if the field of public health is to improve on those advances, make the sustainable changes needed to address the social determinants of health and health equity—an "all-hands-on deck" approach is needed. This means ensuring that current and future generations of the public health workforce are competent in the use of law as a tool just like surveillance, epidemiology, and any other tool in the public health toolbox. Each chapter in this book aims to help do that.

# REFERENCES

Burris, S., Ashe, M., Levin, D., Penn, M., & Larkin, M. (2016). A transdisciplinary approach to public health law: The emerging practice of legal epidemiology. *Annual Review of Public Health, 37*, 135–148. https://doi.org/10.1146/annurev-publhealth-032315-021841

Centers for Disease Control and Prevention. (1999). Ten great public health achievements—United States, 1900-1999. *Morbidity and Mortality Weekly Report, 48*(12), 241–243.

Centers for Disease Control and Prevention. (2019). *PHLP, Health equity law.* https://www.cdc.gov/phlp/publications/topic/healthequity.html

Council on Education for Public Health. (2016). *Accreditation criteria schools of public health & public health program.* https://media.ceph.org/wp_assets/2016.Criteria.pdf

Executive order 2020-01D. (2020, March 9). *Governor declaring a state of emergency.* https://governor.ohio.gov/wps/portal/gov/governor/media/executive-orders/executive-order-2020-01-d

Garfield, L. (2017, April 4). *This fascinating time-lapse show how New York City's population density changed over 210 years.* https://www.businessinsider.com/new-york-population-changes-2017-4

Gostin, L. O. (2007). A theory and definition of public health law. *Georgetown Law Faculty Publications and Other Works, 95.* https://scholarship.law.georgetown.edu/facpub/95

Gostin, L. O., Monahan, J. T., Kaldor, J., DeBartolo, M., Friedman, E. A., Gottschalk, K., Kim, S. C., Alwan, A., Binagwaho, A., Burci, G. L., Cabal, L., DeLand, K., Evans, T. G., Goosby, E., Hossain, S., Koh, H., Ooms, G., Roses Periago, M., Uprimny, R., & Yamin, A. E. (2019). The legal determinants of health: harnessing the power of law for global health and sustainable development. *Lancet (London, England), 393*(10183), 1857–1910. https://doi.org/10.1016/S0140-6736(19)30233-8

*Jacobson v. Massachusetts,* 197 U.S. 11 (1905)

Liboiron, M. (2013, October 13). *A history of New York City's solid waste management in photographs.* https://discardstudies.com/2013/10/13/a-history-of-new-york-citys-solid-waste-management-in-photographs/

Miller, B. (1998). Fat of the land: New York's waste. *Social Research, 65*(1), 75–99.

Moulton, A. D., Mercer, S. L., Popovic, T., Briss, P. A., Goodman, R. A., Thombley, M. L., Hahn, R. A., & Fox, D. M. (2009). The scientific basis for law as a public health tool. *American Journal of Public Health, 99,* 17–24. https://doi.org/10.2105/AJPH.2007.130278

New York City. (2007, October 29). *Mayor Bloomberg accepts the Julius B. Richmond award from The Harvard School of Public Health.* https://www1.nyc.gov/office-of-the-mayor/news/391-07/mayor-bloomberg-accepts-julius-b-richmond-award-the-harvard-school-public-health#/1

Olsen, K. (2015). What do you do with the garbage? New York City's progressive era sanitary reforms and their impact on the waste management infrastructure in Jamaica Bay. *Long Island History Journal.* http://lihj.cc.stonybrook.edu/2015/articles/olsen/

Rojas, N., Yuen, T., & Johnson, R. (2020). *Health in all policies for a stronger recovery.* https://www.changelabsolutions.org/blog/health-all-policies-stronger-recovery

Sante, L. (1991). *Low life.* Farrar, Strauss, and Giroux.

White Wings. (n.d.). *The White Wings.* http://whitewings.leadr.msu.edu/white-wings/

Zeliadt, N. (2010, July 29). Talking trash during the dog days: A brief history of sanitation in New York City. *Scientific American.* https://blogs.scientificamerican.com/observations/talking-trash-during-the-dog-days-a-brief-history-of-sanitation-in-new-york-city/

# I

# LAW AS THE FOUNDATION FOR PUBLIC HEALTH PRACTICE: CONCEPTS

# The U.S. Legal System and Sources of Authority for Public Health Laws

Lauren Tonti and Aila Hoss

## Learning Objectives

By the end of this chapter, the reader will be able to:

- Identify the governments in the United States and their legal authorities to engage in public health activities.
- Discuss the legal levers available to engage in public health activities.

## Key Terminology

**Case Law:** law made by the judiciary; case law refers to a collection of decisions made by courts that establish authority on a particular topic.

**Dillon's Rule:** express grants of authority to local governments; grants of authority to local governments are specific and should be narrowly interpreted.

**Executive Branch:** the branch of government that executes and enforces law.

**Executive Orders:** legally binding directives issued by a president, governor, or other leader of an executive branch.

**Federalism:** a system of governance where a jurisdiction is governed equally by two levels of government.

**Home Rule:** the degree of autonomy a local government can exercise; in home rule states, local authority exists so long as it is not expressly restricted by the state.

**Judicial Branch:** the branch of government that adjudicates disputes and interprets law.

**Judicial Review:** courts' review of an executive agency's actions when an aggrieved party files a lawsuit to challenge a newly promulgated regulation or issuance of a public health order.

**Jurisdiction:** the area over which a government, court, or other legal entity can exercise its power.

**Legislative Branch:** the branch of government that creates law.

**Legislative Process:** the process by which legislation is proposed and potentially passed.

**Litigation:** criminal or civil actions in a court of law; using legal processes in courts of law to resolve disputes.

**Ordinance:** an example of a local law passed by a county or municipal government.

**Police Powers:** inherent authority that allows states to promote general welfare within their boundaries.
**Regulation:** legally binding instruments made by agencies.
**Rulemaking:** the process of interpreting legislative guidance found in a statute and promulgating new regulations.
**Statute:** a law passed by a legislature and enacted through a constitutional process.

## Public Health Law Competencies

This chapter addresses the following competencies from the Public Health Law Competency Model (PHLCM; Ransom, 2016):

1.1  Define basic constitutional concepts and legal principles framing the practice of public health across relevant jurisdictions.

1.2  Identify and apply public health laws (e.g., statutes, regulations, ordinances, and court rulings) pertinent to practitioner's jurisdiction, agency, program, and profession.

2.3  Recognize the legal authority and limits of critical system partners and others who influence health outcomes.

---

### Spark Questions

1.  Which governmental actors engage in public health practice?
2.  How is law used to advance public health?

---

## INTRODUCTION

Public health law refers both to laws related to governments' public health authority and laws that impact public health (Goodman, 2007; Gostin & Wiley, 2016). This textbook explores public health law in each of these ways. Part I outlines the legal underpinnings of law in public health practice. Parts II and III study applied public health law across different settings.

In the United States, public health is the product of an intricate patchwork of laws, legal structures, authorities, actors, policies, and politics. Law is an intricate part of the patchwork that promotes public health. Law is a tool of public health promotion that operates on the population level (Goodman et al., 2007; Gostin et al., 2019). Actions at the population level have important impacts on both individual and collective health (Burris, 2011; Burris et al., 2002). Legal structures unite within the patchwork to protect and promote the public's health. Modern American society has inherited this fascinating patchwork structure, a product of democratic debate and compromise (Hodge, 1998; Moncrieff & Lawless, 2017), which in turn has allowed innovative public health policies and interventions to develop in "laboratories of democracy" that operate at all levels of governance (Gostin, 2010). The United States is made up of five categories of governments: federal, state, local, territorial, and Tribal. Each government has its own unique source of public health authority, which this chapter introduces and subsequent chapters describe in more detail.

This chapter familiarizes you with the patterns, fabric, and stitching of public health promotion in the U.S. legal system. Specifically, it first briefly orients the balance of powers by outlining **federalism** as a pattern of public health law in the United States. It next identifies the levels at which public health action occurs by describing each of the governmental types in the United States. It then describes the legal mechanisms through which public health law is advanced by these governments. Throughout the chapter, real-world examples highlight the instruments that actively impact health within the U.S. legal system, illustrating the unique shapes and forms public health laws can take. Understanding these foundational principles of the U.S. legal system provides important insight into public health practice. Comprehending the dynamics and intricacies of the U.S. legal system and sources of authority for public health laws will help identify ways to promote health equity.

## GOVERNMENTS AND THEIR STRUCTURES: THE PATTERNS AND FABRIC IN THE PUBLIC HEALTH PATCHWORK

U.S. governance is decentralized by design. The Constitution of the United States helps the cogs and wheels of American governance structures fit together within its system. The Constitution clarifies the balance and scope of authority in the sovereign powers to both a united federal government and individual governments within the union of states (Hodge, 1998). In this distribution of power, public health governance is also decentralized. These models establish patterns of public health law governance. While each government in the United States has authority to promote public health in its **jurisdiction**, the sources and types of legal interventions available can vary (Institute of Medicine [IOM], 2002). As a consequence, many actors (and their actions) simultaneously affect health. Each governmental actor in the U.S. legal system is described in what follows. This section briefly introduces constitutional law principles and the branches of government that make up the patterns and fabric of the public health law patchwork. Constitutional law impacting public health is discussed in more detail in Chapter 2. The important role of agencies and the judiciary in public health is discussed in Chapters 4 and 5, respectively. Let us dive into the fabrics of federal, state, local, Tribal, and territorial governments.

### Federal Government

The nation's founders deliberately adopted federalism, a system of governance where a jurisdiction is governed equally by two levels of government (Legal Information Institute at Cornell University Law School, n.d.-c; Sheppard, 2012). Here, "jurisdiction" refers to the area over which a government, court, or other legal body can exercise its power (Sheppard, 2012).

The federal government is the national governing body of the United States. The authority of the federal government comes from the U.S. Constitution (Gostin & Wiley, 2016). The Constitution grants the federal government express enumerated powers, including the power to tax, spend, and regulate interstate commerce among other things (U.S. Const. art. I, § 8). These powers allow the federal government to allocate funds to support public health and regulate business and commerce between states, which is defined broadly to include a variety of public health activities (Burris et al., 2018, p. 127; Gostin & Wiley, 2016, pp. 95–100). The Constitution also establishes three branches of government: the Legislative, Executive, and the Judiciary (U.S. Const. art. I, II, III). The **legislative branch** makes law, the **executive branch** enforces law, and the judiciary interprets law. In practice, these functions are complicated.

The U.S. Congress is the legislative branch of the federal government. As bodies of directly elected representatives, the two houses of Congress, the House and Senate, draft and pass laws. They do so under specific constitutional authority. Two of the most powerful authorities granted to Congress by the Constitution are the power to tax and spend for the country's general welfare and the power to regulate interstate commerce (for more detail on these powers, see Chapter 2). While these two grants may seem like too few powers, these authorizations allow Congress to create a wide range of laws and incentives that impact and promote health. Perhaps one of the most significant and controversial pieces of health legislation passed by Congress in the last decade is the Patient Protection and Affordable Care Act. Signed into law by President Barack Obama in 2010, this bill overhauled important aspects of the U.S. healthcare system structure and expanded access to healthcare services for millions of Americans.

The office of the president and federal agencies make up the executive branch (Whitehouse.gov., n.d.-b). The Executive branch can propose laws to the legislature, issue **regulations**, enforce laws, and set agendas related to health and healthcare (Whitehouse.gov., n.d.-b).

The president holds specific powers that can be used in the promotion of health, such as the vital responsibility of signing bills approved by both houses of Congress into law (Whitehouse.gov., n.d.-b). The president also retains the power to negotiate treaties that deal with health-related matters, and can appoint agency officials, such as the secretary of Health and Human Services (Whitehouse.gov., n.d.-b). Sometimes, the president can issue **executive orders** directly related to health and healthcare (Whitehouse.gov., n.d.-b). For instance, President Barack Obama issued executive orders establishing both the White House Office of Health Reform (Executive Order 13507, 2009) and the National Prevention, Health Promotion, and Public Health Council (Executive Order 13544, 2010).

The executive branch also includes federal regulatory agencies that influence health by issuing, implementing, and enforcing rules and regulations via delegated authority from Congress, as well as by providing research, funding, and guidance (Gostin & Wiley, 2016). Many of these agencies exist under the auspices of the Department of Health and Human Services (DHHS; U.S. DHHS, 2015). The agencies in existence today under this executive branch each have specific subject matter competencies. For instance, the Food & Drug Administration (FDA) promotes public health and safety by issuing rules and regulations on pharmaceuticals, medical devices, and tobacco products, as well as some food and veterinary products (Burris et al., 2018). The Centers for Disease Control & Prevention (CDC) issues guidance, information, and training on disease prevention and health promotion. In addition to conducting research and funding grants in key public health domains, CDC has authority to monitor the outbreak and spread of illness and responds to public health emergencies (CDC, 2019). The National Institutes of Health (NIH) concentrate on conducting and funding clinical research that advances health (NIH, 2017). In its oversight and regulation of Medicare and Medicaid programs, the Centers of Medicare and Medicaid Services (CMS) finance medical care for specific populations (U.S. DHHS, 2015). The Substance Abuse and Mental Health Services Administration (SAMHSA) focuses on behavioral health issues in the nation, promoting access to and availability of services and resources for individuals at risk of or living with substance use and mental health disorders (SAMHSA, 2020). The Indian Health Service (IHS) administers health programs and services to American Indians and Alaska Natives (IHS, n.d.). These agencies, and many others, work together under the umbrella of the DHHS to advance the health of all.

Federal district courts, circuit courts, and the U.S. Supreme Court make up the **judicial branch**. While much direct public health regulation is left to other branches of government, the judicial branch and its various member courts also play important roles. In their interpretation of law and resolution of disputes, these courts serve both as barriers against rights infringement, as well as forums for civil redress (Stier & Nicks, 2007).

The judicial branch ensures that rights are protected and that actors stay within their constitutional scopes of authority. *Jacobson v. Massachusetts* (1905) illustrates the Supreme Court's decisive role in public health with its evaluation of an individual's right to refuse a required vaccination. It weighed an individual's right against the public good of protecting the community against smallpox during an outbreak of the disease in Boston, therein examining the lawful scope of a state's vaccination mandate. Ultimately, the Court ruled that the vaccination requirement was within the scope of the authority of the Commonwealth of Massachusetts, and while Jacobson was not forced to be vaccinated, he was forced to pay a fine instead. *Whole Woman's Health v. Hellerstedt* provides an example of the Supreme Court ruling that a state overstepped its authority in promulgating an abortion-related restriction. At issue in the case was a Texas law mandating that physicians who perform abortions must also have admitting privileges at hospitals nearby, and requiring abortion clinics be equipped with ambulatory surgical centers. The Court determined that these requirements violated constitutional protections. Today, courts are also the arenas of many challenges to state and local governments' alleged overextension of public health authorities, as a flurry of cases have been filed to challenge or halt COVID-19 measures like business closures, restrictions on religious gatherings, or other exercises of executive authority during this public health emergency (Association of State and Territorial Health Officials [ASTHO], 2020).

At the same time, courts are forums of civil litigation, where members of society seek redress for wrongs related to health. Courts are forums where strategic litigation and tort law play out, thereby indirectly regulating public health through the tort system (Gostin, 2010; Gostin et al., 2017). **Litigation** targets individuals and businesses to incentivize accountability, compensate for harms, deter harmful behavior, and reduce risks of harm (Gostin, 2010). For example, the 1998 tobacco Master Settlement Agreement (MSA) is the result of strategic litigation against the four largest tobacco industries in the United States for their marketing of cigarettes (Gostin, 2010, p. 216; Lester & Cork, 2020). Forty-six state attorneys general along with four territories, the Commonwealth of Puerto Rico, and the District of Columbia sued America's leading tobacco companies (Philip Morris Incorporated, R.J. Reynolds Tobacco Company, Brown & Williamson Tobacco Corporation, and Lorillard Tobacco Company) asking for compensation for the cost of care of individuals afflicted with or dying from tobacco-related illnesses. The settlement agreement terms protected the tobacco companies from states' past and future legal challenges involving smoking-related illnesses or death. In exchange for this immunity, the tobacco companies would make indefinite annual payments to states and territories, and abide by specific cigarette promotion and marketing restrictions (Gostin & Wiley, 2016, p. 259; Lester & Cork, 2020). The MSA, the largest civil settlement in American history, remains in place to this day.

## BOX 1.1 THE RIGHT TO HEALTH AND HEALTH EQUITY

**What is the "Right to Health?"** Article 12 of the International Covenant on Economic, Social and Cultural Rights (ICESCR), an international treaty, recognizes "the right of everyone to the enjoyment of the highest attainable standard of physical and mental health" (United Nations General Assembly, 1966, Article 12). The right obliges states to protect, respect, and fulfill the right to health, which should entail the availability, accessibility, and acceptability of quality healthcare for all (Committee on Economic, Social, and Cultural Rights Committee, 2004). Today, many treaties and national constitutions recognize a right to health (Tobin & Barrett, 2020).

> **Brazil:** "Health is the right of all and the duty of the National Government and shall be guaranteed by social and economic policies aimed at reducing the risk of illness and other maladies and by universal and equal access to all activities and services for its promotion, protection and recovery" (Constitution of the of the Federative Republic of Brazil, Title VIII, Chapter II, Article 196; Prado, 2014).

> **Italy:** "The Republic safeguards health as a fundamental right of the individual and as a collective interest, and guarantees free medical care to the indigent" (Constitution of the Italian Republic, Article 32).

> **Kenya:** "Every person has the right . . . to the highest attainable standard of health, which includes the right to health care services, including reproductive health care" (Constitution of Kenya, 2010, Chapter 4, Part 2, Section 43[1][a]).

> **Portugal:** "1. Everyone has the right to the protection of health and the duty to defend and promote health. 2. The right to the protection of health shall be fulfilled: a) By means of a universal and general national health service [. . .]. b) By creating economic, social, cultural and environmental conditions that particularly guarantee the protection of childhood, youth and old age; by systematically improving living and working conditions, and promoting physical fitness and sport at school and among the people; and also by developing the people's health and hygiene education and healthy living practices.

3. In order to ensure the right to the protection of health, the state is charged, as a priority, with: a) Guaranteeing access by every citizen, regardless of his economic situation, to preventive, curative and rehabilitative medical care [. . .]" (Constitution of the Portuguese Republic, PART I, TITLE III, CHAPTER II, ARTICLE 64[1-3]).

**Is there a constitutional right to health in the United States?** There is no explicit right to health at the federal level of government (Yamin & Carmalt, 2013). The U.S. Constitution does not contain an explicit right to health, for the document has traditionally been interpreted as one that protects the populace "from" governmental interference, rather than one that obliges the government "to" act or provide a service (Gostin, 2010).

At the state level, some states have enshrined health considerations in their constitutions. Usually, states do not promote a "positive" right to health, or in other words, an obligation to guarantee health or healthcare. Rather, constituents are free to pursue their own health individually. Even if states do not explicitly mention health in their constitutions, courts could interpret a constitutional duty to protect health from state constitutions (Leonard, 2010, p. 1366). Of states that have explicitly enshrined a duty to protect health, these duties are often limited by service restrictions under the duty, or otherwise reserve the right for specific populations, such as those who are living with mental illness, low-income, or imprisoned (Leonard, 2010). Many states have tried and failed to adopt state constitutional amendments for positive individual rights to health (Leonard, 2010).

The following examples illustrate many diverse forms health interests take in state constitutions.

**Mississippi:**
"It shall be the duty of the legislature to provide by law for the **treatment and care of the insane**; and the legislature may provide for the **care of the indigent sick in the hospitals** in the state" (MISS. CONST. ART. IV, § 86).

**Illinois:**
"We, the People of the State of Illinois . . . in order to provide for the **health**, safety and welfare of the people . . . do ordain and establish this Constitution for the State of Illinois" (ILL. CONST. PMBL.).

"Each person has the right to a **healthful environment**. Each person may enforce this right against any party, governmental or private, through appropriate legal proceedings subject to reasonable limitation and regulation as the General Assembly may provide by law" (ILL. CONST. ART. XI § 2).

**Hawaii:**
"The State shall provide for the protection and promotion of the **public health**" (HAW. CONST. ART. IX, § 1).

"The State shall have the power to provide financial assistance, **medical assistance** and social services for persons who are found to be in need of and are eligible for such assistance and services as provided by law" (HAW. CONST. ART. IX, § 3).

"The State shall have the power to promote and maintain a **healthful environment**, including the prevention of any excessive demands upon the environment and the State's resources" (HAW. CONST. ART. IX, § 8).

**Montana:**
"Section 3. Inalienable rights. All persons are born free and have certain inalienable rights. They include the right to a clean and **healthful environment** and the rights of pursuing life's basic necessities, enjoying and defending their lives and liberties, acquiring, possessing and protecting property, and seeking their safety, **health** and happiness in all lawful ways. In enjoying these rights, all persons recognize corresponding responsibilities" (Mont. Const. Art. II § 3).

Subsequent chapters in this textbook highlight health inequities experienced by different communities. As you learn more, consider what impact a constitutional right to health could mean in preventing or addressing health inequities.

## State Governments

Any powers not expressly enumerated by the federal government are reserved for the states (U.S. Const. amend. X). States also possess **police powers,** an inherent authority predating the Constitution that allows states to promote general welfare within their boundaries (Gostin & Wiley, 2016). Police powers include "the inherent authority of the state . . . to enact laws and promulgate regulations to protect, preserve, and promote the health, safety, and morals, and general welfare of the people" (Gostin, 2000, p. 2980). These police powers establish that states, not the federal government, take the lead in public health prevention and response (Burris et al., 2018; Gostin & Wiley, 2016). State constitutions provide for the structure of state governments (Goodman et al., 2007 p. 56; Kincaid, 1988, p. 18). Like their federal counterpart, state governments are made up of three branches—legislative, executive, and judiciary—although the organization of each branch varies from state to state (Whitehouse.gov., n.d.-a)

The opioid crisis presents examples of public health activity in every branch and at every level of state government. Like the U.S. Congress, state legislatures create laws, often through a bicameral **legislative process,** that can impact health. In response to the opioid use disorder and overdose epidemic, legislatures across the country have been debating and passing laws to reduce the harms linked to opioid use disorder and overdose (Lieberman & Davis, 2020). All 50 states (plus the District of Columbia) have now passed legislation to increase access to naloxone, a drug that can be used to help reverse opioid overdoses in emergencies among community members (Davis, 2018). An overwhelming majority of state legislatures also passed overdose Good Samaritan laws that protect individuals who report overdoses from arrest or other criminal consequences.

In the executive branch, state governors can issue executive orders that directly impact public health. These orders can establish investigatory commissions to study health problems, create public health programs, direct state public health agencies, increase awareness about a public health issue, establish funding, or free resources in the event of public health emergencies, among other functions (Gakh et al., 2013, 2019). Governors' executive orders have been valuable in the fight against the opioid epidemic. As early as 2011, the governor of Ohio issued an executive order that expanded the use of medication-assisted Treatments, like methadone, used in opioid dependence therapy (Executive Order 2011-06K). In 2017, the Arizona governor enhanced opioid surveillance and reporting of suspected overdoes, deaths, naloxone administrations, and incidences of neonatal withdrawal in the state via executive order (State of Arizona Executive Order 2017-04). In 2017, the then-governor of Illinois established an Opioid Prevention and Intervention Task Force via executive order to address opioid-related health issues in the state (State of Illinois Executive Order 2017-04, 2017), and in 2020 the current governor strengthened the initiative by issuing an executive order creating a a steering committee to support and coordinate those efforts (State of Illinois Executive Order 2020-02, 2020).

State agencies are usually part of the state's executive branch. Each state has a health department responsible for a variety of public health activities (CDC, n.d.). The Indiana State Department of Health, for example, has a mission to "promote, protect, and improve the health and safety of all Hoosiers" (Indiana Department of Health, n.d.). It engages in a variety of activities, including disease surveillance and prevention (Indiana State Department of Health, n.d.). Depending on the state, state boards of health can provide advisory opinions or advance policies (Hughes et al., 2011). The exact structure of these state-level health departments can vary from state to state (ASTHO, 2017, p.17). Some states' public health governance structures are more centralized, with state employees in control of public health decision-making and administrating local health units. Others operate under decentralized structures, where local governments take the lead on public health decision-making and administration. Still others share the responsibilities, or otherwise have a form of mixed centralized and decentralized governance to handle the relationship between state and local public health authorities (ASTHO, 2017, pp. 18, 21). Country-wide, state health departments and boards of health worked to study, monitor, and report on overdoses. These local entities also launched educational campaigns, led harm-reduction programs, and made funding available for overdose prevention efforts. (Maryland Department of Health, n.d.; National Association of County and City Health Officials [NACCHO], 2019; Raja & Higgins, 2019; Washington State Department of Health, n.d.)

As in the era of tobacco litigation, state, local, and Tribal governments have used the judiciary as a forum to challenge opioid manufacturers for their contributions to the national opioid use disorder and overdose epidemic (Carr et al., 2018). An alliance of state attorneys general and head legal officers in states or territories challenged Purdue Pharma, along with other major opioid manufacturers. The state of Oklahoma prevailed against Purdue Pharma, Johnson & Johnson, and other opioid manufacturers after challenging in court the companies' violation of Oklahoma's nuisance law by engaging in unlawful marketing and sales practices that fueled the addiction of thousands of Americans (*State of Oklahoma, ex. rel. Hunter v. Purdue Pharma, L.P., et al.*, 2019). Other governments, including Tribal and local governments, have also pursued litigation. Please see Box 1.2 for examples of state action to address opioid use disorder in every branch of government.

---

### BOX 1.2 THE OPIOID USE DISORDER AND OVERDOSE EPIDEMIC: STATE ACTION IN EVERY BRANCH OF GOVERNMENT

This box presents examples of state interventions within each branch of government to reduce opioid-related harms.

#### LEGISLATIVE:

##### Good Samaritan Law

"...a person who, in good faith, seeks medical assistance for a person who is experiencing a drug or alcohol overdose or other medical emergency or who seeks such assistance for himself or herself, or who is the subject of a good faith request for such assistance may not be arrested, charged, prosecuted or convicted, or have his or her property subjected to forfeiture, or be otherwise penalized . . ." (Nev. Rev. Stat. Ann. § 453C.150).

##### Naloxone Access

"Authorization to prescribe, dispense and administer opioid antagonist; immunity from liability and professional discipline [. . .]

2. A person who, acting in good faith and with reasonable care, prescribes or dispenses an opioid antagonist pursuant to subsection 1, is not subject to any criminal or civil liability or any professional disciplinary action for:
   (a) Such prescribing or dispensing; or
   (b) Any outcomes that result from the eventual administration of the opioid antagonist.

3. Notwithstanding any other provision of law:
   (a) Any person, including, without limitation, a law enforcement officer, acting in good faith, may possess and administer an opioid antagonist to another person whom he or she reasonably believes to be experiencing an opioid-related drug overdose.
   (b) An emergency medical technician, advanced emergency medical technician or paramedic, as defined in chapter 450B of NRS, is authorized to administer an opioid antagonist as clinically indicated" (Nev. Rev. Stat. Ann. § 453C.100).

## EXECUTIVE:

## EXECUTIVE ORDER ESTABLISHING THE GOVERNOR'S OPIOID PREVENTION AND INTERVENTION TASK FORCE

"**WHEREAS**, Illinois is in the midst of a public health and safety crisis caused by the opioid epidemic and characterized by an alarming rate of opioid overdose deaths; and

**WHEREAS**, opioid overdoses have recently claimed the lives of far too many Illinois residents; and

**WHEREAS**, opioid overdoses are expected to kill more than 1,900 people in the state of Illinois in 2017, more than one and a half times the number of homicides and nearly twice the number of fatal motor vehicle accidents; and

**WHEREAS**, opioid overdoses can be prevented and lives can be saved; and

**WHEREAS**, we recognize that substance use disorder is a disease, that individuals with substance use disorder come from diverse backgrounds and live in every part of our State, and furthermore, that recovery from substance use disorder is possible; and

**WHEREAS**, the toll that substance use disorder takes on individuals, families, friends, and communities must drive us to do all that we can to reduce its impact and help Illinois residents lead healthy, successful, and productive lives; and

**WHEREAS**, we must come together to build on the existing work and successful initiatives of State agencies, stakeholder coalitions, and community partners to contain the opioid epidemic; and

**WHEREAS**, Illinois needs a comprehensive plan to address opioid misuse and reduce overdose deaths in the State; and

**WHEREAS**, Illinois State agencies have different expertise, capabilities, and data that, when shared, can better inform a coordinated statewide response to the opioid overdose epidemic;

**THEREFORE**, I, Bruce Rauner, Governor of Illinois, by virtue of the executive authority vested in me by Section 8 of Article V of the Constitution of the State of Illinois, do hereby order as follows:

## I. CREATION
There is hereby established the Governor's Opioid Prevention and Intervention Task Force ("Task Force").

## II. PURPOSE
The purpose of the Task Force shall be to develop, approve, and implement a comprehensive Opioid Action Plan to: (1) prevent the further spread of the opioid crisis;

(2) treat and promote the recovery of individuals with opioid use disorder; and (3) respond effectively to avert opioid overdose deaths. The Task Force shall set a statewide goal for the Opioid Action Plan and formulate a set of evidence-based strategies in furtherance of this overall goal. The Task Force shall also coordinate with the Illinois Opioid Crisis Response Advisory Council and other key stakeholders to formulate a detailed implementation plan, including specific activities and metrics, for the execution of the strategies set forth in the Opioid Action Plan [. . .]." (Ill. Exec. Order No. 2017-05 (Sept. 6, 2017))

## STATE HEALTH AGENCY:

*Authority of Department of Health and Human Services to study drug overdoses; report.*
"1. The Department of Health and Human Services may engage in efforts to ascertain and document the number, trends, patterns and risk factors related to fatalities caused by unintentional opioid-related drug overdoses and other drug overdoses.
2. The Department of Health and Human Services may publish an annual report that:
    (a)  Presents the information acquired pursuant to subsection 1; and
    (b)  Provides information concerning interventions that may be effective in reducing fatal and nonfatal opioid-related drug overdoses and other drug overdoses, including, without limitation, the use of opioid analgesic drugs that contain abuse-deterrent mechanisms and access to such drugs." (Nev. Rev. Stat. Ann. § 453C.130).

*Authority of Department of Health and Human Services to award grants.*

"The Department of Health and Human Services may, within the limits of available money, award grants for:
1.  Educational programs for the prevention and recognition of and responses to opioid-related drug overdoses and other drug overdoses;
2.  Training programs for patients who receive opioid antagonists and for the families and caregivers of such patients concerning the prevention and recognition of and responses to opioid-related drug overdoses and other drug overdoses;
3.  Projects to encourage, when appropriate, the prescription and distribution of opioid antagonists; and
4.  Education and training programs on the prevention and recognition of and responses to opioid-related drug overdoses and other drug overdoses for members and volunteers of law enforcement agencies and agencies that provide emergency medical services and other emergency services." (Nev. Rev. Stat. Ann. § 453C.140).

## JUDICIARY:

Excerpt from *State of Oklahoma, ex. rel. Hunter v. Purdue Pharma, L.P., et. al:*
"The challenged conduct here is Defendants' misleading marketing and promotion of opioids. The State claims that Defendants engaged in a false, misleading, and deceptive marketing campaign designed to convince Oklahoma doctors, patients, and the public at large that opioids were safe and effective for the long-term treatment of chronic, nonmalignant pain. The greater weight of the evidence shows that Defendants did, in fact, engage in such false and misleading marketing and the law is clear that such conduct qualifies as the kind of act or omission capable of sustaining liability under Oklahoma's nuisance law [. . .] (*State ex rel. Hunter v. Purdue Pharma L.P.,* 2019)

## Local Governments

States delegate authority to local governments, such as city or county governments. (Briffault, 1990; Gostin & Wiley, 2016). The number and structure of local governments vary from state to state (Gostin & Wiley, 2016, p. 177), but, in total, there are over 3,000 local governments in the United States (U.S. Census Bureau, 2017). States delegate local governmental authority through state constitutions or state legislation (Gostin & Wiley, 2016, p. 177), and can centralize authority at the state level or decentralize authority at the local level (Burris et al., 2018, p. 25). These governmental structures that allocate authority are referred to as **home rule** and **Dillon's rule**, respectively (Gostin & Wiley, 2016, p. 179). Home rule refers to the degree of autonomy a local government can exercise (Gostin & Wiley, 2016, p. 178). In home rule states, local authority exists so long as not expressly restricted by the state (Vanlandingham, 1968, p. 270). For example, a Topeka **ordinance** that raised the minimum age of tobacco sales from 18 to 21 in the home rule state of Kansas was upheld by the Kansas Supreme Court when challenged (Public Health Law Center, 2020). Similarly, when adversaries challenged the city of Houston's smoke-free ordinances banning smoking in public places like bars and restaurants, courts ruled that smoking regulation was part of the city's home rule authority (Public Health Law Center, 2020). States that have adopted Dillon's rule must expressly grant authority to local governments (*Hunter v. City of Pittsburgh*, 1907, p. 178). For example, in Vermont, a Dillon's rule state, the Vermont Supreme Court invalidated the city of Montpellier's ordinance reducing boating, fishing, and swimming on Berlin Pond, the city's water source, for the sake of pollution reduction and public drinking water protection because the state had not granted authority over the pond to the city (Public Health Law Center, 2020). Home rule and Dillon's rule can operate simultaneously in some states (Gostin & Wiley, 2016, p. 179).

Local governments in most states include counties and municipalities (National League of Cities, 2016a). Through the roles of mayor or county commissioner, city or county council, and city courts, local governments reflect the respective executive, legislative, and judicial structures of their state and federal counterparts (National League of Cities, 2016b), though local governance structures can be complex and the separation of powers less distinct at local levels (Kazis, 2018, p. 1157). As administrative departments (Burris et al., 2018, p. 138), local health departments perform executive functions (NACCHO, 2019). Local health departments can serve cities, counties, or larger regions (Burris et al., 2018, p. 27). For example, the Tulsa Health Department is the primary public health agency serving Tulsa County, Oklahoma (Tulsa Health Department, n.d.-b). The Tulsa Health Department is advised by the Tulsa City-County Board of Health (Tulsa Health Department, n.d.-a). The services provided by local health departments vary substantially, but most provide immunizations, preventive health services, communicable disease control, food safety promotion, and education (Burris et al., 2018, p. 25; Gebbie & Rosenstock, 2003). In many ways, local governments are vital to the nation's public health system (Burris et al., 2018, p. 11).

Local boards of health are local-level administrative bodies that direct public health activities at the community level. These activities can include **rulemaking**, reviewing regulations, advising elected officials, developing and prioritizing policies, providing recommendations, coordinating with health departments, conducting disease and epidemiological surveillance, performing health services like immunizations, conducting population health activities, and advancing legislative agendas (NACCHO, 2020; Public Health Law Center, 2015). A 2019 survey by NACCHO reported that 70% of local health departments have local boards of health (NACCHO, 2020). Members of boards of health can be elected or appointed (NACCHO, 2016). The authority of local boards of health to perform these activities varies, though the root of the authority can be traced back to statutory grant (Public Health Law Center, 2015).

## BOX 1.3 AUTHORITY AND SCOPE OF LOCAL BOARDS OF HEALTH ACTIVITY

### EXAMPLE: IOWA

### IA CODE § 137.103 (2016) LOCAL BOARDS OF HEALTH—JURISDICTION

1. A city board shall have jurisdiction over public health matters within the city.
2. A county board shall have jurisdiction over public health matters within the county.
3. A district board shall have jurisdiction over public health matters within the district.

### IA CODE § 137.104 (2016) LOCAL BOARDS OF HEALTH—POWERS AND DUTIES

Local boards of health shall have the following powers and duties:
1. A local board of health shall:
   a. Enforce state health laws and the rules and lawful orders of the state department.
   b. Make and enforce such reasonable rules and regulations not inconsistent with law, the rules of the state board, or the Iowa public health standards as may be necessary for the protection and improvement of the public health.
   [. . .]
   (4) Before approving any rule or regulation the local board of health shall hold a public hearing on the proposed rule. Any citizen may appear and be heard at the public hearing. A notice of the public hearing, stating the time and place and the general nature of the proposed rule or regulation shall be published in a newspaper having general circulation as provided in section 331.305 in the area served by the local board of health.
   c. Employ persons as necessary for the efficient discharge of its duties. [. . .]
2. A local board of health may:
   a. Provide such population-based and personal health services as may be deemed necessary for the promotion and protection of the health of the public and charge reasonable fees for personal health services. A person shall not be denied necessary services within the limits of available resources because of inability to pay the cost of such services.
   b. Provide such environmental health services as may be deemed necessary for the protection and improvement of the public health and issue licenses and permits and charge reasonable fees in relation to the construction or operation of nonpublic water supplies or private sewage disposal systems.
   c. Engage in joint operations and contract with colleges and universities, the state department, other public, private, and nonprofit agencies, and individuals or form a district health department to provide personal and population-based public health services.
   d. By written agreement with the council of any city within its jurisdiction, enforce appropriate ordinances of the city relating to public health.

### IOWA ADMINISTRATIVE CODE CHAPTER 641—77.3 (137) LOCAL BOARDS OF HEALTH—ROLES AND RESPONSIBILITIES

Public health is responsible for safeguarding the community's health. This goal is pursued through three core functions: assessment, policy development and assurance.

77.3(1) Assessment: Regularly and systematically collect, assemble, analyze, and make available information on the health of the community, including statistics on health status, community health needs, personal health services, and epidemiologic and other studies of health problems. A local board of health may perform the following essential public health services:

a. Monitor health status to identify community health problems;
b. Diagnose and investigate health problems and health hazards in the community; and
c. Evaluate effectiveness, accessibility, and quality of personal, population-based, and environmental health services.

77.3(2) Policy development: Exercise responsibility to serve the public interest in the development of comprehensive public health policies. This core function can be accomplished by promoting use of a scientific knowledge base in decision-making about public health and by taking the lead in public health policy development.

a. A local board of health may perform the following essential public health services:
(1) Develop policies and plans that support individual and community health efforts; and
(2) Research new insights and innovative solutions to health problems and health threats.
b. A local board of health shall perform the following essential public health services:
(1) Enforce laws and regulations that protect public health and enforce lawful orders of the department;
(2) Make and enforce reasonable rules and regulations not inconsistent with the law or the rules of the state board as may be necessary for the protection and improvement of the public health; and
(3) Employ persons as necessary for the efficient discharge of the board's duties. [. . .].

## Tribal Governments

Tribes are sovereign nations that have existed in what is now referred to as the United States since time immemorial. As sovereign nations, Tribes have the authority to make laws and govern their communities. This authority is not based on any federal law but instead inherent in Tribes' long history as distinct governments. Their authority extends over both their people and their land. Federal law, however, recognizes Tribal sovereignty across treaties, case law, and **statutes**, among other sources. There are 574 federally recognized Tribes with a nation-to-nation relationship with the United States, more than 80 state-recognized Tribes with a government-to-government relationship with a state, and many Tribes that do not have federal or state recognition under the law but remain politically and culturally significant for their members, communities, and the country (National Conference of State Legislatures, 2020).

Each Tribe has a unique history and culture that informs the structure and scope of its government and laws. In the context of public health, Tribes, like all sovereign nations, have the authority to promote the health and welfare of their people. This is exercised across Tribal law, which can include constitutional law, case law, codes, and cultural law (Hoss, 2019, pp. 126–132). Tribal law contemplates a variety of public health issues, including infectious disease control, motor vehicle safety, and emergency preparedness (Hoss, 2019, pp. 127–129). Tribal public health authority, the provision of healthcare across Indian country, and jurisdictional considerations among Tribes, states, and the federal government are discussed in more detail in Chapter 14.

## Territorial Governments

Colonization and international conflict have resulted in the United States overseeing over a dozen territories (Immerwahr, 2016), five of which are home to permanent residents (American

Samoa, Guam, the Northern Mariana Islands, Puerto Rico, and the U.S. Virgin Islands) (ASTHO, 2017, p. 119; Lin, 2019, p. 1251). Unlike states and Tribes, the federal law does not recognize the territories as having sovereign powers ("Territorial Federalism," 2017). The United States asserts authority over territories under the Territorial Clause of the U.S. Constitution: "The Congress shall have power to dispose of and make all needful rules and regulations respecting the territory or other property belonging to the United States" (U.S. Const. art. IV § 3, cl. 2). The Supreme Court has interpreted this clause to grant Congress extremely broad authority to legislate on any issue regarding territories, retaining power to change or repeal territorial legislatures' laws (Lin, 2019, p. 1285; Van Dyke, 1992, p. 459). Outside of limited delegate or resident representative positions, however, territories do not have elected representation in both houses of Congress (Van Dyke, 1992, pp. 445, 469).

Under federal law, incorporated territories, like the former Hawaii and Alaska territories, were destined for statehood and were bound by the U.S. Constitution ("Territorial Federalism," 2017). Unincorporated territories, like American Samoa, Guam, and the U.S. Virgin Islands, are not bound by the U.S. Constitution, whose application varies depending on the territory and issue (Burnett & Marshall, 2001; Langton, 2016). Previously unincorporated territories, Puerto Rico and the Northern Mariana Islands are commonwealths, established by agreement between the territory and the United States (Van Dyke, 1992). As commonwealths, Puerto Rico and the Northern Mariana Islands can self-govern, subject to certain limitations (Van Dyke, 1992).

Each of the inhabited territories are bound by its Organic Act or Commonwealth Act (passed by the U.S. Congress), the territorial Constitution (approved by Congress), or both ("Introduction" 2017, p. 1623; Van Dyke, 1992). Each territory has an executive, legislative, and judicial branch (Library of Congress, n.d.-a, n.d.-b, n.d.-c, n.d.-d, n.d.-e) and engages in public health activities. Guam's Organic Act requires its governor to "establish, maintain, and operate public-health services in Guam, including hospitals, dispensaries, and quarantine stations, at such places in Guam as may be necessary, and he shall promulgate quarantine and sanitary regulations for the protection of Guam against the importation and spread of disease" (48 U.S.C. § 1421[g][a], 2012). Unique from its federal and state counterparts, the Puerto Rico Constitution guarantees the right to health: "right of every person to a standard of living adequate for the health and well-being of himself and of his family, and especially to food, clothing, housing and medical care and necessary social services" (Puerto Rico Const. art II, § 20).

Territorial (or "insular") health agencies operate differently from those of U.S. states (ASTHO, 2017, p. 120). In territories, health agencies are integrated into the healthcare systems, and provide both clinical and public health services to the territory's residents. Territorial health officials often report directly to the territory's governor, instead of a minister or department head (ASTHO, 2017, p. 120). According to ASTHO, 28% of insular health agencies had a board of health in 2016, and a governor appointed 71% of health officials (ASTHO, 2017, pp. 121, 122). Many territorial health agencies perform the same core activities as those in states. Given insular territories' susceptibility to natural disasters, these agencies also dedicate resources to disaster preparedness and response.

## LEGAL INTERVENTIONS: THE STITCHING IN THE PUBLIC HEALTH PATCHWORK

Each of the governments thus described possess authority to pass laws and other legally binding instruments. These legally binding instruments can be seen as legal interventions that stitch together the patchwork of public health. These interventions act as levers that stakeholders can push to promote health and can serve as highly effective tools within a public health professional's toolbelt. Here we describe some legal interventions and how they can impact public health.

---

### BOX 1.4 WHAT IS LAW?

Black's Law Dictionary, the leading legal dictionary, defines law as:

- set of rules or principles dealing with a specific area
- regime that orders human activities and relations through systematic application
- aggregate of legislation, judicial precedents, and accepted legal principles; the body of authoritative grounds of judicial and administrative action.

**Statutes** are laws enacted by a legislative body (Sheppard, 2012; Tobacco Control Legal Consortium, 2013). The legislative process varies depending on the jurisdiction. In general,

---

### BOX 1.5 WRITTEN FORMS OF LAW

#### Legislation

The term "legislation" can refer to both 1.) the *process* of creating a law and 2.) the *body of laws* created through the process (Sheppard, 2012). The term can be used to refer to legislation at each level of governance: Congressional statutes, State Acts or statutes, or local ordinances.

#### Bill

A "bill" is a draft version of a law (Sheppard, 2012). A member of the legislature can draft a bill proposing a law. The draft bill will be submitted for a legislative body's consideration, debate, and potential passage (Sheppard, 2012; U.S. Congress, n.d.).

#### Act

An "act" can be considered a legislature's decree of law on a certain topic; the term for legislation or a statute (Sheppard, 2012). It is a product of a legislature that is incorporated into a law (Legal Information Institute at Cornell University Law School, n.d.-a).

#### Statutes

"Statutes" are laws passed by legislatures and enacted via a constitutional process (Tobacco Control Legal Consortium, 2013). Statutes go into effect on either their date of enactment or another specified date within the statute. Statutes can be passed at both the federal and state levels. Congress enacts federal statutes. State legislatures pass statutes that apply state-wide.

#### Regulation

In the U.S. context, "regulations" usually refer to rules created and issued by an executive agency (Sheppard, 2012). In a broader sense of the term, "regulation" refers to the creation and enforcement of rules (Sheppard, 2012).

#### Public Law

A public law is a bill that has successfully passed through both houses of Congress and is enacted as a public law. Public laws apply nationwide,[1] and affect the entire society.[2]

---

1. https://www.senate.gov/reference/glossary_term/public_law.htm
2. https://www.archives.gov/federal-register/laws

federal and state legislative processes include introducing a proposed legislation in the form of a bill, reviewing and amending the bill across each chamber of the legislation, and approving the final language by vote (Heitshusen, 2020). For example, Georgia's statutory code establishes the state Department of Health and authorizes it "to declare certain diseases, injuries, and conditions to be diseases requiring notice and to require the reporting thereof" (Ga. Code Ann., § 31-12-2[a]). The Georgia Department of Health outlines the list of reportable conditions in an agency policy (Georgia Department of Health, n.d.).

**Regulations,** also called "rules," are legally binding instruments established by agencies. The legislative branch can delegate some of its authority to agencies to make rules based on the agency's expertise (Gostin & Wiley, 2016). Often, statutes delegate broad authority to agencies to allow them to determine the best course of action in their regulations (IOM, 2011). Thus, regulations are generally more detailed to ensure the individuals or entities regulated understand how to comply with the rule (Burris et al., 2018). For example, in the Family Smoking Prevention and Tobacco Control Act of 2009, Congress gave the FDA primary regulatory authority over tobacco products (21 U.S.C. 387a[a]). The legislation amended the existing definition of tobacco product under the law and allowed the FDA to determine which products met the definition: "This subchapter shall apply to all cigarettes, cigarette tobacco, roll-your-own tobacco, and smokeless tobacco and to any other tobacco products that the Secretary by regulation deems to be subject to this subchapter." (21 U.S.C. § 387a[b]). In 2016, the FDA exercised this authority by establishing regulations that deemed e-cigarettes, cigars, cigarillos, pipe, and hookah tobacco as under its statutory jurisdiction. (Deeming Tobacco Products, 2016). In practice, agencies often have a lot of discretion in the rule-making process (Ruhl & Robisch, 2016, p. 101). However, agency regulations must be within the scope of the legislation that authorized the rule-making (Gostin & Wiley, 2016, p. 172). The federal and state rule-making processes are both unique and complex but generally include notices to the public of the proposed rule and opportunities for public comment (Carey, 2019; Changelab Solutions, 2015a).

**Ordinances** are examples of *local laws* passed by local or municipal governments, like city councils, county boards of supervisors, or other forms of municipal governance (Legal Information Institute at Cornell University Law School, n.d.-d). Ordinances, which are legally binding, usually apply only to the local jurisdiction to which they pertain (Tobacco Control Legal Consortium, 2013). As an example, zoning ordinances are frequently used by local governments to promote health (Changelab Solutions, 2012). Zoning is a system of land development that divides and designates certain land for residential, commercial, or industrial uses. Zoning can limit pollution-causing industries in residential areas. It can also be used to regulate food environments surrounding schools, by controlling how near or far from schools fast food restaurants can be located (Changelab Solutions, 2013).

**Executive orders** are legally binding directives issued by a president, governor, or other leader of an executive branch (Duncan, 2010; Sheppard, 2012). At the federal level, executive orders govern the conduct of federal executive agencies (Duncan, 2010, pp. 335–336). At the federal level, executive orders are signed by the president and published with the Federal Register (n.d.; Duncan, 2010). At other levels of government, executive orders can apply more broadly depending on the jurisdiction (Changelab Solutions, 2015b). State gubernatorial executive orders have increasingly been used to support public health activities (Gakh et al., 2013). As an example, Health in All Policies, a social determinant of health-informed strategy for policy-making calling for the assessment of a proposed governmental action's health impact, is sometimes implemented via executive order (Changelab Solutions, 2015b, p. 18; Pepin et al., 2018). Similarly, some states also allow departments of health leadership to issue public health orders (ASTHO, 2017, p. 22). Public health orders are particularly prevalent in cases of public health emergencies. Michigan law allows the director of the state's Department of Public Health to issue emergency orders prohibiting gatherings during an epidemic (M.C.L.A. 333.2253[1]). The COVID-19 pandemic offers numerous examples of the use of executive orders and public health orders by state governments (Colorado Department of Public Health & Environment, n.d.; New Mexico Department of Health, n.d.; Ohio Department of Public Health, 2021).

**Case law**, or law made by the judiciary, is relied upon by the U.S. legal system in keeping with its tradition as a common law jurisdiction (Legal Information Institute at Cornell University Law School, n.d.-b). Case law, created when two or more parties resolve a dispute in a court of law, refers to a collection of decisions rendered by courts that establish authority on a particular topic (Legal Information Institute at Cornell University Law School, n.d.-b). For instance, U.S. courts have developed case law on mandatory vaccinations, beginning with *Jacobson*, and have held that mandatory vaccinations in school and other settings do not violate constitutional rights to religious freedom or state rights to public education (Gostin, 2010, p. 327). In interpreting law, protecting rights, and preserving constitutional structures, the judicial branch writes/develops a body of case law that stakeholders can look to/use as a guide for cases dealing with similar fact patterns or legal issues (Gostin & Wiley, 2016, p. 81). Case law establishes precedents that can be used to navigate future health-related issues and challenges.

**Litigation** can be a powerful tool to achieve public health goals (Gostin, 2010; Parmet & Daynard, 2000). As mentioned earlier in this chapter, strategic litigation can be used to advance health not only to defend against encroachment on rights by state actors, but also as a strategy to obtain health objectives by using courts to check the actions of individuals, businesses, or other entities (Gostin, 2010, p. 195). Litigation is not exclusively for private entities. Regulators can also use litigation to enforce their rules (Parmet & Daynard, 2000). Beyond tobacco and opioids, litigation has been used in a variety of public health areas, including environmental protection (e.g., drinking water pollution, toxic lead levels, asbestos presence), pharmaceutical and medical products (e.g., hazardous drug marketing), and consumer goods (e.g., the safety of children's toys; motor vehicle safety (*Howard v Ford Motor Company*, 2000; Vernick et al., 2003); validity of sugar-sweetened beverage taxes (Gostin & Wiley, 2016, p. 228; Roache et al., 2017). For more detail on litigation as a legal intervention, see Chapter 5.

## CONCLUSION

The patchwork components of the U.S. legal system have important implications for health. This chapter highlighted how these actors unite in pursuit of a common societal goal: optimal health. The relationships between federal, state, Tribal, and territorial governmental structures illustrate the patterns through which stakeholders can work toward health promotion. The legal interventions used to stitch healthy behaviors, activities, and environments into society vary across jurisdictions, some more delicate, some more durable. But no matter the governance level or intervention, the best health outcomes often occur where multiple actors at multiple levels work together toward a common health goal. Choosing effective combinations of actors and interventions within the U.S. legal system can promote positive, long-lasting health.

## CHAPTER REVIEW

### Review Questions

1.   Which governments engage in public health activities? From where does this authority come?
2.   What legal levers exist to advance public health?

### Essay Question

Read the following Pennsylvania district court case: *Cigar Association of America et al. v. City of Philadelphia et al.* (available at www.paed.uscourts.gov/documents/opinions/20D0581P.pdf). Since the court found the local government could not enforce the e-cigarette law, are there other measures the local government could take to address e-cigarette use in its community?

## Internet Activities

1.   **Covid-19 & Public Health Law:** Find the webpage for your state's executive, legislative, and judicial branch. How has each branch been involved in your state's COVID-19 response? What executive orders, regulations, legislation, or judicial opinions have been passed to respond to the pandemic?
2.   **Shaping the Food Environment:** Berkeley, California, Philadelphia, Pennsylvania, Cook County, Illinois, and Navajo Nation are some of the places in the United States that have enacted taxes on sugar-sweetened beverages or junk foods. Compare and contrast governance mechanisms and specific legal interventions in at least two localities that have enacted sugar-sweetened beverage or junk food taxes. Can you find the research base supporting these interventions? Is there evidence of the effectiveness of these interventions after the taxes go into effect?
3.   **Levels of Marijuana Legalization:** In recent years, numerous jurisdictions have legalized the use of marijuana. At what level of government does marijuana legalization occur? What roles have city or municipal-level governments played in the legalization process? Do you see any conflict between federal and state/local authority on the issue of marijuana legalization? Can you spot any differences between medical marijuana and recreational marijuana legalization?
4.   **Map It Out:** Research the public health law actors and infrastructure in your home state and county. Create a diagram of how these actors and institutions relate to one another. Identify the key public health actors in your community who serve as critical system partners. Be sure your diagram distinguishes between the levels and branches of government.

## REFERENCES

21 U.S.C.A. § 387a.

48 U.S.C. § 1421(g) (2012).

Association of State and Territorial Health Officials. (2017). *ASTHO Profile of State and Territorial Public Health* (Vol. 4). Association of State and Territorial Health Officials. https://www.astho .org/Profile/Volume-Four/2016-ASTHO-Profile-of-State-and-Territorial-Public-Health

Association of State and Territorial Health Officials. (2020). *Report, legal challenges to state COVID-19 orders.* Association of State and Territorial Health Officials. https://www.astho.org/ ASTHOReports/Legal-Challenges-to-State-COVID-19-Orders/10-20-20

Briffault, R. (1990). Our localism: Part I—The structure of local covernment aw. *Columbia Law Review, 90*(1), 7. https://scholarship.law.columbia.edu/faculty_scholarship/13/

Burnett, C. D., & Marshall, B. (Eds.). (2001). *Foreign in a domestic sense: Puerto Rico, American expansion, and the Constitution.* Duke University Press.

Burris, S. (2011). Law in a social determinants strategy: A public health law research perspective. *Public Health Reports, 126*(Suppl. 3), 22–27. https://doi.org/10.1177/00333549111260S305

Burris, S., Berman, M. L., Penn, M. S., & Holiday, T. R. (2018). *The new public health law: A transdisciplinary approach to practice and advocacy.* Oxford University Press.

Burris, S., Kawachi, I., & Sarat, A. (2002). Integrating law and social epidemiology. *The Journal of Law, Medicine and Ethics, 30*(4), 510–521. https://doi.org/10.1111/j.1748-720X.2002.tb00422.x

Carey, M. P. (2019, January 7). *An overview of federal regulations and the rulemaking process.* Congressional Research Service. https://fas.org/sgp/crs/misc/IF10003.pdf

Carr, D., Davis, C. S., & Rutkow, L. (2018). Reducing harm through litigation against opioid manufacturers? Lessons from the tobacco wars. *Public Health Reports, 133*(2), 207–213. https:// doi.org/10.1177/0033354917751131

Centers for Disease Control and Prevention. (n.d.). *State & Territorial Health Department Websites.* https://www.cdc.gov/publichealthgateway/healthdirectories/healthdepartments.html

Centers for Disease Control and Prevention. (2019). *Mission, role, and pledge.* https://www.cdc.gov/ about/organization/mission.htm

Committee on Economic, Social and Cultural Rights Committee. (2004). *General comment 14 (right to health).*

Changelab Solutions. (2012). *Licensing and zoning: Tools for public health.* http://www.change labsolutions.org/sites/default/files/Licensing&Zoning_FINAL_20120703.pdf

Changelab Soltuions. (2013). *Creating a healthy food zone around schools.* https://www.change labsolutions.org/sites/default/files/HealthyFoodZone_FINAL_20130815.pdf

Changelab Solutions. (2015a). *Know the rules: An overview of state agency rulemaking.* https://www.change labsolutions.org/sites/default/files/Know_the_Rules_FINAL_20150709.pdf

Changelab Solutions. (2015b). *Model health in all policies ordinance.* https://www.changelabsolutions .org/sites/default/files/HIAP_ModelOrdinance_FINAL_20150728.pdf

Colorado Department of Public Health & Environment. (n.d.). *Public health & executive orders.* https:// covid19.colorado.gov/public-health-executive-orders

Constitution of Kenya, Ch. 4, Part 2, § 43(1)(a) (2010).

Constitution of the Federative Republic of Brazil, Tit. VIII, Ch. II, art. 196.

Constitution of the Italian Republic, art. 32.

Constitution of the Portuguese Republic, Part I, Tit. III, Ch. II, art. 64(1).

Davis, C. (2018). Legal interventions to reduce overdose mortality: Naloxone access and overdose good Samaritan laws. *The Network for Public Health Law.* https://www.networkforphl.org/wp -content/uploads/2020/01/legal-interventions-to-reduce-overdose.pdf

Deeming Tobacco Products to be Subject to the Federal Food, Drug, and Cosmetic Act, as Amended by the Family Smoking Prevention and Tobacco Control Act; Restrictions on the Sale and Distribution of Tobacco Products and Required Warning Statements for Tobacco Products, 81 Fed. Reg. 28973 (May 10, 2016).

Duncan, J. C., Jr. (2010). A critical consideration of executive orders: Glimmerings of autopoiesis in the executive role. *Vermont Law Review, 35,* 333, 335–336. https://lawreview.vermontlaw.edu/ wp-content/uploads/2012/02/10-Duncan-Book-2-Vol.-35.pdf

Executive Order 13507 of April 8, 2009: Establishment of the White House Office of Health Reform (2009), 3 CFR 13507. https://obamawhitehouse.archives.gov/the-press-office/ executive-order-establishing-white-house-office-health-reform

Executive Order 13544: Establishing the National Prevention, Health Promotion, and Public Health Council (2010), 3 CFR 13544. https://obamawhitehouse.archives.gov/the-press-office/ executive-order-establishing-national-prevention-health-promotion-and-public-health

Federal Register. (n.d.). *Executive orders.* https://www.federalregister.gov/presidential-documents/ executive-orders

Gakh, M., Callahan, K., Goodie, A., & Rutkow, L. (2019). How have states used executive orders to address public health? *Journal of Public Health Management and Practice, 25*(1), 78–80. https://doi. org/10.1097/PHH.0000000000000802

Gakh, M., Vernick, J. S., & Rutkow, L. (2013). Using gubernatorial executive orders to advance public health. *Public Health Reports, 128*(2), 127–130. https://doi.org/10.1177/003335491312800208

Gebbie, K., & Rosenstock, L. (2003). *Who will keep the public healthy?* National Academies Press.

Georgia Code Ann., § 31-12-2.

Georgia Department of Health. (n.d.). *Disease reporting.* https://dph.georgia.gov/epidemiology/ disease-reporting

Goodman, R. A., Hoffman, R. E., Lopez, W., Matthews, G. W., Rothstein, M. A., & Foster, K. L. (Eds.). (2007). *Law in public health practice.* Oxford University Press.

Gostin, L. O. (2000). Public health law in a new century, part II: Public health powers and limits. *Journal of the American Medical Association, 283*(22), 2979–2984. https://doi.org/10.1001/ jama.283.22.2979

Gostin, L. O. (Ed.). (2010). *Public health law and ethics: A reader.* University of California Press.

Gostin, L. O., Hougendobler, D., & Roberts, A. E. (2017). American public health law. *The Oxford Handbook of US Health Law.* http://www.oxfordhandbooks.com/view/10.1093/ oxfordhb/9780199366521.001.0001/oxfordhb-9780199366521-e-44

Gostin, L. O., Monahan, J. T., Kaldor, J., DeBartolo, M., Friedman, E. A., Gottschalk, K., Kim, S. C., Alwan, A., Binagwaho, A., Burci, G. L., Cabal, L., DeLand, K., Evans, T. G., Goosby, E., Hossain, S., Koh, H., Ooms, G., Periago, M. R., Uprimny, R., & Yamin, A. E. (2019). The legal determinants of health: harnessing the power of law for global health and sustainable development. *The Lancet, 393*(10183), 1857–1910. https://doi.org/10.1016/S0140-6736(19)30233-8

Gostin, L. O., & Wiley, L. F. (2016). *Public health law: Power, duty, restraint*. University of California Press.

Hawai'i. Constitution. art. IX.

Heitshusen, V. (2020, November 24). *Introduction to the Legislative Process in the U.S. Congress*. Congressional Research Service. https://fas.org/sgp/crs/misc/R42843.pdf

Hodge, J. G., Jr. (1998). The role of new federalism and public health law. *Journal of Law and Health, 12*, 309. https://engagedscholarship.csuohio.edu/cgi/viewcontent.cgi?article=1227&context=jlh

Hoss, A. (2019). A framework for Tribal public health law. *Nevada Law Journal, 20*(1), 113–144. https://scholars.law.unlv.edu/nlj/vol20/iss1/4/

*Howard v. Ford Motor Company*, No. 763785-2 (Cal. Sup. Ct., October 11, 2000).

Hughes IV, R., Ramdhanie, K., Wasermann, T., & Moscetti C. (2011). State boards of health: Governance and politics. *Journal of Law, Medicine and Ethics, 39*, 37–41. https://doi.org/10.1111/j.1748-720X.2011.00563.x

*Hunter v. City of Pittsburgh*, 207 U.S. 161 (1907).

Illinois Constitution art. XI § 2.

Illinios Constitution Pmbl.

Immerwahr, D. (2016). The greater United States: Territory and empire in US history. *Diplomatic History, 40*(3), 373–391. https://doi.org/10.1093/dh/dhw009

Illinois Department of Public Health. (n.d.). *Prevention & Harm Reduction*. http://www.dph.illinois.gov/opioids/prevention

Indian Health Service. (n.d.). *Agency overview*. https://www.ihs.gov/aboutihs/overview

Indiana Department of Health. (n.d.). *Mission and vision*. https://www.in.gov/isdh/18930.htm

Indiana State Department of Health. (n.d.). *Indiana State Department of Health, Strategic Plan, May 2018–December 2020*. https://www.in.gov/isdh/files/20_STRATEGIC%20PLAN%20docs_7-27%20_FINAL.pdf

Institute of Medicine. (2002). *The future of the public's health in the 21st century—The governmental public health infrastructure*. National Academies Press.

Institute of Medicine. (2011). *For the public health: Revitalizing law and policy to meet new challenges*. National Academies Press.

Introduction: Developments in the law. (2017). *Harvard Law Review, 130*, 1632–1655. https://harvardlawreview.org/2017/04/us-territories-introduction

*Jacobson v. Massachusetts*, 197 U.S. 11 (1905).

Kazis, N. M. (2018). American unicameralism: The structure of local legislatures. *Hastings Law Journal, 96*, 1147–1222. https://repository.uchastings.edu/cgi/viewcontent.cgi?article=3819&context=hastings_law_journal

Kincaid, J. (1988). State constitutions in the federal system. *The Annals of the American Academy of Political and Social Science, 496*(1), 12–22. https://www.jstor.org/stable/1046314?seq=1

Langton, A. K. (2016). The inconsistent limits of the commerce and import-export clauses. *Tax Lawyer, 69*(4), 883–902. https://heinonline.org/HOL/Page?public=true&handle=hein.journals/txlr69&div=37&start_page=883&collection=journals&set_as_cursor=0&men_tab=srchresults

Legal Information Institute at Cornell University Law School. (n.d.-a). *Act*. Wex Legal Dictionary. https://www.law.cornell.edu/wex/act

Legal Information Institute at Cornell University Law School. (n.d.-b). *Case law*. Wex Legal Dictionary. https://www.law.cornell.edu/wex/case_law

Legal Information Institute at Cornell University Law School. (n.d.-c). *Federalism*. Wex Legal Dictionary. https://www.law.cornell.edu/wex/federalism

Legal Information Institute at Cornell University Law School. (n.d.-d). *Ordinance*. Wex Legal Dictionary. https://www.law.cornell.edu/wex/ordinance

Leonard, E. W. (2010). State constitutionalism and the right to health care. *The University of Pennsylvania Journal of Constitutional Law, 12*, 1325–1406. https://scholarship.law.upenn.edu/jcl/vol12/iss5/2

Lester, J. M., & Kerry Cork, K. (2020). *A complex achievement: The tobacco master settlement agreement, looking back to move forward: Resolving health & environmental crises*. Environmental Law Institute.

Library of Congress. (n.d.-a). *American Samoa*. https://guides.loc.gov/law-us-american-samoa

Library of Congress. (n.d.-b). *Guam*. https://guides.loc.gov/law-us-guam

Library of Congress. (n.d.-c). *Northern Mariana Islands*. https://www.loc.gov/law/help/guide/states/us-mp.php

Library of Congress. (n.d.-d). *Puerto Rico.* https://www.loc.gov/law/help/guide/states/us-pr.php

Library of Congress. (n.d.-e). *U.S. Virgin Islands.* https://www.loc.gov/law/help/guide/states/us-vi .php

Lieberman, A. J., & Davis, C. (2020). *Harm reduction laws in the United States.* Network for Public Health Law. https://www.networkforphl.org/wp-content/uploads/2020/12/50-State-Survey -Harm-Reduction-Laws-in-the-United-States-final.pdf

Lin, T. C. (2019). Americans, almost and forgotten. *California Law Review, 107,* 1249. https://www. californialawreview.org/print/americans-almost-and-forgotten/

Maryland Department of Health. (n.d.). *Overdose Prevention in Maryland.* https://bha.health. maryland.gov/OVERDOSE_PREVENTION/Pages/Index.aspx

Michigan Compiled Laws Annotated. 333.2253.

Mississippi Constitution Art. IV, § 86.

Moncrieff, A. R., & Lawless, J. (2017). Healthcare federalism. In I. G. Cohen, A. K. Hoffman, & W. M. Sage (Eds.), *The Oxford Handbook of US Health Law.* Oxford University Press.

Montana Constitution Art. II § 3.

National Association of County and City Health Officials. (2016). *2015 Local Board of Health National Profile.* https://www.naccho.org/uploads/downloadable-resources/Local-Board-of-Health-Profile.pdf

National Association of County and City Health Officials. (2019). *Local Health Department Approaches to Opioid Use Prevention and Response: Florida Department of Public Health.* https:// www.naccho.org/uploads/downloadable-resources/Florida-DOH-Opioids-Success-Story.pdf

National Association of County and City Health Officials. (2020). *2019 National Profile of Local Health Departments.* https://www.naccho.org/uploads/downloadable-resources/NACCHO-2019-Profile-Study-Infographic.pdf

National Conference of State Legislatures. (2020). *Federal and state recognized Tribes.* http://www.ncsl .org/research/state-tribal-institute/list-of-federal-and-state-recognized-tribes.aspx

National Institutes of Health. (2017). *Mission and goals.* https://www.nih.gov/about-nih/what-we-do/ mission-goals

National League of Cities. (2016a). *Cities 101—Forms of local government.* https://www.nlc.org/ resource/cities-101-forms-of-local-government

National League of Cities. (2016b). *Cities 101—Types of local US governments.* https://www.nlc.org/ resource/cities-101-types-of-local-governments

Nev. Rev. Stat. Ann. § 453C.100.

Nev. Rev. Stat. Ann. § 453C.130.

Nev. Rev. Stat. Ann. § 453C.140.

Nev. Rev. Stat. Ann. § 453C.150.

New Mexico Department of Health. (n.d.). *Public health orders and executive orders.* https://cv.nmhealth. org/public-health-orders-and-executive-orders

Ohio Department of Public Health. (2021). *Public health orders.* https://coronavirus.ohio.gov/wps/ portal/gov/covid-19/resources/public-health-orders/public-health-orders

Parmet, W. E., & Daynard, R. A. (2000). The new public health litigation. *Annual Review of Public Health, 21*(1), 437–454. https://doi.org/10.1146/annurev.publhealth.21.1.437

Pepin, D., Winig, B. D., Carr, D., & Jacobson, P. D. (2018). Collaborating for health: Health in all policies and the law. *Journal of Law Medicine and Ethics, 45,* 60–64. https://www.ncbi.nlm.nih .gov/pmc/articles/PMC5523806

Prado, M. M. (2014). Provision of health care services and the right to health in Brazil. In C. M. Flood & A. Gross (Eds.), *The right to health at the public/private divide: A global comparative study.* Cambridge University Press. https://www.cambridge.org/core/books/right-to-health-at-the -publicprivate-divide/provision-of-health-care-services-and-the-right-to-health-in-brazil/ BACF144784DB53A9E593FEA048EE9373

Public Health Law Center. (2015). *State & local public health: An overview of regulatory authority.* https://www.publichealthlawcenter.org/sites/default/files/resources/phlc-fs-state-local-reg -authority-publichealth-2015_0.pdf

Public Health Law Center. (2020). *Dillon's rule, home rule, and preemption.* https://www.public healthlawcenter.org/sites/default/files/resources/Dillons-Rule-Home-Rule-Preemption.pdf

Puerto Rico Constitution art II, § 20.

Raja, K., & Higgins, F. (2019). *Local health department approaches to opioid use prevention and response: An environmental scan*. National Association of County & City Health Officials. https://www .naccho.org/uploads/downloadable-resources/Environmental-Scan-V3-July-2019-FINAL-v2 .pdf

Ransom, M. M. (Ed.). (2016). *Public health law competency model: Version 1.0*. https://www.cdc.gov/ phlp/docs/phlcm-v1.pdf

Roache, S. A., Platkin, C., Gostin, L. O., & Kaplan, C. (2017). Big food and soda versus public health: Industry litigation against local government regulations to promote healthy diets. *Fordham Urban Law Journal, 45*, 1051. https://papers.ssrn.com/sol3/papers.cfm?abstract_id=3190448

Ruhl, J. B., & Robisch, K. (2016). Agencies running from agency discretion. *William & Mary Law Review, 58*, 97, 101. https://scholarship.law.wm.edu/wmlr/vol58/iss1/4/

Sheppard, S. M. (2012). *The Wolters Kluwer Bouvier Law Dictionary, Desk Edition*. Wolters Kluwer.

*State ex rel. Hunter v. Purdue Pharma L.P.*, 2019 Okla. Dist. LEXIS 3486, *36–38.

State of Arizona Executive Order 2017-04, Enhances Surveillance Advisory. https://azgovernor.gov/ sites/default/files/eo_2017-04_0.pdf

State of Illinois Executive Order 2017-05: Executive Order Establishing the Governor's Opioid Prevention and Intervention Task Force (2017). https://www2.illinois.gov/Pages/government/ execorders/2017_5.aspx

State of Illinois Executive Order 2020-02, Executive Order Strengthening the State's Commitment to Ending the Opioid Epidemic (2020). https://www2.illinois.gov/IISNews/21086-Executive _Order_2020-02.pdf

State of Ohio Executive Order 2011-06K (2011). http://worldcat.org/arcviewer/4/OHI/2011/03/04/ H1299259697107/viewer/file1.aspx

Stier, D., & Nicks, D. (2007). Public health and the judiciary. In R. A. Goodman, R. E. Hoffman, W. Lopez, G. W., Matthews, M. A. Rothstein, & K. L. Foster (Eds.), *Law in public health practice*. Oxford University Press. https://oxford.universitypressscholarship.com/view/10.1093/acprof: oso/9780195301489.001.0001/acprof-9780195301489-chapter-4

Substance Abuse and Mental Health Services Administration. (2020). *About us*. https://www .samhsa.gov/about-us

Territorial federalism: Developments in the law. (2017). *Harvard Law Review, 130*, 1632–1655. https:// harvardlawreview.org/2017/04/territorial-federalism

Tobacco Control Legal Consortium. (2013). Laws, policies and regulations: Key terms & concepts. *Public Health Law Center: Tobacco Control Legal Consortium*. https://www.publichealthlawcenter .org/sites/default/files/resources/tclc-fs-laws-policies-regs-commonterms-2015.pdf

Tobin, J., & Barrett, D. (2020). The right to health and health-related human rights. In L. O. Gostin & B. M. Meier (Eds.), *Foundations of global health & human rights*. https://oxford.universitypressscholarship .com/view/10.1093/oso/9780197528297.001.0001/oso-9780197528297-chapter-4

Tulsa Health Department. (n.d.-a). *Director/Board of Health*. https://www.tulsa-health.org/about-us/ directorboard-health

Tulsa Health Department. (n.d.-b). *Mission and values*. https://www.tulsa-health.org/mission -and-values

United Nations General Assembly. (1966). International covenant on economic, social and cultural rights. *Resolution 2200A (XXI) of December, 16, 1966*.

U.S. Census Bureau. (2017). *2017 Census of governments—Organization table 3 general-purpose local governments by state: Census years 1942 to 2017* [CG1700ORG03]. https://www.census.gov/data/ tables/2017/econ/gus/2017-governments.html

U.S. Congress. (n.d.). *Glossary of legislative terms*. https://www.congress.gov/help/legislative-glossary

U.S. Constitution amend. X.

U.S. Constitution art. I, II, III.

U.S. Constitution art. I, § 8.

U.S. Constitution art. IV § 3, cl. 2.

U.S. Department of Health and Human Services. (2015). *HHS agencies & offices*. https://www.hhs .gov/about/agencies/hhs-agencies-and-offices/index.html

Van Dyke, J. M. (1992). The evolving legal relationships between the United States and its affiliated U.S.-Flag Islands. *University of Hawai'i Law Review, 14*(2), 445–518. https://heinonline.org/HOL/

Page?public=true&handle=hein.journals/uhawlr14&div=20&start_page=445&collection=jour nals&set_as_cursor=0&men_tab=srchresults

Vanlandingham, K. E. (1968). Municipal home rule in the United States. *William and Mary Law Review, 10*(2), 269–314. https://heinonline.org/HOL/Page?public=true&handle=hein.journals/ wmlr10&div=25&start_page=269&collection=journals&set_as_cursor=0&men_tab=srchresults

Vernick, J. S., Mair, J. S., Teret, S. P., & Sapsin, J. W. (2003). Role of litigation in preventing product -related injuries. *Epidemiologic Reviews, 25*(1), 90–98. https://doi.org/10.1093/epirev/mxg001

Washington State Department of Health. (n.d.). *Opioids.* https://www.doh.wa.gov/Community andEnvironment/Opioids

Whitehouse.gov. (n.d.-a). *State & local government.* https://www.whitehouse.gov/about-the-white -house/state-local-government

Whitehouse.gov. (n.d.-b). *The executive branch.* https://www.whitehouse.gov/about-the-white-house/ the-executive-branch

Yamin, A. E., & Carmalt, J. C. (2013). The United States: Right to health obligations in the context of disparity and reform. *Advancing the Human Right to Health,* 231–241. https:// oxford.universitypressscholarship.com/view/10.1093/acprof:oso/9780199661619.001.0001/ acprof-9780199661619-chapter-17

## Additional Resources

- **Public Health Law Academy**
  https://www.cdc.gov/phlp/publications/topic/phlacademy.html
- **State & Local Public Health**
  https://www.nhpf.org/library/background-papers/BP77_GovPublicHealth_08-18-2010.pdf
- **An Overview of Regulatory Authority**
  https://www.publichealthlawcenter.org/sites/default/files/resources/phlc-fs-state-local-reg -authority-publichealth-2015_0.pdf
- **Major Components and Themes of Local Public Health Laws in Select U.S. Jurisdictions**
  https://www.ncbi.nlm.nih.gov/pmc/articles/PMC2663884/

# 2

# Constitutional Foundations for Public Health Practice

## Key Terms and Principles

Marice Ashe and Fazal Khan

## Learning Objectives

By the end of this chapter, the reader will be able to:

- Distinguish how the government is structured between the federal, state, and local governments.
- Explain the systems of checks and balances between the legislative, executive, and judicial branches of government.
- Analyze the power of the government to protect the public's health and the limits on that power as outlined in the U.S. Constitution.

## Key Terminology

**Cooperative Federalism:** Cooperative federalism is a form of government in which federal, state, and local governments interact cooperatively and collectively to solve common problems.

**Delegation of Authority:** Delegation of authority means division of authority and powers downward to the subordinate levels of government.

**Enumerated Powers:** Enumerated powers are specific powers granted to Congress by the United States Constitution.

**Equal Protection:** Equal Protection means that the government must treat an individual in the same manner as others in similar conditions and circumstances.

**Immutable Characteristic:** An immutable characteristic is a physical attribute that is perceived as being unchangeable, entrenched, and innate.

**Police Powers:** Police powers are the intrinsic authority to exercise reasonable control over persons and property to promote the health, safety, welfare, and morals of the public.

**Procedural Due Process:** Procedural due process is the constitutional requirement that when the government acts in such a way that denies a person a life, liberty, or property interest, the person must be given notice, the opportunity to be heard, and a decision about the denial must be made by a neutral decision-maker.

**Separation of Powers:** Separation of powers means vesting the legislative, executive, and judicial powers of government in separate bodies.

**Substantive Due Process:** Substantive due process is the notion that due process not only protects certain legal procedures, but also protects certain fundamental human rights.

## Public Health Law Competencies

This chapter addresses the following competencies from the Public Health Law Competency Model (PHLCM; Ransom, 2016).

**1.1**  Define basic constitutional concepts and legal principles framing the practice of public health across relevant jurisdictions.

**2.3**  Recognize the legal authority and limits of critical system partners and others who influence health outcomes.

---

### Spark Questions

1. Suppose an incoming president or governor announces an ambitious plan to change how health-care is delivered—how might separation of powers limit the executive branch's ability to carry out this initiative? (*N.F.I.B. v. Sebelius*, 2012).
2. Many states have passed laws that allow for the sale and possession of marijuana, but this substance is still classified as an illegal drug under the federal Controlled Substances Act. If a marijuana dispensary is operating legally under state law (e.g., Colorado), does this business have legal protection from being prosecuted by the federal government? (*Gonzales v. Raich*, 2005).
3. Should states use their police powers to prohibit activities that pose the threat of self-endangerment, but not any harm to third parties? (*Swann v. Pack*, 1975; *Washington v. Glucksberg*, 1997).
4. The COVID-19 outbreak, some states declared gun shops to be essential businesses allowed to remain open while other states did not list gun shops as essential businesses and they had to close. Do you think this inconsistency should be allowed under the 14th Amendment?
5. The U.S. Constitution protects the rights of individuals to practice religion without government interference, but during the COVID-19 outbreak, religious congregations had to close their doors to large gatherings and regular services. Do you think these public health orders violate Constitutional protections? (*Roman Catholic Diocese of Brooklyn v. Cuomo*, 2020; *South Bay United Pentecostal Church v. Newsom*, 2020).

---

## INTRODUCTION

This chapter introduces the structure of the government in the United States and the concept of **separation of powers** among the federal, state, and local governments. Core legal principles are introduced from the U.S. Constitution that frame the authority of the government to enact and enforce laws to protect and promote the public's health. These Constitutional principles are essential for the health advocate and leader to understand because every federal, state, and local law must comply with them. The core principles include the **enumerated powers** of the federal government and the broad plenary powers of state and local governments—which we call **police powers**—to promote and protect the health, safety, and welfare of the population. The principles also include the limits on this government authority—through the Constitutional doctrines of due process and **equal protection**—that ensure individual liberties such as right to travel and freely associate with other persons, the right to practice religion as one chooses, and the right to not be discriminated against) are protected. Throughout this chapter, we explore how these Constitutional principles affect healthy equity and the social determinants of health by analyzing landmark legal decisions that explain how the law ensures basic notions of justice and fairness for all people.

## Structure of Government

The structure of the federal government consists of three main branches: executive, legislative, and judicial. State governments mirror the federal structure; however, states have their own individual constitutions and reserve the right to organize in any manner they choose. States delegate some of their power to lower levels of government such as counties, and cities. Local governments typically take responsibility for police and fire protection, housing services, emergency medical services, transportation, and public works (sanitation, streets, water, etc.).

The head of the executive branch is the president at the federal level and the governor at the state and/or Tribal level, and their primary function is to carry out the laws. At both federal and state levels, the executive branch is the largest of the three as it contains all the administrative agencies (e.g., health, education, transportation, military/national guard, social services, environmental protection). Federal administrative agencies are implicitly authorized by the U.S. Constitution and are created by Congressional legislation (e.g., the Food, Drug, and Cosmetics Act of 1939 created the Federal Drug Administration [FDA]) to enforce these statutes and develop regulations and policies that further the purpose of the statute. States follow a similar process in the creation of their administrative agencies. The legislative branch is made up of elected representatives and its role is to consider matters brought forth by the executive branch or introduced by its own members to create legislation that becomes law. With the exception of Nebraska, all states have a bicameral legislature made up of two chambers: the smaller upper house is called the Senate and the larger lower chamber is often known as the House of Representatives, the Assembly, or House of Delegates.

As in the federal judicial system, state judicial branches are led by the state supreme court, which hears appeals from lower-level district trial and appellate courts. Rulings made in the supreme court become binding law.

## Separation of Powers

The "separation of powers" doctrine describes the functions of the three main branches of government (executive, legislative, and judicial branches) and how the Constitution ensures an interlocking system of "checks and balances" so that no one branch can exceed its Constitutional authority. Thus, an individual can challenge a law enacted by the legislature and enforced by the executive branch by asking the courts (judiciary) to review the legality of a law (legislature) or a government's action (executive).

## Delegation of Authority

Both the federal and state governments delegate authority either to lower levels of government (i.e., federal to state government, or state to local government) or to administrative agencies. States vary widely in what powers they delegate to local governments. At one end of a continuum, the home rule states delegate all powers vested in the state to local governments, while Dillon rule states delegate no state powers to local governments. Most states are arrayed across this continuum, so local governments in every state have varying authorities to protect public health. For example, during the COVID-19 outbreak, six health departments in the San Francisco Bay Area, which enjoy broad public health authority, declared public health emergencies before the state of California. In other regions of the country, local health agencies had to wait for state declarations of emergency before they could issue stay-at-home orders.

The U.S. Supreme Court case *Jacobson v. Massachusetts* discussed throughout this chapter demonstrates the concept of the statutory **delegation of authority** (*Jacobson v. Massachusetts*, 1905). In this case, the Massachusetts state legislature passed a law that delegated the authority to issue mandatory vaccination orders to local boards of health. Thus, the Massachusetts law did not directly require residents to be vaccinated but gave local boards of health—in this instance, it was the Cambridge board of health—the authority to issue vaccination orders for its residents.

This legislative delegation of authority and discretion to an administrative agency is a common feature of public health laws. In modern times, for reasons related to efficiency, practicality, and insufficient subject matter expertise, legislatures also typically do not pass laws that dictate specific courses of action for most public policy issues. Instead, legislatures approve general laws that state a policy goal (e.g., reduce pollution emissions from cars) and then delegate to an administrative body (e.g., the Environmental Protection Agency) the authority to create more detailed regulatory standards and the discretion to take specific enforcement actions pursuant to such regulations.

## Cooperative Federalism

Oftentimes, legal conflicts arise between Tribal nations, states, and the federal government about which level of government has authority on different matters. In general, the federal, state, Tribal, and local levels of governments try to cooperate with each other whenever possible. **Cooperative federalism** is the term used to describe the political relationship between the federal government, the fifty states, and more than 570 Tribal nations to solve common problems. Here are some examples of cooperative federalism in practice:

- Congress appropriates more than $200 million per year to the Centers for Disease Control and Prevention (CDC) to prevent and control the use of tobacco products. The CDC sends almost $75 million of this funding to states and Tribal nations to implement the CDC's tobacco control goals within their jurisdiction (CDC, Office on Smoking and Health, 2019). The states and Tribal nations regrant some of the funding to cities or counties to implement the CDC's goals at the local level.
- The National Highway Traffic Safety Administration does not regulate whether motorcycle helmets must be worn anywhere in the United States; it leaves that decision to the discretion of the states. However, it has issued regulations detailing the minimum performance requirements for any motorcycle helmet allowed to be sold in the United States. So, while the federal government does not regulate whether a motorcycle helmet must be worn, if a state law requires helmets to be worn, those helmets must meet the federal safety standards (https://one.nhtsa.gov/people/injury/pedbimot/NoMigrate/fmvss218.htm).

However, under the Supremacy Clause of the U.S. Constitution, if there is a conflict between a federal law and a state law, the federal law will preempt or supersede the state law regardless of the Tribal or state sovereignty. Likewise, state constitutions have their own version of a supremacy clause and states can preempt the authority of lower levels of government like cities and counties within their jurisdiction. See Chapter 3 for a more detailed discussion about preemption.

## Police Power: The Basis of State Public Health Authority

When Europeans traveled to the New World, they, too, created a governance process to order society and protect the common good of the community. An early example is the Mayflower Compact, which was signed by Pilgrim leaders to "enact, constitute, and frame, such just and equal laws, ordinances, acts, constitutions, and offices, from time to time, as shall be thought most meet and convenient for the general good of the colony." Eventually, each of the original 13 colonies and all the cities and towns within them had some form of government in place such as an executive (e.g., a governor or a mayor), legislatures (e.g., state legislatures and city councils) composed of elected individuals that passed laws, and a judicial system that interpreted the laws and settled disputes.

When the U.S. Constitution was debated, drafted, and signed, colonial leadership necessarily voided any loyalty or obligations they had to Europe, called themselves "states" rather than "colonies," and voted to give some of their sovereign authority to the newly formed federal government they called the "United States." The new states did not give this new federal government complete power over the states, rather they created a list of limited or "enumerated powers" for the federal government. For example, Article I, Section 8 of the U.S. Constitution gives Congress the power to tax and to spend the money raised by taxes, to provide for the nation's defense and general welfare, and to regulate commerce between the states and with foreign governments.

Any power that was not listed in the Constitution as being given to the federal government was reserved by the new states who retained all the rest of governmental authority to themselves. The states further protected their authority through the 10th Amendment to the Constitution, which says, "The powers not delegated to the United States by the Constitution, nor prohibited by it to the States, are reserved to the States by it, or the people." The 10th Amendment essentially means that when the original 13 colonies became states by joining the United States, they retained—on a state by state basis—a significant degree of sovereignty to enact and enforce laws that each state independently determined would further the health and welfare its residents. Each of the 37 other states that eventually joined the United States also enjoys such authority.

We call the authority of the individual states to pass and enforce the laws and regulations to promote the health, safety, and welfare of their residents the "police power" of that state. In *Jacobson v. Massachusetts*, the Court discussed the scope of a state's police power authority to regulate individual behavior to protect public health. In this case, Reverend Henning Jacobson challenged the constitutionality of a Massachusetts law that authorized local boards of health to order all residents to receive smallpox vaccinations. He argued that the Cambridge law—derived from the state's police power authority—violated his individual liberty rights and that he was being forced to submit to an unsafe medical practice. The Court's opinion highlights several key legal issues that are critical to understanding the broad scope of a state's authority to compel individuals to take unwanted action in order to protect community health.

> The authority of the State to enact this statute is to be referred to what is commonly called the police power—a power which the State did not surrender when becoming a member of the Union under the Constitution. According to settled principles, the police power of a State must be held to embrace, at least, such reasonable regulations established directly by legislative enactment as will protect the public health and the public safety.

Reverend Jacobson claimed that the law, which required him to pay a fine or face imprisonment for refusing a vaccination, was, in effect, equivalent to a state-sanctioned assault that he would be punished for resisting. The Court's powerful rejection of Jacobson's claim and support for the Massachusetts law forms the bedrock of public health law ever since.

[T]he liberty secured by the Constitution of the United States to every person within its jurisdiction does not import an absolute right in each person to be, at all times and in all circumstances, wholly freed from restraint. There are manifold restraints to which every person is necessarily subject for the common good. On any other basis, organized society could not exist with safety to its members. Society based on the rule that each one is a law unto himself would soon be confronted with disorder and anarchy. Real liberty for all could not exist under the operation of a principle which recognizes the right of each individual person to use his own, whether in respect of his person or his property, regardless of the injury that may be done to others.

Today, states use their police power to address a broad array of public health issues, from laws requiring vaccinations and motorcycle helmets, to laws regulating access to abortion or how much pollution a car can emit, to laws closing or opening businesses during the COVID-19 outbreak. And, because each of the 50 states retain sovereignty within a federal system, they often exercise their own judgment on how to exercise their police powers. Thus, there is significant variation in public health laws across the nation. Here are some examples of how states differ in their exercising of police power authorities:

- *School vaccination laws*: Alabama allows for religious exemptions from school vaccination laws, but Arkansas does not (Public Health Law, 2015).
- *Motorcycle helmet laws*: California requires all riders to wear helmets, Texas requires riders 20 years of age and younger to wear a helmet, and three states—Illinois, Iowa, and New Hampshire—have no requirements for any riders to wear helmets (National Conference of State Legislatures, 2018).
- *Tobacco control laws*: As of August 2019, 29 states already raised the legal age to smoke tobacco products to 21 years old (Preventing Tobacco Addiction Foundation, 2019). Then in December 2019, the Congress followed the states' lead and passed legislation increasing the legal age to smoke to 21 years throughout the U.S. (Food & Drug Administration, 2020).

## CONSTITUTIONAL REQUIREMENTS TO PROTECT INDIVIDUAL LIBERTIES

While the government has extensive power to regulate individuals, property, and businesses to protect the public's health, government power has meaningful limits on its reach. The Due Process and Equal Protection clauses derive from the Fifth Amendment (which applies to the federal government) and Fourteen Amendment (which applies to state governments) to the Constitution. These amendments protect individuals from discrimination and unreasonable intrusions into their personal liberty guaranteed by the Constitution.

### Due Process

The Fifth and Fourteenth Amendments to the U.S. Constitution state that the government shall not take a person's life, liberty, or property without "due process" of the law. Conceptually, due process has two major components: **procedural due process** and **substantive due process.**

#### Procedural Due Process

Procedural due process requires the government be fair in the methods used to deprive someone of life, liberty, or property. This requires that the government give a person adequate notice of a proposed government action against that person's liberty and give the person an opportunity to be heard at an official hearing before the government action.

Due process applies to a wide variety of government actions, including both criminal and civil hearings. For example, in *Greene v. Edwards* (1980), the public health authority confined Greene involuntarily to a hospital for treatment of active tuberculosis (TB) under West Virginia's TB Control Act. Greene successfully argued that the TB Control Act violated procedural due process because the law deprived him of significant personal liberty without offering the following procedural safeguards.

(1) an adequate written notice detailing the grounds and underlying facts on which commitment is sought; (2) the right to legal counsel; (3) the right to be present, cross-examine, confront and present witnesses; (4) the standard of proof to warrant commitment to be by clear, cogent, and convincing evidence; and (5) the right to a verbatim transcript of the proceeding for purposes of appeal...

Other examples of procedural due process requirements include: disallowing involuntary confinement of a mentally ill person without convincing evidence that the person poses a threat to themselves or others, ensuring that tobacco or alcohol retailers who allegedly sell products to minors can present exculpating evidence at an administrative hearing before their retail license is rescinded, allowing drivers to present evidence to a court about why they should not have to pay a ticket for a traffic violation. In short, any time the government takes action to deprive a person of life, liberty, or property, the government must follow the five-step process outlined in the *Greene* case. However, note that during a declared public health emergency like COVID-19, the government can issue stay at home orders, close businesses and ration property (like personal protective equipment) without any advanced public hearings or other due process protections.

## Substantive Due Process

"Substantive due process" protects certain fundamental rights from government interference. The U.S. Supreme Court identified fundamental rights that are so "implicit in the concept of ordered liberty" and "deeply rooted" in American history and tradition that any government action infringing on these rights is assumed to be invalid unless proven otherwise.

In applying a substantive due process analysis, the Court will first identify whether an asserted right is a "fundamental right" by analyzing whether it is deeply rooted in American history and traditions. The Court first looks to the Bill of Rights (the first 10 Amendments to the Constitution) to identify fundamental rights. For example, in *Roman Catholic Diocese of Brooklyn v. Cuomo*, the Court shed a new light on the scope of police powers, especially in regard to religious liberties protected under the First Amendment to the constitution. To withstand judicial scrutiny, "emergency orders must now describe gatherings to which they apply and the capacity limits they impose in terms that are tailored to specific risks, rather than imposing location- or purpose-specific restrictions on houses of worship or religious services." (Wiley, 2020)

The Court also recognizes several fundamental rights not specifically enumerated in the Constitution, including but not limited to:

- The right to interstate travel: *Crandall v. Nevada* (1868)
- The right to parent one's children: *Pierce v. Society of Sisters* (1925)
- The right to privacy: *Griswold v. Connecticut* (1965), *Roe v. Wade* (1973), and *Lawrence v. Texas* (2003)
- The right to marriage: *Loving v. Virginia* (1967) and *Obergefell v. Hodges* (2015).

For example, in *Bowers v. Hardwick* (1986), the U.S. Supreme Court upheld the constitutionality of a Georgia "anti-sodomy" law which criminalized oral and anal sex between consenting adults. The majority opinion stated that nowhere in the Constitution is there a "fundamental right to engage in homosexual sodomy" so states such as Georgia were free to prohibit such conduct. But 17 years later, in *Lawrence v. Texas*, the Court invalidated a Texas law (along with

13 other similar state laws) that criminalized homosexual conduct on the grounds that the laws violated the fundamental liberty interests of consenting adults who have the right to be free from government interference in choosing how they have intimate sexual relations. In other words, because U.S. Supreme Court decisions can supersede or preempt state laws, if a state law is found to be in conflict with the U.S. Constitution, the state law is invalid.

Despite the core Constitutional principle of protecting fundamental rights, courts recognize during public health emergencies like the COVID-19 outbreak, the government can restrain the expression of individual liberties. For example, stay at home orders infringed on the right to travel and the right to freely associate with others, the prohibition on holding large events infringed on the right to the free exercise of religion, and the business closures infringed on the right to earn a living and care for one's family. But, as mentioned above, the Court has rejected some limits on holding religious services during the COVID-19 pandemic deeming them too restrictive to pass constitutional muster.

## Equal Protection

The Fifth and Fourteenth Amendments to the U.S. Constitution also state that the government shall not deprive any person the "equal protection" of the laws. The Equal Protection doctrine requires that all laws are applied equally and do not discriminate against individuals because of gender, race, religion, nationality, and physical ability. This means that laws must be both written and applied in a manner that does not discriminate against certain groups without a good reason or what courts call a "rational basis." For instance, all states have laws allowing for the isolation of individuals known to have dangerous contagious diseases and for the quarantine of those known to have been exposed to infected persons. The *Jacobson* case describes such a law. These laws enable a form of government "discrimination" based on disease status or exposure during an outbreak, but they are constitutionally permissible because there is a "rational basis" or good reason to separate such people from those who have not been exposed in order to protect the general population.

But, if a law discriminates against an individual based on an **immutable characteristic** where there has been a history of past wrongful discrimination—such as gender, race, religion, nationality, and physical ability—the government must meet a higher burden of "heightened or strict scrutiny" to justify its actions.

The case of *Jew Ho v. Williamson* (1900) was one of the first federal court decisions to limit the authority of government agencies to infringe on individual liberties of U.S. residents because of racial or ethnic discrimination. In response to nine deaths that San Francisco city officials credited to the bubonic plague, in May of 1900, the local board of health adopted a quarantine order that roughly covered the twelve blocks of the affected Chinatown neighborhood to isolate people who may have been exposed to the plague. The quarantine order did not single out any specific group of people based on race or ethnicity. However, the order was highly discriminatory because it was enforced only against ethnic Chinese homes and businesses but not people of European descent even if they lived in the Chinatown neighborhood.

The federal district court stated,

> [T]his court will, of course, uphold any reasonable regulation that may be imposed for the purpose of protecting the people of the city from the invasion of epidemic disease. In the presence of a great calamity, the court will go to the greatest extent, and give the widest discretion, in construing the regulations that may be adopted by the board of health or the board of supervisors. But is the regulation in this case a reasonable one?...

> The court cannot but see the practical question that is presented to it as to the ineffectiveness of this method of quarantine against such a disease as this. So, upon that ground, the court must hold that this quarantine is not a reasonable regulation to accomplish the purposes sought. ... But there is still another feature of this case that has been called to the

attention of the court, and that is its discriminating character; that is to say, it is said that this quarantine discriminates against the Chinese population of this city, and in favor of the people of other races.…

Therefore the court must hold that this ordinance is invalid and cannot be maintained, that it is contrary to the provisions of the fourteenth amendment of the constitution of the United States, and that the board of health has no authority or right to enforce any ordinance in this city that shall discriminate against any class of persons in favor of another.

It also was due to the equal protection doctrine that the Supreme Court invalidated laws that mandated racially segregated public schools. In *Brown v. Board of Education* (1954), the Court stated,

We conclude that, in the field of public education, the doctrine of "separate but equal" has no place. Separate educational facilities are inherently unequal. Therefore, we hold that the plaintiffs and others similarly situated for whom the actions have been brought are, by reason of the segregation complained of, deprived of the equal protection of the laws guaranteed by the Fourteenth Amendment.

Although it has been over six decades since *Brown*, and five decades since the passage of the Civil Rights Act of 1964, in recent years marginalized groups and individuals have continued to challenge what they see as discriminatory exercises of the government's police powers. In *Church of the Lukumi Bababalu Aye v. City of Hialeah* (1993), the U.S. Supreme Court heard a challenge to three city ordinances that banned "animal sacrifice" within city limits under the guise of protecting public health. Since animal sacrifice is an important religious rite in the Santeria faith, members of a Santeria church in this South Florida city argued that the city violated their Constitutional rights by infringing upon their freedom to practice their religious faith.

## BOX 2.1  HEALTH EQUITY

The Due Process and Equal Protection clauses found in the Fifth and Fourteenth Amendments to the U.S. Constitution provide a strong theoretical basis to redress health inequities if the inequities are rooted in the restriction of a fundamental liberty or if the inequities are caused by discrimination related to an immutable characteristic. But as we see in the *Trump v. Hawaii* case, we cannot always count on the courts to interpret Constitutional guarantees in a consistent manner. Public health leaders and advocates can find themselves on the front lines of ensuring all people are protected from discrimination regardless of who they love or whatever their gender, race, or religion. For more on this subject, see Harris, A. and Pamukcu, A. (2019, March 11). The civil rights of health: A new approach to challenging structural inequality. *UCLA Law Review*, Forthcoming, Available at SSRN: https://ssrn.com/abstract=3350597

Like in the *Jew Ho* case, the city argued that ordinances were not discriminatory as they did not reference the Santeria faith and it was incidental that these regulations prevented their religious rites. However, the Court disagreed and showed evidence of official discriminatory intent by city officials against the Santeria Church through numerous hostile statements they made in public meetings. For example, during one public hearing, a city official stated that followers of Santeria "are in violation of everything this country stands for," and the President of the City Council asked other members what the city could do to "prevent the Church from opening." Thus, in *Lukumi* the Court said that blatantly discriminatory statements against minority groups by political office holders can be used as evidence of unconstitutional discriminatory intent.

However, public health necessity may permit some forms of discrimination without violating the Equal Protection Clause. For example, people who have antibodies for COVID-19 may be able safely to return to work, while people without antibodies must keep sheltering at home. This form of discrimination does not distinguish people based on their race, ethnicity or other immutable characteristic, but rather on neutral criteria of the likelihood of harm to oneself or another due to the infectious disease.

## CONCLUSION

The separate and coequal branches of government are designed to ensure a system of checks and balances to prevent abuses of power by any one branch. The government has broad powers to protect the public's health. The U.S. Constitution limits the reach of that power to protect individual liberty, fairness, and equality.

## CHAPTER REVIEW

### Review Questions

1.  If a motorcycle rider has full health insurance and knows the risks of riding without a helmet, does the state have a compelling reason to mandate that the rider wear a helmet?
2.  Is there clear evidence that points to the causes of the opioid addiction epidemic in the United States? Further, how would you propose combatting the spread and deadly effects of this crisis?

### Essay Question

Should states allow parents to opt-out of having their children receive standard vaccinations? Does it make a difference if their objection is based on religious grounds or if it is simply philosophical (nonfaith based)?

### Internet Activities

1.  Find and describe the structure of government in your state. You may want to start by looking at your state's official government website (often, STATE.GOV). Describe the governmental structure. Who is the governor? What administrative agency(ies) oversees public health functions? What is the make-up of the legislative body? Who sits on the state Supreme Court? How is authority delegated to local governments? It might be interesting to do this exercise and ask the same questions for your local government, too.
2.  Find the list of Enumerated Powers in Article 1, Section 8 of the U.S. Constitution. Create a list of all the powers of Congress. What is the "necessary and proper" clause? Identify a Supreme Court case wherein a Congressional statute was upheld under this clause.
3.  Find the Alcohol Policy Information System (APIS). Describe at least five variables for how the alcohol control laws for all 50 states are similar and different from each other.
4.  Suppose there is a new outbreak of the deadly SARS virus, and it is spreading rapidly through a large U.S. city. Do local public health officials have to follow all the *Greene* standards if the Governor has declared a state of emergency?
5.  Find the Bill of Rights and the Supreme Court cases listed previously. Can you describe the test the Supreme Court uses to identify whether a claimed individual right is a fundamental right under the Constitution? Why do you think application of this test sometimes yields inconsistent results, for example in the *Bowers* and *Lawrence* decisions?

6. Find the case *Trump v. Hawaii* (2018) challenging the federal ban on travel from predominantly Muslim countries. In that case, the State of Hawaii claimed that President Trump made blatantly hostile public statements that targeted almost exclusively immigrants from several Muslim-majority countries. Do you agree with the Court that the travel ban was not discriminatory because it was not motivated by religious hostility and it was justified on national security grounds?

## REFERENCES

*Bowers v. Hardwick*, 478 U.S. 186 (1986).

*Brown v. Board of Education of Topeka*, 347 U.S. 483 (1954).

Centers for Disease Control and Prevention, Office for State, Tribal, Local and Territorial Support. (2017). State school immunization requirements and state vaccine laws. Public Health Law. https://www.cdc.gov/phlp/docs/school-vaccinations.pdf (Originally published 2015).

Centers for Disease Control and Prevention, Office on Smoking and Health. (n.d.). *National tobacco control program funding.* https://www.cdc.gov/tobacco/about/osh/program-funding/index.htm

*Church of the Lukumi Babalu Aye, Inc. v. Hialeah*, 508 U.S. 520 (1993).

*Crandall v. Nevada*, 73 U.S. (6 Wall.) 35 (1868).

Food & Drug Administration. (2020, October 6). *Selling tobacco products in retail stores.* https://www.fda.gov/tobacco-products/retail-sales-tobacco-products/selling-tobacco-products-retail-stores

*Gonzales v. Raich*, 545 U.S. 1 (2005).

*Greene v. Edwards*, 263 S.E.2d 661 (W. Va. 1980).

*Griswold v. Connecticut*, 381 U.S. 479 (1965).

Haudenosaunee. (n.d.). *Government.* http://www.kahnawakelonghouse.com/index.php?mid=1

*Jacobson v. Massachusetts*, 197 U.S. 11 (1905).

*Jew Ho v. Williamson*, 103 F. 10 (1900).

*Lawrence v. Texas*, 539 U.S. 558 (2003).

*Loving v. Virginia*, 388 U.S. 1 (1967).

Lindsay F. Wiley, Democratizing the Law of Social Distancing, 19 YALE J. HEALTH POL'Y L. & ETHICS (2020). Available at: https://digitalcommons.law.yale.edu/yjhple/vol19/iss3/2

National Conference of State Legislatures. (2021, May 12). *Motorcycle safety overview.* http://www.ncsl.org/research/transportation/motorcycle-safety-overview.aspx

*N.F.I.B. v. Sebelius*, 567 U.S. 519 (2012).

*Obergefell v. Hodges*, 135 S. Ct. 2584 (2015).

*Pierce, Governor of Oregon, et al. v. Society of the Sisters of the Holy Names of Jesus and Mary*, 268 U.S. 510 (1925).

Preventing Tobacco Addiction Foundation. (2019). *State by state.* https://tobacco21.org/state-by-state/

Public Health Law. (2015). *State school immunization requirements and state vaccine laws.* Centers for Disease Control Public Health Law Program. https://www.cdc.gov/phlp/docs/school-vaccinations.pdf

Ransom, M. M. (Ed.). (2016). *Public health law competency model: Version 1.0.* Centers for Disease Control. https://www.cdc.gov/phlp/docs/phlcm-v1.pdf

*Roe v. Wade*, 410 U.S. 113 (1973).

*Roman Catholic Diocese of Brooklyn v. Cuomo*, 592 U.S. __ (2020).

*South Bay United Pentecostal Church v. Newsom*, 590 U.S. __(2020).

*Swann v. Pack*, 527 S.W.2d 99 (1975).

*Trump v. Hawaii*, 138 S. Ct. 2392 (2018).

*Washington v. Glucksberg*, 521 U.S. 702 (1997).

Wiley, L. 20 Yale J. Health Pol'y, L & Ethics (forthcoming, December 2020).

## Additional Resources

- **Public Health Law Academy: Public Health Law: Past & Present**
  https://www.changelabsolutions.org/phla/public-health-law
- **Public Health Law Academy: Structure of Government**
  https://www.changelabsolutions.org/product/structure-government

# 3

# Limitations on Public Health Authority

## Exploring Preemption

Derek Carr, Benjamin D. Winig, and Sabrina Adler

## Learning Objectives

By the end of this chapter, the reader will be able to:

- Discuss the legal concept of preemption and contrast the different types of preemption.
- Articulate when and how preemption can positively or negatively affect public health and health equity.
- Determine how public health professionals can identify preemption.

## Key Terminology

**Ceiling Preemption:** When a higher-level government prohibits lower-level governments from requiring anything more than or different from what the higher-level law requires.

**Express Preemption:** When a law explicitly states that it preempts lower-level lawmaking authority.

**Field Preemption:** When a higher-level government prohibits lower-level governments from passing or enforcing any laws on an issue, reserving the entire area (the field) of regulation to itself.

**Floor Preemption:** When a higher-level government passes a law that establishes a minimum set of requirements and allows lower-level governments to pass and enforce laws that impose more rigorous requirements.

**Implied Preemption:** When a law passed by a higher-level government contains no explicit preemption-related language but is nevertheless found to preempt the authority of a lower-level government.

**Preemption:** A legal doctrine that provides that a higher-level government may limit, or even eliminate, the power of a lower-level government to regulate a certain issue.

**Punitive Preemption:** When a state government not only preempts local laws on a subject but also punishes local officials and local governments that attempt to enact or enforce preempted laws.

**Vacuum Preemption:** When a higher-level government chooses not to enact any substantive regulations on a topic and forbids lower-level governments from doing so, creating a regulatory vacuum.

## Public Health Law Competencies

This chapter addresses the following competencies from the Public Health Law Competency Model (PHLCM; Ransom, 2016).

**1.1** Define basic constitutional concepts and legal principles framing the practice of public health across relevant jurisdictions.

**1.2** Identify and apply public health laws (e.g., statutes, regulations, ordinances, and court rulings) pertinent to a practitioner's jurisdiction, agency, program, and profession.

**2.3** Recognize the legal authority and limits of critical system partners and others who influence health outcomes.

---

### Spark Questions

1. What is one way that state preemption may have a *negative* effect on public health and/or health equity?
2. What is one way that state preemption may have a *positive* effect on public health and/or health equity?

---

### BOX 3.1 PREEMPTION AND HEALTH EQUITY

- A report from the National Employment Law Project found that in 12 jurisdictions where states preempted previously enacted local minimum-wage laws, the affected populations were often disproportionately women and people of color. These communities also had significantly higher poverty rates compared to the U.S. population generally (Huizar & Lathrop, 2019).
- "[M]any state legislatures are exercising their power to preempt local laws in a manner that frustrates racial justice goals and reduces the political self-determination of people of color. ... [However, s]tate legislation can, at times, be an effective tool for limiting the ability of local governments to adopt policies that generate inequality. ... The challenge for racial justice advocates is differentiating between the increasingly common state preemption laws that undermine racial justice goals and those that do the opposite" (Silverstein, 2017, pp. 1–2).

## INTRODUCTION

The legal term **preemption** may have little resonance outside of courts and legislative chambers. But what it describes—the invalidation of state law by federal law, or of local law by state or federal law—has profound significance for public health (Mermin, 2009). Preemption affects everything from the quality of medical devices to the extent of tobacco advertising, from the availability of affordable housing to employment conditions and immigration enforcement. In other words, preemption affects almost everything a public health professional does. Although legal briefs and court opinions about preemption are routinely filled with elaborate and complicated analyses of the issue, outside the courtroom—and particularly inside legislative offices—preemption is mostly a matter of policy and political judgment.

A fundamental question with respect to preemption is which level of government is most appropriate to advance public health and health equity. Public health and movements for social-norm change often start at the local level, with cities and counties serving as "laboratories

## BOX 3.2 LEGAL PRINCIPLES AND FRAMEWORKS

"Preemption" is a legal doctrine allowing a higher level of government to limit or even eliminate the power of a lower level of government to regulate a specific issue (ChangeLab Solutions, 2019). Under the U.S. Constitution's Supremacy Clause, federal law takes precedence over state and local laws (U.S. Const. art. VI, cl. 2). Similarly, cities, counties, and other localities are "creatures of the state," and therefore state law generally takes precedence over local laws ("A municipal corporation … is one of [the state's] creatures, made for a specific purpose, to exercise within a limited sphere the powers of the State. The State may withdraw these local powers of government at pleasure, and may, through its legislature or other appointed channels, govern the local territory as it governs the State at large. It may enlarge or contract its powers or destroy its existence" [*United States v. Baltimore & Ohio Railroad Company*, (1872)]).

Preemption can take several forms, establishing minimum or maximum standards, or create a regulatory void by preventing any regulation on an issue. Higher-level laws may include explicit preemption language or may be interpreted to preempt lower-level laws. The scope of preemption also varies substantially: higher-level laws can preempt an entire area of regulation or only specific components of an issue (ChangeLab Solutions, 2019).

In addition to preemption, protections afforded by the U.S. Constitution and state constitutions—the Due Process Clause, for example—can prevent state and local governments from taking certain actions (U.S. Const. amend. V).

of democracy" to test new and innovative policies (Diller, 2014).[1] The risks of innovation are often best borne out at the local level, where the electorate can more easily register its preferences through the democratic process, and where changes can be made more swiftly.

Today, local governments frequently serve as a locus for policy innovations with the potential to improve community health outcomes and reduce health inequities. These include more traditional public health policies such as those that regulate tobacco and alcohol sales, promote healthy eating, and restrict access to firearms. They also include policies focused on social determinants of health (SDOHs) such as paid sick leave, mandatory inclusionary zoning, and expanded antidiscrimination protections.

Some state legislatures, however, are using preemption with increasing regularity to block local government action (Riverstone-Newell, 2017). Extensive literature has documented this rise in state preemption and warned about its potential to undermine local efforts to protect public health (Pomeranz & Pertschuk, 2017; Pomeranz et al., 2019; Riverstone-Newell, 2017; Schragger, 2018). Preliminary research supports these concerns: states that removed local authority to raise the minimum wage, mandate paid employment leave, or regulate firearms have made smaller gains in life expectancy since the 1980s and now find themselves on par with middle-income countries (Montez, 2017).

When misused, preemption can threaten a state or local government's ability to be representative of and responsive to the people they represent. When a locality is demographically very different—for example, racially or socioeconomically—from the whole state, the state legislature may not reflect either the makeup or the political preferences of the locality. By enacting preemptive state-level laws, the state legislature prevents the locality from addressing specific problems in a manner that best serves those most affected. This can also occur at the federal level, when a state is demographically very different than the country and the federal government preempts state and local regulation of an issue. In some of these cases, preemption may be purposefully discriminatory or have an inequitable effect regardless of intent.

---

[1] See *New State Ice Co. v. Liebmann* (1932). Justice Brandeis' dissent stated: "It is one of the happy incidents of the federal system that a single courageous state may, if its citizens choose, serve as a laboratory; and try novel social and economic experiments without risk to the rest of the country."

Despite its potential for misuse, preemption itself is not inherently adversarial to public health, equity, or good governance. To the contrary, as the Civil Rights Movement took hold, the federal government responded to discriminatory state and local policies with preemptive federal laws. Congress enacted legislation establishing nationwide antidiscrimination protections, including the Civil Rights Act of 1964, the Voting Rights Act of 1965, and the Fair Housing Act (Silverstein, 2017). Although some viewed the preemptive nature of these laws as unduly interfering with state and local authority, subsequent research demonstrated their positive effect on public health and health equity (Hahn et al., 2018; McGowan et al., 2016). Indeed, federal civil rights legislation exemplifies the use of preemption to foster more equitable systems, institutions, and health outcomes.

Accordingly, preemption is not an inherently positive or negative tool. With respect to public health, health equity, and SDOHs, preemption has often thwarted potentially beneficial local innovations. At other times, however, preemptive laws have set strong standards, either at the federal or state levels, that reach people in jurisdictions where such laws might not have been enacted otherwise. For example, the federal menu-labeling rule requires certain chain restaurants around the country to label calories on their menus (21 U.S.C. § 343(q)(5)(H); 21 C.F.R. § 101.11). Customers in states that never would have enacted menu-labeling requirements will nonetheless reap the benefits of that policy. However, the resulting trade-off is that no state or locality may enact different or stronger standards for menu labeling in those same restaurants (21 U.S.C. § 343-1[a][4]). The varying effects of preemption on health and health equity make it important to frame any social norm, public health, or policy change effort around the advancement of public health and equity, and then to assess how preemption might factor into accomplishing that goal.

## FEDERAL AND STATE LEGAL FRAMEWORK

### Federal, State, and Local Regulatory Authority

Chapter 2 addresses the sources from which different levels of government derive their authority to create and enforce laws that affect public health and health equity, and limitations on those powers. Understanding preemption requires consideration of these authorities and limitations. As the "supreme law of the land," the U.S. Constitution defines the power of the federal government and distributes power between the federal and state governments. Under the Constitution's "Supremacy Clause," federal law takes precedence over lower-level laws (U.S. Const. art. VI, cl. 2). The federal government has "limited powers," meaning it has only those powers enumerated by the Constitution such as to tax, spend, and regulate interstate commerce (16A Am. Jur. 2d Constitutional Law § 214). This allows the federal government to make and enforce some laws relating to public health and equity.

States and local governments have greater flexibility to enact laws to protect public health and equity. The U.S. Constitution's 10th Amendment reserves to states all legal authority not specifically granted to the federal government (U.S. Const. amend. X). States have what is known as "police power," which encompasses the power of states—and, by delegation, local governments—to promote the public health, safety, and general well-being of the community (16A Am. Jur. 2d Constitutional Law § 332; *Jacobson v. Commonwealth of Massachusetts*, 1905). The police power is a plenary power of the state, meaning that states can choose how much, if any, of this power to share with local governments (56 Am. Jur. 2d Municipal Corporations, Etc. § 13; Schragger, 2018). Thus, whereas the U.S. Constitution is the source of states' police power, local governments must rely on states for this authority.[2]

The degree to which local governments have autonomous powers varies greatly by state. Some states give local governments extensive autonomy, known as "home rule authority"

---

[2] See, e.g., *Payne v. Massey* (1946). "Municipalities are creatures of our law and are created as political subdivisions of the state as a convenient agency for the exercise of such powers as are conferred upon them by the state. They represent no sovereignty distinct from the state and possess only such powers and privileges as have been expressly or impliedly conferred upon them. All acts done by them must find authority in the law of their creation."

(56 Am. Jur. 2d Municipal Corporations, Etc. § 109). In those states, local governments can directly enact laws without relying on a specific delegation of power from the state legislature. Home rule limits the degree of state interference in local affairs but does not eliminate it (Schragger, 2018). In contrast, local governments in other states—known as "Dillon's Rule states"—may exercise only those powers explicitly granted to them by the state legislature (§ 4:11.Delegation of powers by legislature—Municipal powers under Dillon's Rule, 2 McQuillin Mun. Corp. § 4:11 [3d ed.]; § 10:10.Scope of powers—Dillon's Rule, 2A McQuillin Mun. Corp. § 10:10 [3d ed.]).

## Preemption as a Limitation on State and Local Authority

Regardless of the general scope of a state or local government's legal authority, its ability to enact public health laws or regulations may be affected by the laws of higher-level governments. Generally, regardless of whether there is explicit preemption, a government cannot do anything that *conflicts* with a higher-level government law (*Massachusetts Crosby v. Nat'l Foreign Trade Council*, 2000). For example, federal law prohibits the sale of all flavored cigarettes except for menthol cigarettes (21 U.S.C. § 387g[a][1][A]). A state law authorizing the sale of fruit-flavored cigarettes would conflict with federal law and thus federal law would preempt (i.e., invalidate) the state law. Similarly, if a state law prohibits the sale of menthol cigarettes, the state law would preempt a conflicting local law authorizing the sale of menthol cigarettes.

### What Are the Types of Preemption?

Preemption can take many forms. Depending on the type of preemption, lower-level governments may be prevented from enacting any laws on a certain issue or they may be unable to pass certain types of laws affecting that issue.

Higher-level governments commonly enact laws establishing minimum standards but allow lower-level governments to decide whether to exceed those standards. This type of preemption is referred to as **floor preemption** because the higher-level government (e.g. Congress or the state legislature) is setting a base level, which lower-level governments (i.e., states or localities) cannot go below but may choose to exceed. For example, the federal Fair Labor Standards Act establishes a national minimum wage but allows states and localities to establish a higher minimum wage (Fair Labor Standards Act of 1938, 29 U.S.C. §§ 206[a], 218[a]).

Conversely, higher-level governments can preempt lower-level governments' laws that impose additional requirements or limitations. This type of preemption is known as **ceiling preemption** because lower-level governments may not exceed the standards established in the higher-level law. The federal law regulating warning labels on cigarette packages, for example, expressly prohibits states and localities from imposing additional warning requirements (15 U.S.C. § 1334). Likewise, although the federal minimum wage law establishes a floor, many state minimum wage laws preempt localities from establishing a higher minimum wage (National Employment Law Project, 2017).

A final form of preemption, sometimes referred to as **vacuum preemption,** occurs when a higher-level government chooses not to enact regulations on an issue but still forbids lower-level governments from regulating that issue, creating a regulatory void. For example, Iowa state law preempts local governments from requiring that employers provide paid sick leave to employees even though Iowa state law does not regulate paid sick leave (Iowa Code § 331.304(12)).

### How Does Preemption Occur?

Preemption can occur in several ways. **Express preemption** occurs when a law explicitly states that it preempts lower-level lawmaking authority, whereas **implied preemption** occurs when a law contains no explicit preemption-related language but nevertheless is found to preempt state or local authority (ChangeLab Solutions, 2019). For example, implied preemption may occur when a higher-level law sets forth a comprehensive scheme of regulation on an issue, leaving no room for lower-level governments to regulate. Implied preemption may also be found when a lower-level law poses an obstacle to or frustrates the purpose of a higher-level law (*Geier v. Am. Honda Motor Co.*, 2000).

## What Is the Scope of Preemption?

Preemption can be broad or narrow. **Field preemption** occurs when a higher-level government prohibits a lower-level government from passing or enforcing *any* laws on an issue, reserving the entire area of regulation to itself (Mermin, 2009). Alternatively, a higher-level government can choose to preempt only lower-level laws affecting *specific components* of an issue (Mermin, 2009). South Dakota, for instance, largely preempts the field of tobacco control, including local regulations on the distribution, marketing, promotion, and sale of tobacco products (S.D. Codified Laws § 34-46-6). California, in contrast, preempts only local taxation of tobacco products (Cal. Rev. & Tax. Code § 30111).

## How Do You Identify Preemption?

Lower-level governments can identify express preemption by reviewing the plain language of higher-level laws. Express preemption clauses do not always use the term "preemption," however. Other words or phrases that may demonstrate preemptive intent include "exclusive," "supersede," "matter of statewide concern," "occupy the field," "uniform," "and sole authority" (ChangeLab Solutions, 2020). A preemptive higher-level law may also specify that lower-level laws must be consistent with, not exceed, nor be more stringent or restrictive than the higher-level law (ChangeLab Solutions, 2020). Implied preemption is more difficult to spot because the higher-level law does not include any explicit language indicating a preemptive intent—even courts at times have trouble determining whether preemption is present if it is not explicit. Identifying implied preemption requires examining other sources such as court decisions and legislative intent (§ 24:57.Requisites for validity—Conformity or conflict with state law—Implied preemption, 6A McQuillin Mun. Corp. § 24:57 [3d ed.]).

## Additional Limitations on State and Local Authority

In addition to preemption, other legal principles can operate to limit state and local action. For example, both the U.S. Constitution and state constitutions afford individuals certain due process protections prior to infringing on an individual's autonomy or property interests, such as by mandating vaccination or suspending a professional or business license (*Holm v. Iowa Dist. Court for Jones Cty.*, 2009; *Jacobson v. Commonwealth of Massachusetts*, 1905). These protections can be substantive, requiring the government to provide a sufficient justification, such as a legitimate public health rationale, or procedural, requiring the government to provide a fair process such as an impartial decision rendered after providing an individual notice and an opportunity to be heard (16B Am. Jur. 2d Constitutional Law § 953).[3] Chapter 2 discusses due process in greater detail.

Other constitutional provisions may also preclude a state or local government from taking certain actions. The First Amendment, for instance, is increasingly used to invalidate public health laws such as prohibiting tobacco advertisements near schools (*Lorillard Tobacco Co. v.*

---

[3] *Cleveland Bd. of Educ. v. Loudermill* (1985). "The point is straightforward: the Due Process Clause provides that certain substantive rights—life, liberty, and property—cannot be deprived except pursuant to constitutionally adequate procedures."

*Howard v. Grinage* (1996). "In short, substantive due process prohibits the government's abuse of power or its use for the purpose of oppression, and procedural due process prohibits arbitrary and unfair deprivations of protected life, liberty, or property interests without procedural safeguards."

*Reilly*, 2001). Several states impose limitations on local government authority to raise and spend revenue, often referred to as "tax and expenditure limitations," such as requiring voter approval for new or increased taxes (Wen et al., 2018). Finally, some states and localities authorize voter initiatives and referendums and restrict the ability of governments to modify or repeal laws enacted through such processes (42 Am. Jur. 2d Initiative and Referendum § 1).[4]

## NEW PREEMPTION

The tug-of-war over the distribution of power among federal, state, and local governments is nothing new. The history of the tobacco control movement is rife with examples of industry using state-level preemption to stop local efforts to expand tobacco control laws (Public Health Law Center, 2018). Traditionally, however, preemption was used as a legislative and judicial tool to resolve problems that arose when different levels of government adopted conflicting laws on the same subject. The preemption analysis in these scenarios generally sought to balance uniformity in laws across jurisdictions with the value of locally tailored policies (Briffault et al., 2019).

In recent years, however, states have increasingly used preemption to prevent communities from enacting laws that could reduce inequities and enhance community health, instead seeking to protect the power and financial interests of established political or commercial entities (Schragger, 2018). Many of these more recent preemptive efforts appear motivated by "ideological or practical opposition to specific measures" rather than a need for uniform statewide regulation (Johnson, 2016). Indeed, model legislation crafted by the American Legislative Exchange Council, an organization whose members include corporations and state legislators, has served as a driving force promoting state preemption across subject areas (Riverstone-Newell, 2017). These more recent preemptive laws—referred to as "New Preemption"—differ from traditional preemption laws in form, substance, and application, more commonly employing vacuum preemption to operate as a blunt deregulatory tool (Briffault, 2018a).

New Preemption has also been characterized by the proliferation of state legislation that not only prohibits local governments from regulating an area but also penalizes local officials and local governments from enacting, or even attempting to enact, potentially preempted local policies (Briffault, 2018b). For example, several states have adopted laws that would subject local officials to fines, civil liability, and removal from office for passing or enforcing local gun safety regulations (Ariz. Rev. Stat. Ann. § 41-194.01, Fla. Stat. § 790.33). Some of these **punitive preemption** laws also seek to punish local governments by withdrawing state funding. Arizona, for instance, can withhold all state funds from any local government that does not repeal local laws, on any subject, that are subject to state preemption (Ariz. Rev. Stat. Ann. § 41-194.01).

## PREEMPTION IN ACTION

In June 2018, the California legislature enacted a law preempting any new or increased local sugary drink taxes until 2031 (Keep Groceries Affordable Act of 2018, Cal. Rev. & Tax Code §§ 7284.12, 7284.16). This preemptive legislation, which occurred in a state known for strong local authority and where four local jurisdictions had already adopted sugary drink taxes, is part of a larger story. Earlier in the year, the beverage industry and other special interests had qualified a ballot proposition for the November 2018 election that would have devastated state

---

[4] See, e.g., *People v. Kelly* (2010). "We begin with the observation that [t]he purpose of California's constitutional limitation on the Legislature's power to amend initiative statutes is to protect the people's initiative powers by precluding the Legislature from undoing what the people have done, without the electorate's consent."

and local government finances (Koseff, 2018). The proposition, however, served as a bargaining chip to obtain preemption of local sugary drink taxes. Knowing that local jurisdictions were reliant on the types of revenues at risk should the proposition pass, the beverage industry offered to rescind the proposition in exchange for state legislation prohibiting localities from enacting sugary drink taxes. State legislators made clear that they did not support preempting local sugary drink taxes, but felt they had no choice other than to accept the deal to avoid the proposition's potentially devastating effects on California cities and counties (O'Connor & Sanger-Katz, 2018). The legislature easily passed the bill and the beverage industry removed the proposition from the ballot. Now, state law preempts local governments in California from enacting any new or increasing any existing sugary drink taxes. As a result, California cities and counties, several of which were actively pursuing sugary drink taxes, now lack the authority to adopt an evidence-based policy proven to improve public health and raise revenues to support initiatives to combat health inequities.

## SEMINAL AND HISTORICAL CASES

### Cipollone v. Liggett Group, Inc., 505 U.S. 504 (1992)

The Federal Cigarette Labeling and Advertising Act (FCLAA) expressly preempts states and local governments from requiring cigarette health warnings beyond those mandated by federal law (15 U.S.C. § 1334). In 1992, the U.S. Supreme Court held this preemption clause prohibits most lawsuits based on cigarette advertisements' failure to include sufficient health warnings but does not preempt lawsuits based on tobacco companies' efforts to mislead the public about the dangers of smoking (*Cipollone v. Liggett Group, Inc.*, 1992). In limiting FCLAA's preemptive scope, the Supreme Court relied on the statute's plain language and the "presumption against preemption of state police powers" (*Cipollone v. Liggett Group, Inc.*, 1992).

### City of Cleveland v. State of Ohio, 989 N.E.2d 1072 (Ohio Ct. App. 2013)

In April 2011, the city of Cleveland adopted an ordinance prohibiting local grocery stores and restaurants from selling foods containing artificial trans-fat. The state legislature subsequently adopted legislation to block (i.e., preempt) Cleveland's ability to regulate food ingredients. In response, the city sued the state arguing that the preemptive legislation violated Cleveland's home rule authority. The court agreed with Cleveland, finding that the state legislature's action was an unconstitutional attempt to preempt the city from exercising its home rule powers. Home rule is discussed in detail in Chapter 1.

### U.S. Smokeless Tobacco Manufacturing Company LLC v. City of New York, 708 F.3d 428 (2d Circ. 2013)

In 2009, New York City adopted an ordinance restricting the sale of flavored tobacco products except in a tobacco bar. The tobacco industry responded by filing a lawsuit arguing that the federal Family Smoking Prevention and Tobacco Control Act (TCA) preempted the New York City ordinance (*U.S. Smokeless Tobacco Mfg. Co., LLC v. City of New York*, 2010). The federal Second Circuit Court of Appeals held that the TCA does *not* preempt New York City's ordinance. The court reasoned that the TCA reserves exclusive authority to regulate tobacco *manufacturing* but explicitly allows (i.e., does not preempt) state and local governments to enact more stringent *sales* restrictions (*U.S. Smokeless Tobacco Mfg. Co., LLC v. City of New York*, 2013). Other federal courts that have examined this issue have reached the same conclusion (*Indeps. Gas &*

*Serv. Stations Associations, Inc. v. City of Chicago*, 2015; *National Association of Tobacco Outlets, Inc. v. City of Providence*, 2013).

## CONCLUSION

Preemption is when a higher-level government limits or even eliminates the authority of a lower-level government to regulate a certain issue. Preemption can establish minimum standards (floor preemption), maximum standards (ceiling preemption), or a regulatory void (vacuum preemption). State legislatures are using preemption with increasing regularity to prevent local regulation across a range of areas related to public health and the SDOHs. Although preemption has most often been used to block local public health laws, it is not inherently adversarial to public health, health equity, or good governance. The inconsistent effects of preemption on health and equity make it important to frame any policy change effort around the advancement of public health and health equity, and then to assess how preemption might factor into accomplishing that goal.

## CHAPTER REVIEW

### Review Questions

1.  The federal government has total authority over state and local affairs.
    True/False

2.  Local governments have authority to enact laws regardless of what state law says.
    True/False

3.  Preemption is always harmful to public health and health equity.
    True/False

4.  To determine whether a higher-level law preempts an issue, what should you consider?
    a.  Plain language of the law
    b.  Legislative intent
    c.  Case law
    d.  A and B
    e.  A, B, and C

### Discussion Questions

1.  What is one example of *ceiling preemption* likely to harm public health and/or health equity? An example likely to advance health equity?
2.  What is one example of *floor preemption* likely to harm public health and/or health equity? An example likely to advance health equity?
3.  What is one example of *vacuum preemption* likely to harm public health and/or health equity? An example likely to advance health equity?

### Internet Activities

1.  Determine whether your state preempts specific public health or social determinant of health issue areas. Identify which ones, if any, are preempted.
2.  How do major population centers in your state differ demographically from the state as a whole? How might these differences affect preemption and its impact on public health and health equity?

# REFERENCES

§ 10:10.Scope of powers—Dillon's Rule, 2A McQuillin Mun. Corp. § 10:10 (3d ed.).

§ 24:57.Requisites for validity—Conformity or conflict with state law—Implied preemption, 6A McQuillin Mun. Corp. § 24:57 (3d ed.).

§ 4:11.Delegation of powers by legislature—Municipal powers under Dillon's Rule, 2 McQuillin Mun. Corp. § 4:11 (3d ed.).

15 U.S.C. § 1334.

16A Am. Jur. 2d Constitutional Law § 214.

16A Am. Jur. 2d Constitutional Law § 332.

16B Am. Jur. 2d Constitutional Law § 953.

21 C.F.R. § 101.11.

21 U.S.C. § 343(q)(5)(H).

21 U.S.C. § 343-1(a)(4).

21 U.S.C. § 387g(a)(1)(A).

42 Am. Jur. 2d Initiative and Referendum § 1.

56 Am. Jur. 2d Municipal Corporations, Etc. § 13.

56 Am. Jur. 2d Municipal Corporations, Etc. § 109.

Ariz. Rev. Stat. Ann. § 41–194.01.

Briffault, R. (2018a). *The challenge of the new preemption.* Columbia Public Law Research Paper No. 14-580. https://scholarship.law.columbia.edu/faculty_scholarship/2090

Briffault, R. (2018b). *Punitive preemption: An unprecedented attack on local democracy.* Local Solutions Support Center.

Briffault, R., Davidson, N. M., & Reynolds, L. (2019). *The new preemption reader: Legislation, cases, and commentary on the leading challenge in today's state and local government law.* West Academic.

California Revenue & Tax. Code § 30111.

ChangeLab Solutions. (2019, June). *Fundamentals of preemption.* https://www.changelabsolutions.org/product/understanding-preemption

ChangeLab Solutions. (2020). *Assessing and addressing preemption: A toolkit for local policy campaigns.* https://www.changelabsolutions.org/product/assessing-addressing-preemption

*Cipollone v. Liggett Group, Inc.,* 505 U.S. 504 (1992).

*Cleveland Board of Education v. Loudermill,* 470 U.S. 532, 105 S. Ct. 1487, 84 L. Ed. 2d 494 (1985).

Diller, P. A. (2014). Why do cities innovate in public health? Implications of scale and structure. *Washington University Law Review, 91,* 1219–1291. https://openscholarship.wustl.edu/cgi/viewcontent.cgi?referer=&httpsredir=1&article=6092&context=law_lawreview

Fair Labor Standards Act of 1938, 29 U.S.C. §§ 206(a), 218(a).

Florida Statute § 790.33.

*Geier v. American Honda Motor Company,* 529 U.S. 861 (2000)

Hahn, R. A., Truman, B. I., & Williams, D. R. (2018). Civil rights as determinants of public health and racial and ethnic health equity: Health care, education, employment, and housing in the United States. *Social Science and Medicine Population Health, 4,* 17–24. https://doi.org/10.1016/j.ssmph.2017.10.006

*Holm v. Iowa District. Court for Jones Cty.,* 767 N.W.2d 409 (Iowa 2009), as amended (July 6, 2009).

*Howard v. Grinage,* 82 F.3d 1343, 1349 (6th Cir. 1996).

Huizar, L., & Lathrop, Y. (2019, July). *Fighting wage preemption: How workers have lost billions in wages and how we can restore local democracy.* National Employment Law Project. https://s27147.pcdn.co/wp-content/uploads/Fighting-Wage-Preemption-Report-7-19.pdf

*Independents Gas & Service Stations Associations, Inc. v. City of Chicago,* 112 F. Supp. 3d 749 (N.D. Ill. 2015).

Iowa Code § 331.304(12).

*Jacobson v. Commonwealth of Massachusetts,* 197 U.S. 11 (1905).

Johnson, O. C. A. (2016). The local turn: Innovation and diffusion in civil rights law. *Law and Contemporary Problems, 79,* 115–144. https://scholarship.law.columbia.edu/cgi/viewcontent.cgi?article=2089&context=faculty_scholarship

Keep Groceries Affordable Act of 2018, Cal. Rev. & Tax Code §§ 7284.12, 7284.16.

Koseff, A. (2018, April 23). Soda, oil companies back initiative to limit taxes in California. *The Sacramento Bee.* https://web.archive.org/web/20181122041913/https://www.sacbee.com/news/politics-government/capitol-alert/article209446084.html

*Lorillard Tobacco Company v. Reilly,* 533 U.S. 525 (2001).

*Massachusetts Crosby v. National Foreign Trade Council,* 530 U.S. 363 (2000).

McGowan, A. K., Lee, M. M., Meneses, C. M., Perkins, J., & Youdelman, M. (2016). Civil rights laws as tools to advance health in the twenty-first century. *Annual Review of Public Health, 37,* 185–204. https://doi.org/10.1146/annurev-publhealth-032315-021926

Mermin, T. (2009). *Preemption: What it is, how it works, and why it matters for public health.* National Policy & Legal Analysis Network to Prevent Childhood Obesity, ChangeLab Solutions. http://changelabsolutions.org/publications/preemption-memo

Montez, J. K. (2017). Deregulation, devolution, and state preemption laws' impact on US mortality trends. *American Journal of Public Health, 107*(11), 1749–1750. https://doi.org/10.2105/AJPH.2017.304080

*National Association of Tobacco Outlets, Inc. v. City of Providence,* R.I., 731 F.3d 71 (1st Cir. 2013).

National Employment Law Project. (2017). *Fighting preemption: The movement for higher wages must oppose state efforts to block minimum wage laws.* https://www.nelp.org/publication/fighting-preemption-local-minimum-wage-laws

*New State Ice Company v. Liebmann,* 285 U.S. 262 (1932).

O'Connor, A., & Sanger-Katz, M. (2018, June 27). *California, of all places, has banned soda taxes. How a new industry strategy is succeeding.* https://www.nytimes.com/2018/06/27/upshot/california-banning-soda-taxes-a-new-industry-strategy-is-stunning-some-lawmakers.html

*Payne v. Massey,* 145 Tex. 237 (1946).

*People v. Kelly,* 47 Cal. 4th 1008, 222 P.3d 186 (2010).

Pomeranz, J. L., & Pertschuk, M. (2017). State preemption: A significant and quiet threat to public health in the United States. *American Journal of Public Health, 107*(6), 900–902. https://doi.org/10.2105/AJPH.2017.303756

Pomeranz, J. L., Zellers, L., Bare, M., Sullivan, P. A., & Pertschuk, M. (2019). State preemption: Threat to democracy, essential regulation, and public health. *American Journal of Public Health, 109*(2), 251–252. https://doi.org/10.2105/AJPH.2018.304861

Public Health Law Center. (2018, April). *Untangling the preemption doctrine in tobacco control.* https://publichealthlawcenter.org/sites/default/files/resources/Untangling-the-Preemption-Doctrine-in-Tobacco-Control-2018.pdf

Ransom, M. M. (Ed.). (2016). *Public health law competency model: Version 1.0.* https://www.cdc.gov/phlp/docs/phlcm-v1.pdf

Riverstone-Newell, L. (2017). The rise of state preemption laws in response to local policy innovation. *Publius: The Journal of Federalism, 47*(3), 403–425. https://doi.org/10.1093/publius/pjx037

South Dakota Codified Laws § 34-46-6.

Schragger, R. C. (2018). The attack on American cities. *Texas Law Review, 96*(6), 1163–1233. https://texaslawreview.org/the-attack-on-american-cities

Silverstein, T. (2017). Combating state preemption without falling into the local control trap. *Poverty and Race, 26*(4), 1–2, 9–12. https://prrac.org/combating-state-preemption-without-falling-into-the-local-control-trap

Texas Government Code Ann. § 752.051-7.

U.S. Const. amend. V.

U.S. Const. amend. X.

U.S. Const. art. VI, cl. 2.

*U.S. Smokeless Tobacco Manufacturing Company, LLC v. City of New York,* 708 F.3d 428 (2d Cir. 2013).

*U.S. Smokeless Tobacco Manufacturing Company, LLC v. City of New York,* 703 F. Supp. 2d 329 (S.D.N.Y. 2010).

*United States v. Baltimore & Ohio Railroad Company,* 84 U.S. 322 (1872).

Wen, C., Xu, Y., Kim, Y., & Warner, M. E. (2018). Starving counties, squeezing cities: Tax and expenditure limits in the US. *Journal of Economic Policy Reform, 23*(2), 101–119. https://doi.org/10.1080/17487870.2018.1509711

## Additional Resources

- **Equity First: Conceptualizing a Normative Framework to Assess the Role of Preemption in Public Health**
  https://www.changelabsolutions.org/product/equity-first-approach-assessing-preemption
- **Assessing & Addressing Preemption: A Toolkit for Local Policy Campaigns**
  https://www.changelabsolutions.org/product/assessing-addressing-preemption
- **Public Health Law Academy Preemption Training**
  https://www.changelabsolutions.org/product/preemption-public-health
- **ChangeLab Solutions Understanding Preemption**
  https://www.changelabsolutions.org/product/understanding-preemption
- **Local Solutions Support Center**
  http://www.supportdemocracy.org
- **Grassroots Change**
  https://grassrootschange.net
- **Partnership for Working Families: Mapping State Interference**
  https://www.forworkingfamilies.org/preemptionmap

# 4

# Regulating Public Health

## Administrative Law

Priscilla Keith and Heather A. Walter-McCabe

## Learning Objectives

By the end of this chapter, the reader will be able to:

- Define and characterize administrative law and its impact on public health practice.
- Describe the framework for federal, state, and local administrative law.
- Explain the role of federal and state Administrative Procedure Acts.
- Understand the process of judicial review.
- Highlight key administrative law cases.

## Key Terminology

**Administrative agency:** "An organization within the executive branch of government, with the authority to implement and administer legislation" (ChangeLab Solutions, 2020).

**Delegation:** Powers and authority granted from one governmental entity to another (Gostin & Wiley, 2016).

**Due process:** A fundamental protection of fairness and reasonableness guaranteed by the due process clause of the Fifth and Fourteenth Amendments to the United States Constitution.

**Enabling act:** Legislation passed at the federal or state level granting specific authority to an administrative agency to act for a specific purpose (Gostin & Wiley, 2016).

**Federalism:** The legal structure which governs the distribution and allocation of powers between the federal and state governments in the United States (Gostin & Wiley, 2016; Hodge, 2016).

**Promulgate:** The process by which an agency puts forth and files an administrative rule (Administrative Procedures Act).

**Regulation:** A rule promulgated by an administrative agency with the binding effect of law (Koyuncu, 2008).

## Public Health Law Competencies

This chapter addresses the following competencies from the Public Health Law Competency Model (PHLCM; Ransom, 2016):

**1.1**  Define basic constitutional concepts and legal principles framing the practice of public health across relevant jurisdictions.

**1.2**  Identify and apply public health laws (e.g., statutes, regulations, ordinances, and court rulings) pertinent to practitioner's jurisdiction, agency, program, and profession.

**2.2**  Identify law-based tools and enforcement procedures available to address day-to-day (nonemergency) public health issues.

---

### Spark Question

Which branch of government is responsible for creating, implementing, and enforcing regulations?

---

## INTRODUCTION

Administrative law is a branch of law governing the creation and operation of **administrative agencies**. Of special importance are the powers granted to administrative agencies, the substantive rules that such agencies make, and the legal relationships between such agencies, other government bodies, and the public at large.

Administrative law includes laws and legal principles which govern the administration and **regulation** of government agencies (both federal and state). Agencies are delegated power by Congress (or in the case of a state agency, the state legislature), to act as agencies responsible for carrying out certain rights of the Congress. Agencies are created through their own enabling statutes, allowing them to establish new laws and/or promulgate regulations, and thus, creating the respective agencies to interpret, administer, and enforce those new laws. Administrative agencies are created to protect a public interest rather than to vindicate private rights, and administrative law can impact health equity (See Box 4.1). Some of the most well-known

---

**BOX 4.1  AN ILLUSTRATION OF ADMINISTRATIVE LAW AND HEALTH EQUITY**

Administrative interpretation of a statute, through the promulgation of rules, can have an impact on health equity. For example, agency interpretation of the nondiscrimination clause of the Patient Protection and Affordable Care Act (ACA) has an impact on the lesbian, gay, bisexual, transgender, and queer (LGTBQ) population.

Section 1557 of the ACA includes a provision prohibiting discrimination in health programs or activities. The goal of this nondiscrimination clause was to provide more equitable access to healthcare and decrease health disparities. This provision is interpreted by a rule promulgated in 2016 by the U.S. Department of Health and Human Services (DHHS) that explicitly interpreted the law to include protections for persons regardless of sexual orientation and gender identity. In 2019, the DHHS promulgated a new rule (42 CFR 438) explicitly interpreting the statute to not cover gender identity. It remains to be seen what disparate impact this may have on the health of persons in the transgender community. Changes in the administrative interpretation of the rule allow for potential acts that affect the ability of transgender persons to access health services.

agencies are the Environmental Protection Agency, the Food and Drug Agency (FDA), the Department of Transportation, and the U.S. Department of Health and Human Services (DHHS).

The terms "regulations" and "rules" are often used interchangeably, but regulations are, in fact, the rules that are authorized by the **enabling act.** See Table 4.1 for an example of an Indiana statute authorizing the health department to "establish a program to certify individuals as

## TABLE 4.1 ILLUSTRATION OF REGULATORY INTERPRETATION OF A STATE STATUTE

| STATE STATUTE PROVIDING AUTHORITY TO THE DEPARTMENT OF HEALTH | STATE REGULATION RESULTING FROM THE STATUTE |
| --- | --- |
| IC 16-19-3.1-1 Program for Certification of Qualified Inspectors; Rules; List<br>Sec. 1. (a) The state department shall, in order to protect the public health, establish a program to certify individuals as qualified inspectors to perform decontamination of a site that has been contaminated by the illegal manufacture of controlled substances.<br>(b) The state department shall do the following concerning qualified inspectors:<br>  (1) Adopt rules under IC 4-22-2 concerning the following:<br>    (A) Training, testing, and certification of qualified inspectors to perform decontamination on sites that have been contaminated by the illegal manufacture of controlled substances.<br>    (B) The inspection and remediation of sites used in the illegal manufacturing of a controlled substance.<br>  (2) Maintain a list of individuals certified as qualified inspectors.<br>  (3) Remove individuals who no longer meet the certification requirements from the list described in subdivision (2).<br>*As added by P.L.111-2018, SEC.10.* | 410 IAC 38 Inspection and Cleanup of Property Contaminated With Chemicals Used in the Illegal Manufacture of a Controlled Substance<br>Rule 4. Listing by the Department as a Qualified Inspector<br>Sec. 4. (a) The department will maintain a current list of all persons who have been found by the department to have met the requirements of section 2 of this rule.<br>(b) The purpose of the qualified inspector list is to allow owners of contaminated properties, local health departments, and other persons to:<br>  (1) locate qualified inspectors; and<br>  (2) verify that a person is qualified to inspect and clean up contaminated properties.<br>(c) Listing of a person on the qualified inspector list does not convey a property right.<br>(d) The qualified inspector list will be available to the public as follows:<br>  (1) In person or by mail at Indiana State Department of Health, Environmental Public Health, Room N855, 100 North Senate Avenue, Indianapolis, Indiana 46204-2251.<br>  (2) By telephone at (317) 233-7173 in Indiana.<br>  (3) Electronically on the department's Web site at http://www.in.gov/isdh<br>(e) The department will review each application for completeness. When the person or persons identified in the application have demonstrated that all criteria of this rule have been met, the department will place that person or persons on the qualified inspector list.<br>(f) The department will remove a person from the qualified inspector list who submits a written request for removal from the list to the address in section 3(b) of this rule.<br>(g) The department may remove a person from the qualified inspector list if the person demonstrates a failure to meet one (1) or more of the requirements of this article.<br>(h) The department may return a person to the qualified inspector list when the condition that caused the department to remove that person from the list has been corrected. *(Indiana State Department of Health; 410 IAC 38-4-4; filed Feb 21, 2007, 1:56 p.m.: 20070321-IR-318060125FRA; readopted filed Aug 5, 2013, 2:08 p.m.: 20130904-IR-318130240RFA; errata filed Jun 22, 2018, 10:19 a.m.: 20180704-IR-410180270ACA; readopted filed Nov 13, 2019, 3:14 p.m.: 20191211-IR-410190391RFA) NOTE: Transferred from the Department of Environmental Management (318 IAC 1-4-4) to the Indiana State Department of Health (410 IAC 38-4-4) by P.L.111-2018, SECTION 17, effective July 1, 2018.* |

qualified inspectors to perform decontamination of a site that has been contaminated by the illegal manufacture of controlled substances" (Ind. Code Ann. § 16-19-3.1-1 (West, 2018)).

## Due Process

**Due process** is an important view in administrative law proceedings. It has both substantive and procedural elements to it. The foundation of due process is to afford individuals with fairness and protection from arbitrary and capricious government action. Moreover, it ensures that when the government wishes to take one's life, liberty, or property, the government gives a person adequate notice of the reasons for the government's actions and a hearing, possibly a trial, for the person to challenge what the government has done or plans to do.

The Administrative Procedures Act (APA) was enacted to ensure fairness and due process in executive agency actions or proceedings involving rule-making and adjudications. As such, due process requires agencies to use the *least restrictive means* or *less drastic means* to achieve its purpose, particularly if the enactment of a law restricts a fundamental personal liberty. This test applies even when the government has a legitimate purpose in adopting the particular law.

With regard to adjudications, an administrative law judge (ALJ) serves as the judge and trier of fact who presides over administrative hearings. ALJs have the power to administer oaths, make rulings on evidentiary objections, and render legal and factual determinations.

## Administrative Law in a Federalist System

The legal system in the United States operates under the concept of **federalism.** It is critical to understand how administrative agencies operate under this framework. The U.S. Constitution creates powers which are reserved for the federal government leaving the remaining powers to the states. States create their own statutes and public health regulations as well as systems of local government to which they may delegate authority to act. The following section describes the way administrative agencies operate for public health within the different levels of government.

### Federal Administrative Law

This chapter concentrates on administrative law in the United States. For more information on constitutional law and its impact on the topics reserved to the federal government, see Chapter 2. Administrative law at the federal level is governed by the APA. The APA details the process by which federal rule-making takes place and ensures that rules are created fairly, publicly, and in compliance with the **delegation** of authority given by Congress. This process ensures due process of law. If an agency does not follow the process for rule-making or attempts to create rules outside of the subject matters delegated to the agency by Congress, the APA creates a process to challenge the resulting rules (Gostin & Wiley, 2016).

In order to **promulgate** a rule which has the force of law, the proposed rule must be published in the federal register with a public comment period (prior notice) with a statement of the purpose and basis for the rule. Written comments must be considered with the agency's rationale for response. The consideration process creates a record for use in cases where the final rule is challenged. Once the public comments have been considered and response created, the final rule is published in the Federal Record and the rule is implemented (Gostin & Wiley, 2016). Once the process is complete, the final rule is added to the Code of Federal Regulations and has the full force of law.

### State Administrative Law

Each state has its own version of an APA; therefore, it is important to look for and understand what is required in any state within which you work. State APAs, as with their federal counterparts, serve to protect due process and ensure transparent regulatory processes. State regulatory agencies cover a wide variety of subject areas. Though many public health–related regulations will originate in the state public health agency, state environmental agencies, planning agencies, departments of insurance, and others agencies can all originate regulation that could have an impact on the public's health. State agencies, as with federal agencies, are limited to the powers and topics that have been delegated to them, at the state level by the state's legislative body. If agencies seek to regulate topics outside their prevue or beyond the scope of powers given to them by the legislature, it is likely that, if the regulation is challenged, the court will fail to uphold the regulation.

## Local Administrative Law

Local agencies have the authority delegated to them by the state. Local levels of governance are useful to ensure that public health interventions can be tailored to the specific needs of the local community. States have different approaches to local governments. All states have county levels of government, but there is a wide range of county size and numbers between different states. Some states create city- and town-level governments in addition to the county governments. These governmental entities can also create law that impacts public health.

The extent to which local actors govern in public health can be influenced by the state legislature's perspective on the concept of home rule. States which embrace the concept of home rule seek to have laws originate as close to the impacted community as possible, generally at the local level. States may also be influenced by Dillon's Rule. Judge Dillon, after whom the rule is named, believed that any question regarding the ability of the local government to rule in an area should be judged by a narrow interpretation of local powers, thus limiting local public health authority. For more information on home rule, see Chapters 1 and 3.

Local public health agencies are sources of a variety of innovative public health policies. For example, tobacco laws and healthy food policies have originated in localities and later become prevalent in state-level legislation and regulation. The balance between the various levels of governance continues to be varied and changing across the United States.

## ENFORCEMENT AND JUDICIAL DEFERENCE

Administrative agencies have the power to enforce compliance with regulations. Agencies use tools such as fines and license revocation to require compliance with regulatory mandates. Agencies at the federal, state, and local level may use processes such as annual inspections or license renewals in order to monitor compliance. Federal and state APAs provide processes to challenge an agency's decision. The agency's process, when fully exhausted, results in a final decision of the agency. When an individual or business believes that the agency has made a faulty decision or regulated outside the permits of its enabling act, they may challenge the decision or regulation in court (Gostin & Wiley, 2016).

## Judicial Review

When courts review a regulation, it is called "judicial review." An entity seeking to challenge an administrative action must exhaust all administrative remedies provided through the agency prior to seeking intervention of the courts. The court will examine the regulation to determine whether or not the agency acted within the legal authority granted through the enabling statute. The APA specifically provides for courts to overturn administrative regulations when those actions are "arbitrary, capricious, or an abuse of discretion" (APA, 1966). The courts generally defer to the determination by an agency unless it is clearly erroneous or inconsistent with the statute. As described previously, agencies promulgate rules in areas requiring technical expertise and courts make rulings consistent with recognizing this expertise.

Courts use what is known as a "Chevron Test," a two-step process first described by the U.S. Supreme Court in the *Chevron U.S.A., Inc. vs National Resources Defense Council, Inc.* (1984). First, the court looks to see if the legislature provided specific and unambiguous guidance on the topic, sometimes called an "intelligible principle," to guide the agency actions. If so, as long as the agency acted within those guidelines, the regulation meets this standard. If the guidance is not clear, the court will move to step two determining if the agency's interpretation was reasonable and not arbitrary or capricious. If so, the court does not determine whether or not the agency was correct in its determination, only that it is not clearly erroneous. Where the legislative delegation of power was broad, the courts defer under the concept that the legislature intended to give deference to the expertise of the agency. Given the structure of judicial review, the result is a court system which gives wide deference to agency action where the agency is acting under the powers delegated to it (Gostin & Wiley, 2016).

A seminal public health law case, *Jacobson v. Massachusetts,* was an early case requiring the U.S. Supreme Court to determine how much deference to give a public health agency. In *Jacobson* the local public health agency created a mandate to receive the smallpox vaccination or pay a fine. Mr. Jacobson challenged the regulation. The court set a standard that provided wide deference to the agency, including allowing the delegation of power from a state to a local agency, and has been widely cited in subsequent cases questioning the use of public health agency powers. During the COVID-19 pandemic of 2020, a large number of courts examined the powers granted to public health agencies (*In re: Abbott*, 954 F.3d 772 (5th Cir. 2020); *In re: Rutledge,* No. 20-1791, 2020 WL 1933122, at five (8th Cir. Apr. 22, 2020; see generally Wiley & Vladek, 2020). A number of courts declined to use the standard set in *Jacobson* and instead required public health agencies to meet a higher standard in that their activities must be enacted using the least restrictive means available. At this time it is unclear what the long term impact of these cases will be on public health agency jurisprudence, but for those interested in public health administrative law, it will be important to continue to watch the courts for any trends which might created heightened scrutiny for public health agency actions.

## KEY ADMINISTRATIVE LAW CASES

As previously discussed in the Judicial Review section, *Chevron v. NRDC, 467 US 837 (1984)* established the extent to which a federal court, in reviewing a federal government agency's action, should defer to the agency's interpretation of a statute that the agency has been delegated to administer, also known as the Chevron deference.

Although the Supreme Court in *Chevron* ruled in favor of showing deference to an agency's interpretation of a statute, it created an exception to the Chevron's ruling in *FDA v. Brown & Williamson Tobacco Corp.*, 529 US 120 (2000). The FDA attempted to regulate tobacco products under the Food, Drug and Cosmetic Act, subsequently promulgating regulations governing tobacco's promotion, labeling and accessibility to minors. The goals of the regulations were to reduce minors' current use of tobacco, the use of tobacco in future generations as well as the reduction of tobacco related deaths. Respondents challenged the agency's interpretation and moved for summary judgement on the grounds that the FDA lacked jurisdiction to regulate tobacco products because they did not market their product with claims of therapeutic use. The District Court upheld the FDA's authority to regulate tobacco. On Appeal, the Circuit Court reversed the District Court's ruling, holding that Congress had not granted the FDA jurisdiction to regulate tobacco products. The Supreme Court, affirming the District Court's ruling, held that the FDA did not have jurisdiction to regulate tobacco citing Congress's intent to exclude tobacco products from the FDA's jurisdiction. Justice O'Connor, using the *Chevron* deference, argued that *FDA v. Brown & Williamson* merited an exception to normal proceedings under *Chevron*. She wrote "*Chevron* deference is premised on the theory that a statute's ambiguity constitutes an implicit delegation from Congress to the agency to fill in the statutory gaps. In extraordinary cases, however, there may be reason to hesitate before concluding that Congress has intended such an implicit delegation. This is hardly an ordinary case."

It should be noted that the Supreme Court's ruling was superseded by the Family Smoking Prevention and Tobacco Control Act, which granted the FDA the authority to regulate tobacco products. It was signed into law on June 22, 2009.

The Supreme Court in *U.S. v. Mead Corporation 533 U.S. 218 (2001)* narrowed the scope of application for the Chevron deference to agency regulations and adjudicatory actions. In *Mead*, the Harmonized Tariff Schedule of the United States (HTSUS) authorizes the U.S. Customs Service to classify and fix the rate of duty on imports under the rules and regulations issued by the secretary of the treasury. The secretary provides for tariff rulings before the entry of goods by regulations authorizing "ruling letters' setting tariff classifications for particular imports. For several years, the Mead Corporation had imported day planners duty-free; however, the Customs Headquarters Office issued a ruling letter that classified the day planners as bound diaries subject to a tariff. As a result, the Mead Corporation filed suit in the Court of International Trade, which granted the Government summary judgement. Mead appealed the decision. The U.S. Court of Appeals for the Federal Circuit ruled that letters should not be given judicial deference since they are not subject to notice-and-comment rule-making, and do not carry the force of law. The ruling was appealed to the Supreme Court. The Supreme Court reasoned that administrative implementation of a particular statutory provision failed to qualify for deference under *Chevron* although noting that it may deserve some deference which led the Supreme Court to vacate and remand the decision.

The question of whether or not an agency action must be final before it is reviewable by the courts was answered by the Supreme Court in *FTC v. Standard Oil Company of California, 449 U.S. 232 (1980)*. In 1973, the Federal Trade Commission (FTC) filed a complaint with a notice of hearing against eight oil companies which included Standard Oil of California (Soscal) on the grounds that the companies were in violation of the unfair method of competition or unfair deceptive practices in the Federal Trade Commission Act. Standard Oil of California filed a complaint in District Court alleging that the FTC did not have enough evidence to file the original complaint and to commence proceedings to determine if it was in violation of the law. The District Court dismissed the case. The Ninth Circuit Court of Appeals reversed the District Court's decision, holding that it did have authority to review whether the FTC had made a factual determination or issued the complaint solely due to outside pressure. The Supreme Court reversed the decision of the Ninth Circuit Court of Appeals holding that the decision to initiate proceedings was not a final agency action under the Administrative Procedure Act and thus, could not be reviewed until adjudication was complete.

In *Citizens to Preserve Overton Park v. Volpe, 401 US 407 (1971)*, the Supreme Court clarified the requirements and guidelines for judicial review of discretionary agency actions.

The federal government proposed a plan to build a six-lane interstate highway through Overton Park, which would have resulted in the destruction of 26 acres of the park. The secretary of transportation could not approve this plan unless Section 4(f) of the Department of Transportation Act of 1966 were satisfied: 1) there were no feasible and alternative uses for the land; and 2) the program included all possible planning to minimize harm to the park, wildlife, historic sites, and recreational areas. Moreover, the Federal Aid Highway Act of 1968 updated Section 4(f) to include public parks and the natural beauty of the countrysides.

The Citizens to Preserve Overton Park sued the Secretary of Transportation John Volpe, arguing that Volpe did not adhere to Section 4(f) as part of the decision-making process. The U.S. District Court for the Western District of Tennessee and the U.S. Court of Appeals for the 6th Circuit ruled in favor of Volpe. Plaintiffs appealed to the U.S. Supreme Court. Justice Thurgood Marshall, writing the opinion for the Supreme Court, cited that the District Court approved the secretary of transportation's plan that was based on insufficient evidence. The Supreme Court held that the secretary's actions were subject to judicial review pursuant to Section 702 of the Administrative Act. Additionally, the Court ruled that Congress did not seek to limit or prohibit judicial review in this case and the exemption for action "committed to agency discretion" does not apply, as the secretary does have "law to apply," rather than wide-ranging discretion.

The case was remanded to the District Court to conduct a **plenary** review based on all of the available documentation.

## CONCLUSION

Administrative law is an important area that plays a crucial role in public health. Much of the public health responsibility of the federal and state governments is **delegated** to **administrative agencies.** Agencies interpret and utilize this legal authority by **promulgating regulations** that further the purpose for which the agency was formed. Administrative law defines both the authority and limitations within which agencies operate. It is important for public health practitioners and others who work within the field, to have an understanding of agency rule-making, adjudication, and enforcement powers in order to effectively advocate for actions that promote public health.

## CHAPTER REVIEW

### Review Questions

1.  When an agency is acting within its statutory authority, a court may still set aside the agency action if it finds the action is _____, _____, or an _____ _____.
2.  The courts are generally largely deferential to administrative agency decisions.
    True/ False
3.  Which level or levels of government have administrative agencies?
    a.  Federal
    b.  State
    c.  Local
    d.  Federal & State
    e.  All of the above

### Essay Questions

1.  In what ways might the public comment period required for administrative regulations help advance health equity?
2.  What are the two steps of *Chevron* deference used by courts when determining if an agency had authority to act?
3.  Describe the steps an agency must take to promulgate a rule.

### Internet Activities

1.  Explore current regulations: visit http://regulations.gov and use the search bar to find regulations that have been published in the Federal Register. You can also use the "advanced search" option to search for regulations by topic area, agency, date, etc. Try searching for proposed rules that are open for public comment by selecting the "open for comment" check box. Explore opportunities to comment on proposed rules that are of interest to you!

2.  Research the Congressional Review Act (CRA). How many times has the CRA been used to invalidate a rule since it went into effect in 1996?
3.  Look up your state's administrative procedures act. Generally, you will be able to find it by typing in your state with administrative procedures act or check your state government website. Who may seek judicial review of agency actions? What types of actions are immediately reviewable? What process must agencies follow when engaging in rule-making? What requirements are imposed on the notice and comment process?

## REFERENCES

Adminstrative Procedures Act, 5 U.S.C. sect. 706(2) (1966). https://open.defense.gov/Portals/23/Documents/Regulatory/apa.pdf

ChangeLab Solutions. (2020). *The ABC's of administrative law in public health practice.* https://www.changelabsolutions.org/product/abcs-administrative-law-public-health-practice

*Chevron U.S.A. Inc. v. Natural Resources Defense Council Inc.* (U.S. Supreme Court 1984).

*Citizens to Preserve Overton Park, Inc. v. Volpe*, 401 (U.S. Supreme Court 1971).

Controlled Substances Site Decontamination and Qualified Inspector Certification, Ind. Code Ann. § 16-19-3.1-1 (West, 2018).

*Federal Trade Commission v. Standard Oil Company of California*, 449 U.S. 232 (1980).

*Food and Drug Administration v. Brown & Williamson Tobacco Corp.*, 529 US 120 (2000).

Gostin, L. O., & Wiley, L. F. (2016). *Public health law: Power, duty, restraint.* University of California Press.

*Jacobson v. Massachusetts* (U.S. Supreme Court 1905).

Koyuncu, A. (2008). *Administrative law and public health.* Springer.

Ransom, M. M. (Ed.). (2016). *Public health law competency model: Version 1.0.* https://www.cdc.gov/phlp/docs/phlcm-v1.pdf

*U.S. v. Mead Corp.*, 533 (Supreme Court of the United States 2001).

Wiley, L. F., & Vladek, S. I. (2020). Coronavirus, civil liberties, and the courts: The case against "suspending" judicial review. *Harvard Law Review Forum, 133*(9), 179–198. https://harvardlawreview.org/2020/07/coronavirus-civil-liberties-and-the-courts/

### Additional Resources

- **Online training on Structure of Government: Public Health Law Academy**
  https://www.changelabsolutions.org/product/structure-government
- **Online training on Administrative Law Parts 1 and 2: Public Health Law Academy**
  https://www.cdc.gov/phlp/publications/topic/phlacademy.html

# 5

# Litigation and Public Health

Christopher Ogolla, Emily Allender, Troy Viger, and Lena Amanti Yueh

## Learning Objectives

By the end of this chapter, the reader will be able to:

- Discuss the role of epidemiology in assisting the judge and the jury in the courtroom.
- Analyze how epidemiology can support large-scale modern litigation such as in cases against pharmaceutical companies targeting the opioid crisis.
- Choose specific public health law cases covering areas such as obesity, food poisoning, opioids, and bleach poisoning.
- Articulate the difference between public health litigation and public health law.
- Illustrate the differences between civil and criminal sanctions in public health litigation.

## Key Terminology

**Bleach poisoning:** The chlorine in bleach can poison individuals if overexposed. Bleach poisoning can occur from injection, inhalation through the nose or mouth, or ingestion if the chlorine is in liquid form (https://emergency.cdc.gov/agent/chlorine/basics/facts.asp).

**Dialysis:** A treatment for when a person's kidneys fail to perform certain natural functions. Dialysis treatment helps to remove waste, salt, and extra water from the body as well as regulate certain necessary chemicals in the person's blood such as potassium and sodium (https://www.kidney.org/atoz/content/dialysisinfo).

**Federal Tort Claims Act:** A 1946 federal statute that permits private parties to sue the United States in federal court for most torts committed by persons acting on behalf of the United States.

**Negligence:** In the legal context, a failure to behave with reasonable care that someone of ordinary prudence would have exercised under the same or similar circumstances.

**Obesity:** According to the Centers for Disease Control and Prevention (CDC), overweight and obesity are both labels for ranges of weight that are greater than what is generally considered healthy for a given height (https://www.cdc.gov/ncbddd/disabilityandhealth/obesity.html).

**Opioid:** A substance used to treat moderate to severe pain (https://www.cancer.gov/publications/dictionaries/cancer-terms/def/opioid).

## Public Health Law Competencies

This chapter addresses the following competencies from the Public Health Law Competency Model (PHLCM; Ransom, 2016).

**1.1** Define basic constitutional concepts and legal principles framing the practice of public health across relevant jurisdictions.

**1.2** Identify and apply public health laws (e.g., statutes, regulations, ordinances, and court rulings) pertinent to a practitioner's jurisdiction, agency, program, and profession.

**2.3** Recognize the legal authority and limits of critical system partners and others who influence health outcomes.

---

### Spark Question

How can epidemiology support large-scale modern litigation such as in cases against pharmaceutical companies targeting the opioid crisis?

---

## INTRODUCTION

Public health students interested in the study of law may wonder what legal knowledge would add to their careers as public health practitioners. Concomitantly, law students interested in dual degrees in law and public health may wonder what and how public health education can enhance their legal careers. The answer may lie, not "in the wind" as Bob Dylan famously put it, but in public health litigation. Indeed, Professors Wendy Parmet and Richard Daynard observed that "one of the most remarkable developments of the last three decades (1970–2002) has been the increasing use of litigation as a public health tool" (Parmet & Daynard, 2000). They further note that "increasingly, individuals and organizations concerned about public health have sought to use litigation to further their goals" (Parmet & Daynard, 2000).

Examples of public health litigation span wide areas of public health practice such as **obesity**, lead poisoning, alcohol-induced injuries and deaths, use of legal and illegal drugs, vaccines, motor vehicle safety, pollution, and smoking. Indeed, tobacco litigation has been one of the most widely successful litigations in public health.[1]

This chapter addresses litigation in public health by looking at recent cases and disputes of some of the major public health issues like **opioids**, food, drinks and obesity, and foodborne outbreaks. The chapter, however, does not discuss tobacco and vaccine injury cases (*University of St. Thomas Law Review*, 2010), even though these are some of the major areas of litigation in public health. This is because there is a vast amount of literature already published elsewhere and in this book. For example, see chapter 6 for a discussion of vaccination law; see chapter 12 on global health law, which include a discussion of the framework convention on tobacco control. For an in-depth discussion of tobacco litigation, see Mitchell Hamline School of Law, Public Health Law Center, Tobacco Control Act Cases, https://publichealthlawcenter.org/content/tobacco-control-act-cases.

## WHAT IS PUBLIC HEALTH, PUBLIC HEALTH LAW, AND PUBLIC HEALTH LITIGATION?

To understand public health litigation, one needs to understand public health and public health law. The World Health Organization (WHO) defines public health as "the art and science of

---

[1] "From a plaintiff's viewpoint, some recent tobacco litigation has been wildly successful" (McMenamin & Tiglio, 2006).

preventing disease, prolonging life and promoting health through the organized efforts of society" (WHO, n.d.). The CDC Foundation defines it as "the science of protecting and improving the health of people and their communities" (CDC Foundation, n.d.). Put succinctly, public health is "what we, as a society, do collectively to assure the conditions for people to be healthy" (Institute of Medicine, 1988). Public health law has been defined as:

> the authority of the state or other actors to assure the health of a population, including the study of the powers and duties of the state or other actors to assure the health of a population, the limitations on the power of the state to constrain the autonomy, privacy, liberty, proprietary, or other legally protected interests of individuals in order to assure the health of a population, and the limitations on the duties of the state to assure the health of a population (Gostin, 2008, p. 4).

Public health litigation differs from public health law in three major respects. First, whereas public health law focuses mostly on communities and populations, public health litigation relies on using litigation to help those affected by public health problems, be they individuals or groups. Second, public health law is undergirded by state action. Indeed, the definition of public health law just cited includes the word "state" several times. This means the legislatures and administrative bodies are heavily involved in the enactment and enforcement of public health laws. Public health litigation, on the other hand, includes both state and nonstate actors seeking remedies in courts of law. The disputes in public health litigation may be directly related to public health law, or not. For example, a law seeking to ban cigarette advertising may have a public health purpose, but because it attempts to regulate commercial speech, if challenged, a court will apply First Amendment law to determine whether the law is constitutional. Third, unlike public health law, the principal goal of public health litigation is mostly to recover money damages. Put differently, the benefits of public health litigation inure primarily to individuals who file lawsuits, i.e., the plaintiffs (assuming they prevail).

Finally, public health litigation can be critically important when it comes to "enforcing the rights of low-income people to access health care" (National Health Law Program, n.d.). See Box 5.1.

## BOX 5.1 HEALTH EQUITY AND LITIGATION

1. Although there is no constitutional right to healthcare in the United States, litigation does have a positive effect on health equity through enforcement of other "statutory health rights." For example, courts, through Title VI of the Civil Rights Act of 1964, play a critical role in ensuring that there is no discrimination based on race, color, and national origin in programs and activities receiving federal funds, including Medicare and Medicaid.
2. Litigation can also be used to hold defendants liable in cases dealing with the social determinants of health, like education, environment, and housing. For example, the Flint Michigan water crisis has spawned several lawsuits regarding the health risks associated with drinking the Flint River water. In one such case, *Guertin v. State of Michigan (2019)*, the Court noted that "knowing the Flint River water was unsafe for public use, distributing it without taking steps to counter its problems, and assuring the public in the meantime that it was safe is conduct that would alert a reasonable person to the likelihood of personal liability."

## Examples of Recent Litigations in Public Health

### Opioids

One of the most recent forms of public health litigation has involved the opioid crisis. As a background, the opioid epidemic affects people in all demographics from all areas of life, including teenagers, seniors, veterans, and the LGBTQ community. From 1999 to 2017, more than 70,000 people have died from drug overdoses. Approximately 65% of the more than 70,000 drug overdose deaths in 2017 involved an opioid (CDC, n.d.). In 2017, the states with the reported highest rates of death due to drug overdoses were West Virginia (57.8 per 1000,000), Ohio (46.3 per 100,000), Pennsylvania (44.3 per 100,000), the District of Columbia (44.0 per 100,000), and Kentucky (37.2 per 100,000; Scholl et al., 2019). Other states experiencing significant increase in drug overdose death rates include Alabama, Arizona, California, Connecticut, Delaware, Florida, Georgia, Illinois, Indiana, Louisiana, Maine, Maryland, Michigan, New Jersey, New York, North Carolina, South Carolina, Tennessee, and Wisconsin (CDC, 2018).

The opioid lawsuits have been filed mostly by states and, to a lesser extent, the federal government, against those selling drugs (legally or illegally), pharmacists (*United States v. Tobin*, 2012), physicians who overprescribe opioids, and manufacturers. For example, from 1998 to 2006, there were a total of 986 lawsuits against physicians "involving the prescribing of opioid analgesics." About 80% of these physicians "pled guilty or no contest to at least one of the criminal charges brought against them" (Goldenbaum et al., 2008).

State governments have pursued both criminal and civil sanctions. Among the jurisdictions that have used criminal law to address the crisis are Kentucky, which increased penalties for heroin trafficking (Kentucky House Bill 333, 2017), and Florida, which enacted a law that charges drug dealers with murder if their customers overdose on opioids (Florida Stat. Title XLVI § 893.135, 2017).

The federal government has been very aggressive in using criminal law to combat the crisis. For example, in April 2019, the Department of Justice announced charges against 31 doctors, seven pharmacists, eight nurse practitioners, and seven other licensed medical professionals for illegal prescription and distribution of opioids and other dangerous narcotics (U.S. Department of Justice, 2019).

### Civil Lawsuits

There have been several civil lawsuits and settlements regarding the manufacture and distribution of opioids. In May 2019, "West Virginia and drug distributor McKesson Corporation announced a $37 million settlement of a lawsuit over the company's role in the opioid epidemic" (Bernstein, 2019a). In the same year, Teva Pharmaceuticals agreed to a settlement of $85 million in a lawsuit brought by the Oklahoma attorney general. The lawsuit alleged that the company, one of the largest manufacturers of generic drugs, contributed to the state's epidemic of opioid painkillers (Waldrop & Drash, 2019). In March 2017, Purdue Pharma agreed to a $270 million out-of-court settlement with the state of Oklahoma, where the company faced its first trial on deceptively pushing powerful painkillers and misrepresenting the drugs' safety (Bernstein, 2019b). Despite the settlements, there are still several opioid lawsuits winding their way through both state and federal courts. These lawsuits will shed light on not only the liability or nonliability of pharmaceutical companies for the opioid crisis, but also, and more importantly for our purposes, the effectiveness of public health litigation.

### Food, Drinks, and Obesity

Litigation concerning food and drinks has been led primarily by local governments against the food and beverage industries. In return, the industries have sued to stop the local regulations on various grounds,[2] resulting in a back and forth fight in the courts. The underlying public health concern in food litigation is obesity and diabetes. According to the CDC, "more than one-third of U.S. adults are obese and frequent fast-food consumption has been shown to contribute to weight gain" (Fryar & Ervin, 2013, p. 1). In fact, between 2013 and 2016, the latest time period for which we have data, 36.6% of adults consumed fast food on a given day (Fryar et al., 2018). Regarding diabetes, the CDC lists it as among the 10 leading causes of death in 2016 (Herrone, 2018).

Among the oft-cited cases in food litigation related to obesity are *Pelman ex. Rel. Pelman v. McDonald's Corporation,* ( 2005) and *New York Statewide Coalition of Hispanic Chambers of Commerce v. New York City Department of Health and Mental Hygiene,* (2014), both from New York City. In *Pelman,* the plaintiffs sued McDonald's Corporation alleging deceptive trade practices in which McDonald's advertised its meals as healthy, although the foods contained additives that were detrimental to plaintiffs' health. Because of eating McDonald's food two to three times a week, the plaintiffs alleged that they developed "obesity, diabetes, coronary heart disease, high blood pressure, elevated cholesterol intake, related cancers, and/or other detrimental and adverse health effects…" (*Pelman ex. rel Pelman v. McDonald's Corp,* 2005). The trial court dismissed the plaintiffs' case noting that they failed to show a causal connection between their consumption of McDonald's food and their alleged injuries. The Second Circuit Court of Appeals reversed that decision, finding that the plaintiffs' allegations stated a claim against McDonald's Corporation for violation of New York's deceptive trade practices law.

In New York Statewide Coalition of Hispanic Chambers of Commerce, the New York Court of Appeals invalidated a soda ban that barred food service establishments from selling certain sugary drinks in containers larger than 16 ounces. The New York City Board of Health had imposed the ban with the goal of combating rising obesity rates in the city. The appellate court found that under the State's separation of powers doctrine, the Board of Health had exceeded its authority of protecting the public's health by enacting the ban.

The implications of these two cases for public health litigation are twofold. First, a plaintiff must be able to establish a causal connection between the alleged consumption and their injuries. Second, there is likely to be tremendous pushback against laws designed to control behavior, especially where personal responsibility is concerned. Thus, controlling obesity requires a constellation of factors including diet, exercise, regulation, personal responsibility, medical treatments, and knowledge of family genes and history, to mention but a few. Litigation alone is unlikely to be effective.

## Foodborne Outbreaks

Closely related to food, drink, and obesity cases are cases regarding foodborne outbreaks. In response to a foodborne disease outbreak, it is important that public health officials have the discretion to determine what actions to take. These actions are based on an assessment of the available epidemiologic data, traceback data (to find a common point of contamination), and food- and environmental-testing data. When there is sufficient evidence linking illness to a contaminated food, public health officials may warn the public regarding those foods. These warnings have sometimes been the subject of litigation.

## Public Health Investigation

*Salmonella* is a bacterium that commonly causes foodborne illness in humans. *Salmonella* Saintpaul (SS) is a rare strain of *Salmonella.* SS can enter the bloodstream and cause serious health complications, including death. In late May of 2008, the New Mexico Department of Health notified the CDC that a number of local residents had been infected with this bacterium, and

---

[2] "Monster Beverage Corp. has asked a federal court to halt efforts by San Francisco City Attorney Dennis Herrera to place restrictions on its popular energy drinks, arguing such regulations are a federal matter" (Esterl, 2013).

even more reports trickled in from Texas (*Seaside Farm, Inc. v. United States*, 2016). By June, the CDC was investigating 145 incidents and 23 hospitalizations across 16 states. By July, SS was linked to 1,220 infections across 42 states (*Seaside Farm, Inc. v. United States*, 2016).

Initially, the CDC discovered a strong statistical association between the infections and eating raw tomatoes, which was also supported by a historical association. With this information, the CDC notified the Food and Drug Administration (FDA) that tomatoes were the "leading hypothesis" for the source of the outbreak (*Seaside Farm, Inc. v. United States*, 2016). Relying largely on this notification, the FDA issued a warning to the public (titled "FDA Warns Consumers Nationwide Not to Eat Certain Types of Raw Red Tomatoes") that specified certain types of tomatoes as the likely source of the outbreak. The warning also provided a list of states, including South Carolina, whose tomatoes were not associated with the outbreak. Following this warning against tomatoes, the CDC continued its investigation and traced SS to jalapeños and serrano peppers from Mexico. The FDA then withdrew its warning and announced tomatoes were no longer associated with the outbreak.

## Federal Tort Claims Act

Generally, under the doctrine of sovereign immunity, private parties are not permitted to sue government entities. The **Federal Tort Claims Act** (FTCA) provides a limited waiver of this immunity for suits against the federal government (28 U.S.C. §§ 1346[b], 2671-2680; West, 2013). Under the FTCA, the United States is liable for injury, loss of property, personal injury, or death caused by the negligent or wrongful act or omission of any federal government employee acting within the scope of their employment.

The FTCA insulates the federal government from liability, however, when the government is performing a "discretionary function" (28 U.S.C. § 2680[a]; West, 2006). A discretionary act is one where the government is permitted to exercise judgment or choice and where public policy considerations are implicated (*Seaside Farm, Inc. v. United States*, 2016). In other words, the government has discretion when there is no "federal statute, regulation, or policy [that] specifically prescribes a course of action for an employee to follow" (*Seaside Farm, Inc. v. United States*, 2016). The purpose of the discretionary function exception is to "'protect the government from liability that would seriously handicap efficient government operations'" and to prevent courts from second-guessing government decisions based on social, economic, and political policy (*Seaside Farm, Inc. v. United States*, 2016).

## Litigation

In May 2011, Seaside Farm, a South Carolina tomato grower, sued the United States under the FTCA, claiming that the FDA negligently issued a contamination warning in response to the SS outbreak, which caused the producer to lose more than $15 million in crop value (*Seaside Farm, Inc. v. United States*, 2016).

The District Court dismissed the case and Seaside appealed to the Fourth Circuit Court of Appeals. The Fourth Circuit upheld the dismissal based on the discretionary function exception. Among the Court's findings were that: (1) the FDA's decision to issue a contamination warning was a prototypical exercise of discretion under 21 U.S.C. § 375(b), which allows the FDA to disseminate information about food "in situations involving, *in the opinion of the [Commissioner]*, imminent danger to health" (emphasis added); (2) the FDA's decision to warn consumers was grounded in the agency's public health mission to ensure that food is safe; and (3) the discretionary function exception applies irrespective of whether Seaside believed the agency did not investigate the outbreak or interpret evidence in a reasonable manner (*Seaside Farm, Inc. v. United States*, 2016).

The Court considered the burden that would result if the FDA had to ensure that a contamination warning was based on perfect information, particularly during a developing health crisis, as in this case. Further, the Court recognized the massive tort liability that might ensue if a warning were delayed, resulting in serious or grave injuries to consumers. Additionally, the

Court understood that the government delegates broad discretion to the FDA in an emergency situation because every public health emergency is different, and no boilerplate warning exists to account for the vast unknown variables of a pathogenic outbreak. In this case, the FDA used discretion to evaluate available information, determine the total nature of a health threat, and settle on a course of action.

Seaside tried inviting the Court to engage in the very judicial second-guessing that the discretionary function exception forbids (*Seaside Farm, Inc. v. United States*, 2016). The Court noted that if it allowed Seaside to pursue its case, the "law of tort [would] distort one of the most critical ... governmental functions, that of safeguarding the public health and welfare" (*Seaside Farm, Inc. v. United States*, 2016). In its ruling in favor of the U.S. government, the Court's decision affirmed that there is a zone of protection within which public health officials can act to protect the public's health without fear of being held liable for the effects those decisions may have.

## CRIMINAL LAW

Public health litigation can also occur in the criminal context. Criminal prosecutors at the federal, state, and local levels prosecute individuals and companies whose actions negatively affect the public's health. One particular prosecution occurred in Texas and involved a licensed vocational nurse who killed five **dialysis** patients and sickened many others by intentionally injecting bleach into their IVs.

Kimberly Saenz was employed at DaVita Healthcare Dialysis Clinic in Lufkin, Texas. There were a number of strange occurrences during the month of April 2008, notably, "the number of deaths the clinic was experiencing was alarming and unexplainable" (*Saenz v. State*, 2015).

The case came to the attention of public health authorities when a paramedic wrote an anonymous letter to the state health department. The letter asked the department to investigate the dialysis clinic because paramedics were making so many trips to the clinic. When the state health inspectors were at the clinic days later, patients undergoing dialysis reported that they saw Saenz injecting bleach into the dialysis tubing of some patients. Thereafter, the CDC, the state health department, and the local police began an investigation of the incidents at the clinic (*Saenz v. State*, 2014).

A number of public health expert witnesses were crucial to Saenz's ultimate conviction by a jury. A forensic chemist at the FDA analyzed the dialysis lines and syringes used on some of the victims and testified that bleach was found in the lines. A bio-analytical chemist, in collaboration with the CDC and the local health department, compared blood samples of dialysis clinic patients who had experienced an adverse event and those who had not. The bioanalytical chemist found high levels of a biomarker indicating exposure to chlorine (which is found in bleach) in the blood of the victims and no evidence of the biomarker in the blood of the control patients. A CDC physician and toxicologist reviewed the FDA's analysis, the bio-analytical chemist's analysis, and the medical histories of the victims, and testified that the victims were injected with bleach (*Saenz v. State*, 2014).

These experts were able to help show beyond a reasonable doubt that Saenz caused the injuries and deaths of the dialysis clinic patients. A jury found her guilty of capital murder and aggravated assault. Saenz is currently serving a sentence of life in prison without the possibility of parole (*Saenz v. State*, 2014).

## CONCLUSION

This chapter discussed litigation in public health by looking at recent cases and disputes on some of the major public health issues like opioids, food, drinks and obesity, and foodborne outbreaks and investigations. Three salient points emerge from this discussion. First, public health students would benefit greatly from understanding legal principles just as law students would benefit from understanding public health principles. Although an attorney involved in litigation in public health need not have a public health degree, it helps to know the language of public health. Second, public health litigation occurs in both civil and criminal contexts. For example, criminal prosecutors at the federal, state, and local levels prosecute individuals and companies whose actions negatively affect the public's health. Third, when it comes to litigation, it is safe to say, as illustrated by the cases cited here, that public health is "now at the table." That is, the judiciary is now a frequently considered avenue in settling public health disputes (Kromm et al., 2009).

## CHAPTER REVIEW

### Review Questions

1. In the case involving the *Salmonella* outbreak, if the court had ruled that the FDA was negligent in issuing the contamination warning, what effect do you think that ruling would have had on public health officials? Do you think these effects would extend beyond just foodborne outbreak investigations?
2. What are other potential examples of how public health investigations can help solve individual criminal cases?

### Essay Question

In light of the recent public health outbreaks, including but not limited to Severe Acute Respiratory Syndrome (SARS) in February 2003, Middle East Respiratory Syndrome (MERS) in 2012, Ebola Virus Disease (EVD) in 2014, Opiod Epidemics in 2017, and Corona Virus Disease (Covid-19) in 2019, do you see public health litigation gaining strength in the courts and wider recognition among the American public? Put differently, will public health litigation become the norm?

### Internet Activities

1. Go to the National Institute on Drug Abuse website (https://www.drugabuse.gov/drug-topics/opioids/opioid-summaries-by-state) and search for opioid involved overdose death rates per 100,000 people. Which states have the most opioid deaths? Which have the least? Can you think of a reason why?
2. Visit the National Prescription Opiate Litigation Documents website (https://www.industrydocuments.ucsf.edu/drug/collections/national-prescription-opiate-litigation-documents/). Review the documents and answer the following:
   - Who are the parties?
   - What are the plaintiffs alleging?

## REFERENCES

28 U.S.C. § 2680(a); (West, 2006).
28 U.S.C. §§ 1346(b), 2671-2680; (West, 2013).
Bernstein, L. (2019a, May 2). West Virginia reaches $37 million opioid settlement with drug shipper McKesson. *The Washington Post*.
Bernstein, L. (2019b, May 16). Five more states take legal action against Purdue Pharma for opioid crisis. *The Washington Post*.

Centers for Disease Control and Prevention. (2018). *Multiple cause of death 1999–2017 on CDC wide-ranging online data for epidemiologic research (CDC WONDER).* http://wonder.cdc.gov

Centers for Disease Control and Prevention. (n.d.). *Understanding the epidemic.* https://www.cdc.gov/drugoverdose/epidemic/index.html

Centers for Disease Control and Prevention Foundation. (n.d.). *What is public health?* https://www.cdcfoundation.org/what-public-health

Columbia Broadcasting System, Dallas Forth Worth (2018, August 2). Texas nurse accused of killing patients with bleach IVs. https://dfw.cbslocal.com/2012/03/05/texas-nurse-accused-of-killing-patients-with-bleach-ivs/Id

Esterl, M. (2013, April 30). Monster sues to halt efforts to curb drinks. *The Wall Street Journal.*

Florida Stat. Title XLVI § 893.135 (2017).

Fryar, C. D., & Ervin, R. B. (2013, February). Caloric intake from fast food among adults: United States, 2007–2010. *Centers for Disease Control and Prevention, National Center for Health Statistics Data Brief # 113.*

Fryar, C. D., Hughes, J. P., Herrick, K. A., & Ahluwalia, N. (2018, October). Fast food consumption among adults in the United States, 2013–2016. *Centers for Disease Control and Prevention, National Center for Health Statistics Data Brief # 322.*

Goldenbaum, D. M., Christopher, M., Gallagher, R. M., Fishman, S., Payne, R., Joranson, D., Edmondson, D., McKee, J., & Thexton, A. (2008). Physicians charged with 231 analgesic-prescribing offenses. *Pain Medicine, 9,* 737–747. https://doi.org/10.1111/j.1526-4637.2008.00482.x

Gostin, L. (2008). A theory and definition of public health law. In L. O. Gostin & L. F. Wiley (Eds.), *Public health law: Power, duty, restraint* (2nd ed.). University of California Press.

*Guertin v. State,* 912 F.3d 907, 933 (6th Cir. 2019).

Herrone, M. (2018, July 26). Deaths: Leading causes for 2016. *National Vital Statistics Report, 67*(6), 1–77. https://www.cdc.gov/nchs/data/nvsr/nvsr67/nvsr67_06.pdf

Institute of Medicine. (1988). *The future of public health.* National Academies Press.

Kentucky House Bill 333 (signed by Governor, 2017, October 4)

Kromm, J. N., Frattaroli, S., Vernick, J. S., & Teret, S. P. (2009). Public health advocacy in the courts: Opportunities for public health professionals. *Public Health Reports, 124,* 889–894. https://doi.org/10.1177/003335490912400618

McMenamin, J., & Tiglio, A. (2006). Not the next tobacco: Defenses to obesity claims. *Food and Drug Law Journal, 6,* 445–518. https://www.jstor.org/stable/26660886?seq=1#metadata_info_tab_contents

National Health Law Program. (n.d.). https://healthlaw.org/our-work/litigation

Parmet, W. E., & Daynard, R. A. (2000). The new public health litigation. *Annual Review of Public Health, 21,* 437–454. https://doi.org/10.1146/annurev.publhealth.21.1.437

*Pelman ex. rel Pelman v. McDonald's Corp,* 396 F.3d 508, 509 (2d Cir. 2005).

Ransom, M. M. (2016, April). *Public health law competency model. Version 1.0.* CDC. http://www.cdc.gov/phlp/docs/phlcm-v1.pdf

*Saenz,* 479 S.W.3d.

*Saenz v. State,* 421 S.W.3d 725, 734-35 (Tex. App. 2014).

*Saenz v. State,* 479 S.W.3d 939, 941 (Tex. App. 2015).

Scholl, L., Seth, P., Kariisa, M., Wilson, N., & Baldwin, G. (2019). Drug and opioid-involved overdose deaths—United States, 2013-2017. *MMWR Morbidity and Mortality Weekly Report, 67*(5152), 1419–1427. http://dx.doi.org/10.15585/mmwr.mm675152e1

*Seaside Farm, Inc. v. United States,* 842 F.3d 853, 856 (4th Cir. 2016).

Texas nurse accused of killing patients with bleach IVs. (2012). https://dfw.cbslocal.com/2012/03/05/texas-nurse-accused-of-killing-patients-with-bleach-ivs

*United States v. Tobin,* 676 F.3d 1264 (11th Cir. 2012).

*University of St. Thomas Law Review,* 23, 157–185 (2010).

U.S. Department of Justice. (2019, April 17). Appalachian Regional Prescription Opioid (ARPO) strike force takedown results in charges against 60 individuals, including 53 medical professionals. https://www.justice.gov/opa/pr/appalachian-regional-prescription-opioid-arpo-strike-force-takedown-results-charges-against

Waldrop, T., & Drash, W. (2019). Drugmaker Teva to pay $85 million to settle Oklahoma opioid lawsuit. CNN.https://www.cnn.com/2019/05/26/health/drugmaker-teva-to-pay-85-million-to -settle-oklahoma-opioid-lawsuit/index.html

World Health Organization. (n.d.). *Public health services*. http://www.euro.who.int/en/health-topics/ Health-systems/public-health-services

## Additional Resources

- CDC. (2008, August 28). Multistate Outbreak of *Salmonella* Saintpaul Infections Linked to Raw Produce. https://www.cdc.gov/salmonella/2008/raw-produce-8-28-2008.html
- Casey Barton Behravesh et al. (2011, March 10). 2008 outbreak of *Salmonella* Saintpaul infections associated with raw produce. *New England Journal of Medicine, 364*(10), 918–927. https:// www.ncbi.nlm.nih.gov/pubmed/21345092
- Robert Roos, Center For Infectious Disease Research and Policy (CIDRAP). (2008, June 4). Tomatoes suspected in multistate *Salmonella* outbreak. https://www.cidrap.umn.edu/news -perspective/2008/06/tomatoes-suspected-multistate-salmonella-outbreak
- CBS News. (2012, April 2). Kimberly Saenz, ex-nurse convicted of bleach killings, sentenced to life in prison. https://www.cbsnews.com/news/kimberly-saenz-ex-nurse-convicted-of-bleach -killings-sentenced-to-life-in-prison/
- Gary Bass. (2015, August 26). Fourth Court of Appeals upholds Kimberly Saenz' capital murder conviction. https://www.ktre.com/story/29885248/fourth-court-of-appeals-upholds-kimberly -saenz-capital-murder-conviction/

# II

## LAW IN THE EVERYDAY PRACTICE OF PUBLIC HEALTH: CASE STUDIES

6

# Vaccination Law Across the Life-Course

Alexandra Bhatti, Stacie P. Kershner, and Shade O. Olowookere

## Learning Objectives

By the end of this chapter, the reader should be able to:

■ Recognize the value and importance of vaccines and vaccination as well as the role of herd immunity in preventing the spread of vaccine-preventable illnesses.
■ Identify the legal authority for vaccination in the United States at the federal and state levels.
■ Describe the laws regulating vaccination including vaccine research/innovation, development, funding, surveillance, administration, requirements, and injury compensation.
■ Apply the balancing test between individual rights and the public good to vaccination.

## Key Terminology

**Eliminated:** Absence of naturally occurring cases and continued transmission of an infectious disease in a certain geographical area for at least 12 months.
**Epidemic:** Disease occurrence in excess of the expected levels in a certain geographical area or specific population.
**Eradicated:** Complete, worldwide end of an infectious disease such that no additional transmission of the disease occurs.
**Federalism:** The way in which government power is divided between the federal and state governments.
**Herd immunity:** A form of indirect protection of a community from an infectious disease that occurs when a large enough percentage of a population has become immune to an infection, thus providing a measure of protection for individuals who are not immune. This may also be referred to as "community immunity".
**Immunization:** The process by which a person is made immune to an infectious disease. Sometimes this term is used interchangeably with "vaccination".
**Life-course vaccination:** A comprehensive approach to vaccination that aims to ensure all individuals receive the full benefits of vaccination based upon not only their age and health, but also the changing circumstances throughout their lives.
**Outbreak:** Appearance of a disease within a geographic area or among a specific population.
**Pandemic:** An epidemic occurring worldwide, or over a very wide area, crossing international boundaries, and usually affecting a large number of people.

The authors would also like to acknowledge and thank Marice Ashe, JD, MPH for her invaluable assistance in reviewing and editing this chapter.

**Preemption:** Legal theory in which a higher authority of law will displace the law of a lower authority of law when the two authorities conflict.

**Scope of practice:** Actions healthcare practitioners are permitted to undertake in keeping with their professional license.

**Vaccination:** The act of introducing a killed or weakened organism into the body for the purpose of producing immunity to a specific disease.

**Vaccine hesitancy:** the reluctance or refusal to vaccinate despite the availability of vaccines.

## Public Health Law Competencies

This chapter addresses the following competencies from the Public Health Law Competency Model (PHLCM; Ransom, 2016).

**1.1** Define basic constitutional concepts and legal principles framing the practice of public health across relevant jurisdictions.

**1.2** Identify and apply public health laws pertinent to practitioner's jurisdiction, agency, program, and profession.

**2.2** Identify law-based tools and enforcement procedures to address day-to-day (nonemergency) public health issues.

**2.3** Recognize the legal authority and limits of critical system partners and others who influence health outcomes.

---

### Spark Questions

1. What impact do you think vaccination has had on population health over the past 150 years?
2. What role does vaccination play in the health of individual children, adults, and the elderly?
3. What role does vaccination play in community health?

---

## INTRODUCTION

**Vaccination** is recognized as one of the top 10 public health achievements of the 20th century in the United States (Centers for Disease Control and Prevention [CDC], 1999). With the World Health Organization declaring that, *"Immunization is a global health and development success story,"* and worldwide it is estimated to prevent two to three million deaths annually. (World Health Organization [WHO], 2020). The COVID-19 **pandemic** is a reminder of the critical role vaccination plays in reducing **outbreaks**, deaths, and illnesses, associated with infectious diseases. Vaccination relies on maintaining specified levels of immunity within the population. **Herd immunity**, or community immunity, is the interruption of the spread of disease because a large enough proportion of the community is immune to the disease, whether through vaccination or having developed immunity from having been previously exposed to the disease. The "herd immunity threshold" (see Figure 6.1) refers to the percentage of the population that must be vaccinated to maintain herd immunity and differs for each vaccine-preventable disease (Metcalf et al., 2015). Law and broader policy play a critical role in maintaining high herd immunity thresholds, maximizing the number of people who are vaccinated for each of the 18 vaccine-preventable diseases (VPDs), and minimizing the morbidity and mortality caused by those diseases in the United States (Moulton et al., 2007).

This chapter provides an overview of vaccination as an essential health service and public health intervention as well as recent trends associated with vaccination in the United States. It then explores the legal framework for vaccination, including the source and scope of legal authority for vaccination efforts at the state and federal levels, as well as limitations on government intervention when balanced against individual liberties. The chapter also describes key federal and state policies that impact vaccine access, uptake, and coverage rates, which ultimately can influence the incidence of vaccine-preventable diseases.

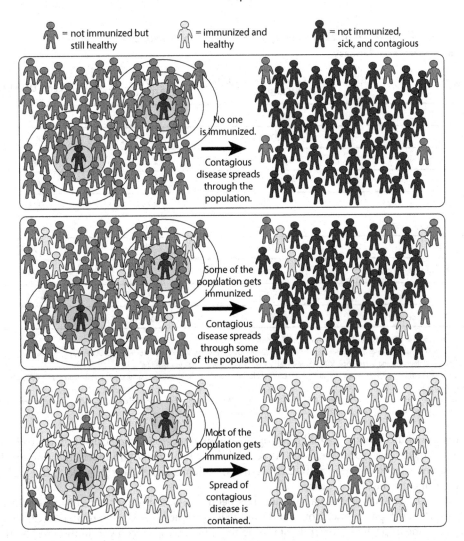

**FIGURE 6.1** Herd, or community, immunity is the result of a high immunization rate.
*Source*: Heleft, L., & Willingham, E. (2014, September 5). What is Herd Immunity?
https://www.pbs.org/wgbh/nova/article/herd-immunity citing The National Institute
of Allergy and Infectious Disease

## HISTORY OF VACCINATION

The development and uptake of vaccination has led to the reduction in VPDs—in fact, smallpox
was **eradicated** and no longer exists outside the laboratory as a result of strategic vaccination efforts (CDC, 1999; Fenner et al., 1988). Edward Jenner is credited with developing modern vaccination. He had observed that milkmaids who were exposed to cowpox did not catch smallpox,
and in 1776 he experimented by taking material from a cowpox lesion of one of the milkmaids
and inoculating an eight-year-old boy with it. When Jenner exposed the boy to smallpox, he
did not catch the disease. Later, Jenner published these results, naming his discovery "vaccination," after the Latin word for cowpox, vaccinia (Riedel, 2005). Smallpox was the first widely
adopted vaccination. Later, in 1979, smallpox was declared eradicated after mass vaccination
efforts and remains today the only human VPD to be eradicated (Greenwood, 2014).

In 1885, about a century after the smallpox vaccine was developed, the next human vaccine
was developed by Louis Pasteur for rabies (Greenwood, 2014). It would not be until the late

**TABLE 6.1 Comparison of 20th Century Annual Morbidity and Currency Morbidity: Vaccine-Preventable Disease**

| DISEASE | 20TH CENTURY ANNUAL MORBIDITY[†] | 2018 REPORTED CASES[††] | PERCENT DECREASE |
|---|---|---|---|
| Smallpox | 29,005 | 0 | 100% |
| Diphtheria | 21,053 | 1 | >99% |
| Measles | 530,217 | 273 | >99% |
| Mumps | 162,344 | 2,251 | 99% |
| Pertussis | 200,752 | 13,439 | 93% |
| Polio (paralytic) | 16,316 | 0 | 100% |
| Rubella | 47,745 | 5 | >99% |
| Congenital Rubella Syndrome | 152 | 0 | 100% |
| Tetanus | 580 | 20 | 97% |
| Haemophilus influenzae | 20,000 | 27* | >99% |

[†]Journal of the American Medical Association (JAMA). 2007; 299(18): 2155–2163.
[††]CDC. National Notifiable Diseases Surveillance System, Week 52 (2018 Provisional Data), Weekly Tables of Infectious Disease Data. Atlanta, GA. CDC Division of Health Informatics and Surveillance, 2019. Available at: www.cdc.gov/nndss/infectious-tables.html
*Haemophilus type b (Hib) < 5 years of age. An additional 11 cases of Hib are estimated to have occurred among the 221 notification of Hib (<5 years with unknown serotype)
*Source*: Centers for Disease Control and Prevention. (2019a). *Comparison of 20th-century annual morbidity and current morbidity: Vaccine-preventable diseases*. https://www.cdc.gov/vaccines/ed/surv/downloads/VPD-morbidity-slide1-mmwr-508.pdf

1940s that scientific knowledge had developed enough to permit large-scale vaccine production and infectious disease–control efforts. As seen in Table 6.1, the overall morbidity due to VPDs has decreased significantly since the 20th century, which is largely attributable to the high up-take of vaccines in the 20th century.

Note, most recently, mass vaccination has been a vital component of response efforts to stem the COVID-19 pandemic. Novel and unique legal issues have arisen related to COVID-19, highlighting the importance for understanding the difference between vaccination research and

## BOX 6.1 MEASLES

- Measles is highly contagious and spreads when someone with the infection coughs or sneezes.
- In an unvaccinated population, 15 people would contract measles from one infected individual.
- Up to 90% of people who are not immune will contract the disease if exposed to it.
- The virus can survive up to two hours outside the body, such as in the air or on a surface.
- People do not experience symptoms until one to two weeks after being exposed and can spread the disease up to four days before and after this rash, possibly without realizing they are sick.
- Complications include pneumonia and other respiratory illnesses and encephalitis, which can cause hearing loss, cognitive delays, and other negative long-term health effects.

*Source*: (CDC, 2015; Metcalf et al., 2015).

development, approval, deployment, and delivery during a declared public health emergency to that of traditional life-course vaccination during non-public health emergencies. This chapter will focus on the latter.

## VACCINE HESITANCY AND RESURGENCE OF VPDs

### Resurgence of VPDs: Measles

If vaccination coverage rates decrease below community immunity thresholds, communities become at increased risk of VPD outbreaks—with the most infectious diseases re-emerging first. In 2019, the US has experienced outbreaks of measles, mumps, and hepatitis A, among other VPDs (CDC, 2019c, 2019e, 2019f), due in part to the hesitancy of parents to have their children vaccinated.

In 2019, 1,292 cases of measles were confirmed in the United States, the greatest number of cases of measles since 1992 (CDC, 2019c). More than 30 states had outbreaks of this highly contagious disease. Before the measles vaccine became available in 1963, measles was considered a childhood rite of passage; each year, an estimated three to four million people in the United States contracted the disease, more than half of whom were children under the age of six and below. Sadly, an average of 500 of these people died annually from complications of the disease. After 1963, measles declined by 95% and was eventually declared **eliminated** in the United States in 2000, with no new naturally occurring cases for a 12-month period (CDC, 2015).

Figure 6.2 demonstrates the recent escalation in the number of reported measles cases in the United States. In 2014, there were 23 outbreaks. Just over half of these cases were attributed to a large outbreak in an unvaccinated Amish community in Ohio. In 2015, 78% of the cases stemmed from an outbreak linked to guests at Disneyland. In Minnesota, 75 cases of measles were identified among a Somali community whose previously high vaccination rates had declined due to fear that measles, mumps, rubella (MMR) vaccination causes autism. Most recently, the majority of measles cases stemmed from a 2018 to 2019 outbreak in New York City, New York State, and New Jersey among an unvaccinated Orthodox Jewish community (CDC, 2019c).

### Reasons for Vaccine Hesitancy and Waning Vaccine Confidence—Challenges Presented

While coverage remains high for most vaccines in the United States, there has been a growing presence of **vaccine hesitancy** that has negatively impacted vaccine coverage rates. Vaccine

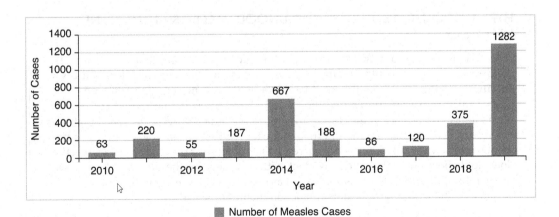

**FIGURE 6.2** Number of measles cases reported by year, 2010–2019 (as of January 31, 2020).

*Source*: Centers for Disease Control and Prevention. (2019c). Measles cases and outbreaks. https://www.cdc .gov/measles/cases-outbreaks.html

hesitancy is the reluctance or refusal to vaccinate despite the availability of vaccines. Numerous sources have documented the negative effects of vaccine hesitancy on individual- and population-level health (McKee & Bohannon, 2016). Vaccine hesitancy is not just about the small but vocal minority of the population that is against vaccination or refuse vaccination. Rather, hesitancy happens along a broad continuum that ranges from vaccine refusal at one end to vaccine acceptance at the other (Dubé et al., 2013). Vaccine hesitancy differs from the "antivaccination movement" by degree, with the latter actively opposing vaccination (Feemster, 2018).

Vaccine hesitancy is complex, and a person's hesitancy may change depending on the context of time, place, and the specific vaccine. Many people have not personally seen or experienced the serious illnesses that vaccines prevent; they may fear the risks of vaccination more than the diseases. Parents may decline or delay vaccines for their children due to these concerns regarding vaccine safety and fear of side effects or vaccine injury, religious or philosophical reasons, or lack of education about or misunderstanding of the risk or threat of VPDs (Glatman-Freedman & Nichols, 2012; McKee & Bohannon, 2016). Increased dialogue regarding freedom from governmental interference have influenced discussions around vaccine policies, such as school-entry requirements (Glatman-Freedman & Nichols, 2012). Vaccine hesitancy may also be influenced by accessibility of vaccinations, including cost.

Addressing vaccine hesitancy is an important issue as there is geographic clustering associated with vaccine refusal and non or underimmunized individuals (Lieu et al., 2015). This means coverage rates in those specific communities may fall below herd immunity thresholds making the community more susceptible to VPDs outbreaks, such as in the recent outbreaks in Ohio, California, Minnesota, and New York previously described. While some states like California and New York have responded to increased vaccine hesitancy and outbreaks of VPDs by implementing stricter school vaccine requirements and removing religious or philosophical exemptions as discussed in detail in what follows, other strategies to reach vaccine-hesitant individuals and non or undervaccinated communities to increase vaccination rates are also needed.

In further responses to the growing vaccine-hesitant community, the CDC has launched the "Vaccinate with Confidence" initiative aimed at strengthening public trust in vaccines by advancing three key priorities: protecting communities, empowering families, and stopping myths (CDC, 2019g).

As the world seeks to restore and strengthen global health security in response to the COVID-19 pandemic, it is imperative to build the public's trust in vaccination and work to ensure people everywhere are protected against the serious, potentially life-threatening diseases for which vaccines already exist.

---

### HYPOTHETICAL CASE STUDY #1: CHILDHOOD VACCINES AND VACCINE HESITANCY

MacKayla is a nurse practitioner in a health clinic. Her next appointment is a well-child visit for four-year-old Ivy. In the past, Ivy's mom Catherine has declined Ivy's vaccines. During the appointment, MacKayla again recommends vaccination, suggests a catch-up vaccination schedule, and advises Catherine that there have been a few instances of measles in the community recently. Catherine tells MacKayla that she has researched vaccines on the internet and after reading several blogs, she does not want Ivy to be vaccinated. Ivy is not currently in childcare or preschool, and Catherine does not believe she will come in contact with anyone with the disease. She refuses further discussion. MacKayla is concerned as she has seen an increase in *"vaccine hesitancy,"* and she is worried about its impact on the public's health.

1. Why might Catherine be hesitant to have Ivy vaccinated?
2. Why is vaccine hesitancy a public health problem? What is the impact to the public's health if some people choose not to vaccinate?

**BOX 6.2** *JACOBSON v. MASSACHUSETTS*, 197 U.S. 11 (1905) AT 29

"There is, of course, a sphere within which the individual may assert the supremacy of his own will and rightfully dispute the authority of any human government, especially of any free government existing under a written constitution. But it is equally true that in every well-ordered society charged with the duty of conserving the safety of its members the rights of the individual in respect of his liberty may at times, under the pressure of great dangers, be subjected to such restraint, to be enforced by reasonable regulations, as the safety of the general public may demand."

## INDIVIDUAL RIGHTS VERSUS PUBLIC GOOD

Early in the 19th century, cities and states in the United States began enacting laws mandating vaccination of private citizens under certain conditions, such as the threat of an outbreak. The Supreme Court case *Jacobson v. Massachusetts* (1905) stems from a legal challenge to one such law. In 1902, Massachusetts was in the midst of a smallpox outbreak. A Massachusetts statute authorized localities to mandate vaccination during outbreaks, and the Board of Health of the town of Cambridge voted to require vaccination of any residents who had not been previously vaccinated since 1897. A Lutheran pastor, Henning Jacobson, refused and was fined five dollars. He then refused to pay the fine and was taken into custody. He argued that the law was unconstitutional, contending that his 14th Amendment rights had been violated and that the state had exceeded its police powers.

The law was upheld by the Massachusetts Supreme Court and then ultimately upheld by the U.S. Supreme Court on appeal. The U.S. Supreme Court articulated several important holdings. First, the Court affirmed the state's authority to use police powers to protect the public's health and the state's ability to delegate authority to localities. The Court also stated that it is outside of the Court's expertise to determine whether a specific initiative is the appropriate method to protect the public's health, instead deferring to the state legislature, which relies on the available medical and scientific information.

Perhaps most importantly, as illustrated in Figure 6.3, the Court established a key legal principle that extends beyond vaccination to public health law more broadly: the balancing of individual rights against the common good. Chief Justice Harlan delivered the opinion of the Court in now-famous words, "[t]here are manifold restraints to which every person is necessarily subject for the common good." Theories of due process and equal protection have advanced, but *Jacobson*

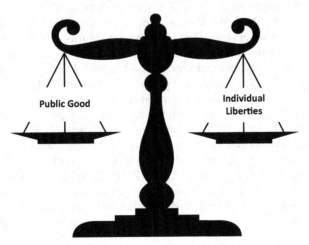

**FIGURE 6.3** The public health balancing act.

is still considered "good law." Public health cases throughout the past century have cited *Jacobson* as precedent and applied this balancing test to determine whether certain government interventions that may infringe on individual rights are constitutionally permissible. Later cases, such as the quarantine case *U.S. v. Shinnick* (1963), extended this test to the federal government as well. While not all public health actions withstand this test or modern principles of due process, vaccination laws continue to be upheld.

## SOURCE OF FEDERAL AND STATE LEGAL AUTHORITY FOR VACCINATION

Under principles of **federalism**, the federal government is limited to "enumerated powers" specifically granted in the Constitution. Prevention and control of communicable diseases specifically and public health more generally are not expressly stated. Legal authority for vaccination is found instead in the federal government's authority under the power to regulate interstate commerce (U.S. Const. art. I, § VIII, Cl. 3) and the power to tax and spend (U.S. Const. art. I, § VIII, Cl. 1). Congress has the power "[t]o regulate Commerce with foreign nations, and among the several states, and with the Indian Tribes." The power to tax and spend gives Congress the ability to raise revenues and fund or defund state and local programs and projects. The federal government promotes vaccination by approving vaccines and monitoring for safety, requiring health insurance to cover the cost of vaccines for certain populations, providing low- and no-cost vaccination programs for specific populations, and compensating individuals for vaccine-related injuries (discussed more fully in what follows).

Authority for state regulation of vaccination is found in the 10th Amendment, which states, "[t]he powers not delegated to the United States by the Constitution, nor prohibited by it to the States, are reserved to the States respectively, or to the people." Thus, states may regulate the health, safety, and welfare of citizens within their borders through what are often referred to as the states' "police powers." Examples of police powers related to vaccination include requiring vaccination for school entry or healthcare workers and maintaining vaccine registries.

## SELECTED FEDERAL VACCINE EFFORTS

### The National Vaccine Plan

Congress enacted the National Childhood Vaccine Injury Act (NCVIA) of 1986 (NCVIA, 1986, U.S.C.A. § §300aa-1 through -34), which has since been amended by the 21st Century Cures Act of 2016, establishing the National Vaccine Program Office (NVPO) within the U.S. Department of Health and Human Services (DHHS). The goals of this office are "to achieve optimal prevention of human infectious diseases through **immunization** and to achieve optimal prevention against adverse reactions to vaccines (NCVIA, 1986, U.S.C.A. § §300aa-1). The NVPO issued the first National Vaccine Plan, a comprehensive strategy for U.S. vaccine initiatives, in 1986 (NCVIA, 1986, U.S.C.A. § §300aa-1). The most recent plan, published in 2021, incorporates stakeholder input and provides direction on the following key goals: "1) foster innovation in vaccine development and related technologies; 2) maintain the highest levels of vaccine safety; 3) Increase knowledge of and confidence in routinely recommended vaccines; 4) Increase access to and use of all routinely recommended vaccines; 5) Protect the health of the nation by supporting global immunization efforts" (OIDP, 2021). As of 2019, NVPO merged with the office of HIV/AIDS and Infectious Disease Policy and is now known as the Office of Infectious Disease Policy and HIV/AIDS (OIDP). While OIDP coordinates federal resources and directs the plan, it relies on collaboration among federal agencies and state, Tribal, and local governments, as well as the pharmaceutical industry, the healthcare system, and other key players, to achieve national vaccine goals.

## Vaccine Development and Approval

Determining which diseases to pursue for vaccine development is a complex question. One factor is whether a disease is considered "high burden." Burden may be determined by the number of people who contract the disease each year, even if the disease is not severe, or by how deadly a disease is, even if not many people contract it (Feemster, 2018). In addition to disease burden and severity of disease, it is important to consider whether treatment options exist for the disease in question. For example, many people contract seasonal influenza each year and while the death rate may be lower than other diseases, there are significant healthcare costs and lost productivity. In contrast, Ebola is deadly but has not affected as many people or as many countries. Both diseases are important for vaccine development (Feemster, 2018).

The Food, Drug, and Cosmetic Act of 1938 (21 U.S.C. ch. 9 § 301 et. seq.) authorizes the U.S. Food and Drug Administration (FDA) to oversee the safety and efficacy of pharmaceuticals, including vaccines. Before a vaccine can be introduced into interstate commerce, it must first go through an extensive vetting process managed by the FDA's Center for Biologics Evaluation and Research (CBER), the precursor of which was created in the early 20th century following the deaths of children given tainted vaccines in order to reduce or prevent future occurrences (FDA, 2018). In non-emergencies, the premarket approval process has the applicant (generally the manufacturer) submit an Investigational New Drug Application (IND) along with any safety and efficacy information and a proposed protocol for the required clinical studies on humans. Rigorous premarket clinical studies are then conducted (FDA, 2018).

After the clinical studies are successfully completed, a team of experts reviews the application and supporting information. The FDA will grant a license for the vaccine only if (1) the vaccine is safe and effective, and (2) the benefits outweigh the risks. After licensing, the FDA continues to monitor production and manufacturing to ensure continued safety, efficacy, purity, and potency by conducting regular inspections (FDA, 2018). A vaccine can take 10 years or longer to move from development to distribution and then is monitored for safety throughout its lifecycle.

## The U.S. Recommended Immunization Schedule

Established under Section 222 of the Public Health Service Act (1944; 42 U.S.C. §217a, as amended), the Advisory Committee on Immunization Practices (ACIP) advises the director of the CDC on vaccine use and administration, including for which age groups the vaccines are recommended and under what circumstances (CDC, 2018b). The ACIP membership comprises 15 voting members; 14 with expertise in vaccinology, immunology, public health, infectious disease, and more, and one consumer representative (CDC, 2018c). In addition to voting members, there are eight above ex officio members who represent other federal agencies and 30 nonvoting organization representatives who bring additional expertise (CDC, 2018c). The ACIP reviews information from a range of organizations with expertise on vaccines, such as the American Academy of Pediatrics. The ACIP then develops or updates recommendations, which the CDC director then reviews and approves. Once published, these recommendations are incorporated into the official Recommended Immunization Schedule and are referred to as "ACIP-recommended vaccines" (Feemster, 2018). See Table 6.2 for the child and adolescent immunizations recommended in the United States.

## TABLE 6.2 Recommended Child and Adolescent Immunizations, United States, 2020

| VACCINES | ABBREVIATIONS |
| --- | --- |
| Diphtheria, tetanus, and acellular pertussis vaccine | DTaP |
| Diphtheria, tetanus vaccine | DT |
| *Haemophilus influenzae* type b vaccine | Hib (PRP-T) |
| | Hib (PRP-OMP) |
| Hepatitis A vaccine | HepA |
| Hepatitis B vaccine | HepB |
| Human papillomavirus vaccine | HPV |
| Influenza vaccines (inactivated) | IIV |
| Influenza vaccine (live, attenuated) | LAIV |
| Measles, mumps, and rubella vaccine | MMR |
| Meningococcal serogroups A, C, W, Y vaccine | MenACWY-D |
| | MenACWY-CRM |
| Meningococcal serogroup B vaccine | MenB-4C |
| | MenB-FHbp |
| Pneumococcal 13-valent conjugate vaccine | PCV13 |
| Pneumococcal 23-valent polysaccharide vaccine | PPSV23 |
| Poliovirus (inactivated) | IPV |
| Rotavirus vaccine | RV1 |
| | RV5 |
| Tetanus, diphtheria, and acellular pertussis vaccine | Tdap |
| Tetanus and diphtheria vaccine | Td |
| Varicella vaccine | VAR |

The ACIP schedule of recommended vaccines is only guidance. States may choose to adopt the recommendations in whole or in part for their vaccination requirements for school entry, as discussed later in this chapter, and healthcare professionals may use this guidance in recommending vaccinations to their patients. Federal and state policy may incorporate the ACIP recommendations, which may influence what vaccines are covered through public and private insurance.

ACIP recommendations may change over time depending on new information and risks associated with a disease (Malone & Hinman, 2007). Risks must be weighed to determine whether certain vaccinations are or continue to be in the public's best interest. For example, one in every 2.4 million people who receive the oral polio vaccine (OPV) develop paralysis associated with the vaccine. When wild poliovirus was circulating in the United States, this was considered an acceptable risk because of the dangers of contracting and spreading wild poliovirus. The last natural polio case in the United States was in 1977. In 1997, it was recommended children instead receive two doses of inactivated polio vaccine (IPV) followed by two doses of OPV. While slightly less effective in preventing the spread of wild poliovirus, there is no risk of paralysis associated with IPV (Malone & Hinman, 2007). In 2000, the ACIP discontinued recommending OPV in the United States (CDC, 2000) and it is being phased out worldwide (World Health Organization Regional Office for Europe, 2016).

## Tracking Adverse Events

Shoulder injury related to vaccine administration (SIRVA) is implicated in Hypothetical Case Study #2. SIRVA is a medical term used to describe any one of various shoulder injuries caused by vaccines such as the flu shot, tetanus shot, or TDaP and DTaP vaccines (Bancsi et al., 2019). Healthcare providers are required to report SIRVA and other potential adverse side effects of vaccines to the Vaccine Adverse Event Reporting System (VAERS, n.d.-a). A joint effort of FDA and CDC launched in 1990, this surveillance system provides an early warning for possible safety concerns of vaccines by helping to detect "unusual or unexpected patterns," such as clustering of bad batches, population groups at risk of certain side effects, administration errors, and so forth (VAERS, n.d.-a). Reporting to VAERS is for information gathering only and is not the same as reporting to the National Vaccine Injury Compensation Program (VICP) described in what follows. VAERS is a passive system and accepts reports of adverse events regardless of seriousness. Some reported adverse events might be coincidental and not related to vaccination (VAERS, n.d.-b).

---

### HYPOTHETICAL CASE STUDY #2

André is a 12-year-old middle school student who is up to date on all of his vaccines according to the ACIP recommendations. Just two days ago, he received his TDaP vaccine at the offices of his family care doctor. Since that time, he has complained to his father about considerable shoulder pain and decreased range of motion. His father calls their family care doctor and reports André's condition. The doctor tells André's father that the pain should resolve on its own within a week or two, but to give him a call back if it does not. Recognizing that there is a possibility that the pain is being caused by a vaccine-related injury, the doctor notes this call in André's records and makes a reminder to follow up.

1. How are potential adverse effects of vaccines reported and surveilled?
2. What legal mechanisms are in place to make claims for vaccination injuries?

---

## Claims and Compensation of Adverse Events

Despite the overall benefit to the public's health, vaccines are not without some risks to the health of individuals. In certain circumstances, vaccines may trigger adverse reactions, such as anaphylaxis, muscle or joint pain, or encephalitis.

In the early 1980s, pharmaceutical companies and healthcare providers expressed concern over the rising costs of defending lawsuits brought by individuals allegedly injured by vaccines. Bolstered by the swine flu scare of the 1970s when a similar injury compensation program was created, they successfully argued to Congress that these lawsuits might discourage vaccine manufacturing and delivery, or increase costs (Parasidis, 2017). Congress established the National Vaccine Injury Compensation Program as part of the NCVIA to avoid shortages, encourage vaccine production, and stabilize costs (Health Resources & Services Administration [HRSA], 2019a).

The VICP is a mechanism to make claims for vaccination injuries outside of the traditional legal system for vaccines routinely administered to children or pregnant women and also seasonal influenza vaccine (HRSA, 2019b). The VICP is a separate program from VAERS and is administered by the HRSA. Under the VICP, industry is granted immunity from certain state tort claims (Parasidis, 2017). Instead, claims are submitted and reviewed by one of eight special masters, appointed by the Court of Federal Claims to four-year terms. The special master

---

**BOX 6.3** *BRUESEWITZ, ET AL. V. WYETH, LLC.,* 131 S.CT. 1068 (2011)

In 1993, Hannah Bruesewitz received the vaccine for diphtheria, tetanus, and pertussis (DTP). She started having seizures hours after her third dose, with 125 seizures in 16 days. There were many other reports of adverse events from this batch of DTP vaccine, which was manufactured by Lederle Laboratories, owned by Wyeth at the time of the case. (Wyeth is now a wholly owned subsidiary of Pfizer.) When Hannah turned 18, her parents filed a claim with the VICP; however, it was dismissed for failure to prove the vaccine caused Hannah's injuries. They then sued in state court in Pennsylvania for product design defects. The case was removed to federal court. The court held that the NCVIA preempts state claims, including design defects. **Preemption** occurs when a higher level of government acts on an issue, limiting a lower level of government's ability to act on the same issue. In some cases, the higher level of government sets a floor, enabling the lower level of government to adopt stricter standards, or a ceiling that the lower level cannot exceed (ChangeLab Solutions, 2013). In the case of vaccination, the federal government has preempted state claims for vaccination injuries due to design defects through enacting the NCVIA and establishing the VICP as an alternative mechanism for vaccine injury claims.

---

considers the evidence and adjudicates the claim. If it is determined that the individual suffered a harm listed on the vaccine injury table within the specified period of time after receiving an eligible vaccine and no unrelated possible cause has been identified, the individual is compensated. If the individual does not agree with the special master's decision or there is no decision within a certain time frame, the individual may appeal to the U.S. Court of Federal Claims (HRSA, 2019b; U.S. Court of Federal Claims, n.d.).

Being awarded compensation is not a determination of anyone's fault and does not prove that the vaccination definitively caused the alleged injury. Approximately 70% of all VICP compensation awards are a result of a negotiated settlement (HRSA, 2019c). In these situations, HHS has not determined a causal link between vaccination and injury (HRSA, 2019c).

---

**BOX 6.4** OMNIBUS AUTISM PROCEEDING

In 1998, Andrew Wakefield published a now-infamous article in *The Lancet,* a prestigious medical journal, linking autism and vaccines. The research was later proven fraudulent and the article retracted (Godlee et al., 2011). In 2010, Wakefield's U.K. medical license was revoked (Burns, 2010). In 2004, the Institute of Medicine (renamed the National Academy of Medicine) released a report analyzing a comprehensive body of research and rejecting the theories that either the vaccine for MMR or vaccines containing thimerosal were a preservative cause of autism (IOM, 2004).

Despite the lack of valid evidence, thousands of claims were filed with the VICP by petitioners alleging that vaccines had caused their children's autism. In 2007, these cases were consolidated into the Omnibus Autism Proceeding. Three test cases were established to advance three theories of "general causation": "(a) that MMR vaccines and thimerosal-containing vaccines can combine to cause autism; (b) that thimerosal-containing vaccines can alone cause autism; and (c) that MMR vaccines alone can cause autism." The cases were assigned by the U.S. Court of Federal Claims to special masters to review all of the evidence and hold hearings. Decisions issued in 2009 and 2010 found no evidence to support a link between autism and MMR or thimerosal (U.S. Court of Federal Claims, Office of Special Masters, 2010).

Individuals may also make a claim "off-table" for injuries not specified on the vaccine injury table; however, to be compensated, the individual must prove the vaccine in fact caused the injury, a much more difficult standard. Other concerns also exist. Critics of the VICP argue claims take longer under the VICP than in a traditional torts case; the government is treating the process as more adversarial than Congress intended; and the special masters vary widely in adjudicating claims (Parasidis, 2017).

Funding for the VICP is provided through the Vaccine Injury Compensation Trust Fund and collected by the Department of Treasury. An excise tax of $0.75 is imposed on each dose (each disease covered is counted as a dose, so a vaccine covering three diseases would be $2.25) (HRSA, 2019a). The CDC reports over 3.4 billion doses of eligible vaccines between 2006 (the first full year that influenza vaccine was included on the table) and 2017 (the most recent year comprehensive data is available). During this time, 6,467 petitions were filed, of which 4,450 were compensated. This is an average of one person compensated for every one million doses of vaccine (HRSA, 2019c).

## Protection of Workers: The Occupational Safety and Health Administration

The Occupational Safety and Health Act of 1970 (29 U.S.C. ch. 15 § 651 et. seq.) established the Occupational Safety and Health Administration (OSHA) to ensure safe and healthy working conditions by creating, implementing, and enforcing protective standards that employers must guarantee in the workplace. The OSHA falls under the Department of Labor and covers most private sector employees in all 50 states, Washington, D.C., and some territories, as well as some public-sector employees (U.S. Department of Labor, n.d.). The OSHA's Bloodborne Pathogens Standard requires that "employers offer the hepatitis B vaccination series to any employee who is reasonably anticipated to have exposure to blood or other potentially infectious materials within 10 working days of initial assignment" (29 CFR 1910.1030[f][2][i]). Employers are required to make the vaccine available at no cost and at a reasonable place and time to their employees (29 CFR 1910.1030[f][1][ii][a] and [b]). However, the OSHA does not require that the employees accept the vaccination. While federal power is limited generally around vaccination law, here is an example where federal law created standards and requirements for certain employers for a specific vaccine.

States create OSHA-approved state plans. In these cases, they must meet the minimum standards set forth by the OSHA but have the authority to be more restrictive and impose higher fines (OSHA, n.d.). Twenty-two states currently have the state plans that cover private sector and state and local government workers, and six states have plans that cover only state and local government workers (OSHA, n.d.).

## SELECTED STATE VACCINE POLICY EFFORTS

### School Vaccination Laws

State laws that require vaccination as a condition for school attendance, including the one highlighted in Hypothetical Case Study #3, are critical components of an effective vaccine delivery system. Massachusetts enacted the first law in the United States conditioning school attendance on vaccination in 1855. Schools are where a large number of children congregate in close proximity and many diseases easily spread, so they present a unique opportunity for vaccination enforcement. Despite a lack of immediate threat of outbreak, the Supreme Court upheld this practice in *Zucht v. King*, 43 S.Ct. 24 (1922), affirming that exclusion of unvaccinated children from public or private schools is a valid exercise of state police powers. The court cited *Jacobson*, stating it is "…settled that it is within the police power of a state to provide for compulsory vaccination" (*Zucht v. King*, 1922, at 176).

While parents have extensive rights to determine how to raise their children, such rights are not unlimited. For example, in a child labor case, parents asserted a law restricting child labor violated their free exercise of religion under the First Amendment. The Supreme Court

---

**HYPOTHETICAL CASE STUDY #3: VACCINATION FOR SCHOOL ATTENDANCE**

Recall Hypothetical Case Study #1. Mom, Catherine, is now preparing to enroll daughter Ivy in kindergarten in the fall, when she will be five. In Ivy's well-child visit, nurse practitioner MacKayla reminds her mom that vaccinations are required for kindergarten attendance in their state. Catherine is still unsure about vaccines and asks whether there is any way she can opt Ivy out of the vaccines required for school. MacKayla explains that their state allows medical exemptions only. Catherine argues that she has a religious objection to vaccination, and it would be a violation of her freedom of religion to require Ivy to be vaccinated in order to go to school.

1. What is the public health support for conditioning school attendance on vaccination?
2. What is the legal authority for conditioning school attendance on vaccination?
3. What exemptions from school vaccination exist? Which are constitutionally required?

---

disagreed and stated that state law could supersede religious and parental rights under the doctrine of *parens patriae* (i.e., the principle that political authority carries with it the responsibility to protect citizens):

> And neither rights of religion nor rights of parenthood are beyond limitation. Acting to guard the general interest in youth's wellbeing, the state, as parens patriae, may restrict the parent's control by requiring school attendance, regulating or prohibiting the child's labor and in many other ways. Its authority is not nullified merely because the parent grounds his claim to control the child's course of conduct on religion or conscience. Thus, he cannot claim freedom from compulsory vaccination for the child more than for himself on religious grounds. The right to practice religion freely does not include liberty to expose the community or the child to communicable disease or the latter to ill health or death. [citations omitted] (*Prince v. Massachusetts*, 321 U.S. 158 [1944] at 167)

Nonetheless, there is considerable variation in state school vaccination laws, including what exemptions are available. Courts have consistently held that only medical exemptions are required and that states may, but are not constitutionally required to, offer nonmedical exemptions. Five states (New York, California, Mississippi, West Virginia, and Maine) have exemptions for medical reasons only. The remainder allow exemptions for religious beliefs against vaccinations, or broader exemptions for philosophical (personal) beliefs against vaccination (National Conference of State Legislatures, 2019). Differences exist among states regarding which vaccinations are required, for what age groups or grades (childcare, elementary, middle or high school, higher education), and what requirements are in place to receive an exemption (CDC, 2017; Yang & Silverman, 2015). States in which administrative policies to obtain vaccine exemptions are more comprehensive have been shown to have lower exemption rates (Blank et al., 2013; Omer et al., 2012; Salmon et al., 2015). Figure 6.4 illustrates school vaccination exemptions for states.

Despite this support, less than half of the states had enacted school vaccination laws by the mid-20th century. In the 1970s, amid early efforts to eliminate measles, research found that school vaccination laws had significant impact: states with laws mandating measles vaccination for school attendance had measles incidence rates 40% to 51% lower than states without these laws. In the late 1970s, the Childhood Immunization Initiative, a campaign to increase vaccination rates, included increasing and improving enforcement of state school vaccination laws. Additional studies demonstrated a correlation between lower incidence rates of measles and states with strictly enforced school vaccination laws, and by 1980, all states had laws requiring vaccination for school attendance (Malone & Hinman, 2007; Orenstein & Hinman, 1999).

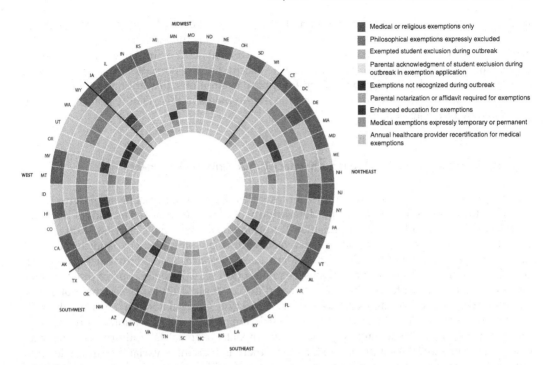

**FIGURE 6.4** Polar graph illustrating state school vaccination exemptions law.

*Source*:  Centers for Disease Control and Prevention. (2017, April 28). *State school and childcare vaccination laws*. https://www.cdc.gov/phlp/publications/topic/vaccinations.html

## Healthcare Facility Vaccination Laws

Some states also require vaccination of employees and patients in healthcare facilities, such as hospitals, long-term care facilities, ambulatory care facilities, and others. States are increasingly requiring healthcare facility employees and patients to have their vaccination status assessed, requiring healthcare facilities to offer specific vaccines, and requiring healthcare facilities to ensure employees or patients are vaccinated against certain VPDs. These laws are disease- and

---

**BOX 6.5** *SPENCE v. SHAH*, 136 A.D.3D 1242, (N.Y. APP. DIV. 2016)

In 2013, the New York Department of Health required that healthcare personnel who had not been vaccinated for influenza wear a surgical mask during influenza season in areas near patients. Four registered nurses and their union challenged the new requirement claiming, in part, that the Department of Health had exceeded its authority and that the requirement was arbitrary. The trial court dismissed the case and the plaintiffs appealed.

The appellate court found that the legislature delegated "broad authority to . . . [the Department of Health] to consider and implement regulations regarding the preservation and improvement of public health, as well as establishing standards in health care facilities that serve to foster the prevention and treatment of human disease" and that the DOH had acted within the scope of its authority. The court did not find that the regulations were arbitrary, but rather that the administrative record demonstrated significant support for the regulation in order to minimize risk of exposure of patients within healthcare facilities to influenza.

facility-specific and sometimes depend on other characteristics, such as age of the patient or employee. For healthcare workers, the influenza vaccination is the most common requirement across facility types and the most challenged (Bhatti et al., 2017). Similar to vaccination requirements related to school entry, exemptions to vaccination are permitted, vary state to state, and can include medical, religious, and philosophical exemptions. In addition to state requirements, facilities may impose additional vaccine requirements in their facility policies but may be limited by union agreements.

## Expanding Vaccine Access Through Pharmacist Authority to Vaccinate

States also determine who may administer vaccines through state **scope of practice** laws (i.e., the state-specific restrictions that determine what tasks healthcare providers may undertake in the course of caring for patients). Traditionally, doctors, physician assistants, nurse practitioners, and nurses can all administer vaccinations, but states may expand the scope of practice for nontraditional healthcare providers, such as pharmacists, to increase patient access to vaccination. There has been widespread adoption of expanded scope of practice laws permitting pharmacists to administer vaccines (Barraza et al., 2017). An assessment of policy changes from 1971 to 2016 showed a total of 627 legislative or regulatory changes, of which 83 resulted in an expansion of practice, three a restriction, and 22 a clarification to a regulation; the remaining did not substantively change or impact pharmacists' authority to vaccinate (Schmit & Penn, 2017). As with other state laws, there is incredible variability in the level of authority pharmacists have, what vaccines they can provide, and to which patients (Barraza et al., 2017).

Expanding patient access to vaccination services through healthcare providers such as pharmacists is critical in rural communities and underserved areas that are sometimes referred to as "medical deserts." In some of these communities, there may be only one primary care provider, and possibly no specialists such as a pediatrician. These communities often experience increased health disparities in comparison to those living in more urban environments (Vanderbilt et al., 2015). One study found that the main barrier to parents in rural Georgia having their children vaccinated against HPV was access to a primary care provider, not vaccine hesitancy. Study respondents "lived in a county with no pediatricians accepting new Medicaid patients and less than one family/general practitioner for every 2,000 residents" (Thomas et al., 2014, at 4). Pharmacists can help to address health disparities by being another access point to vaccination services in communities with limited resources.

## Immunization Information Systems

Immunization information systems (IIS), often referred to as "vaccine registries," are "confidential, population-based, computerized databases that record all vaccine doses administered by participating providers to persons residing within a given geopolitical area," (CDC, 2019d). IIS support vaccination at the point of clinical care by allowing healthcare providers to determine vaccination status of their patients and record vaccinations. IIS are also important at the community level to better understand coverage rates and gaps in the vaccination in the community. The legal framework that supports an IIS is comprised of state and federal policies. Because of this, it is incredibly complex and, in some cases, can pose a barrier to efficient exchange of intrastate and interstate information (Martin et al. 2015).

Privacy, confidentiality, and security of information are important components of IIS, which are established by state laws. A 2011 study related to IIS determined that 66% of states had laws specifically authorizing IIS operation (Martin et al., 2015). While there is tremendous variability in these state laws, they generally include:

- who must report (all vaccine providers, specific provider types),
- whose data is collected (all patients or children under age 18),
- consent (all patients opt in to participate, or all patients are automatically included and opt out to decline participation),
- data sharing (intrastate and interstate sharing),
- what the data can be used for, and
- data retention (how long data is stored in the IIS).

Federal laws such as the Health Insurance Portability and Accountability Act of 1996 (HIPAA) Privacy Rule and the Family Educational Rights and Privacy Act of 1974 (FERPA) interplay with state IIS operation (Martin et al., 2015). The HIPAA is a federal law that protects privacy. IIS must comply with the HIPAA, but reporting of immunizations to an IIS is exempt from the HIPAA Privacy Rule as a public health activity (45 CFR Parts 160 and 164, Subparts A and E). The FERPA is a federal law that protects the privacy of student education records and limits information sharing by school personnel, such as school nurses (20 U.S.C. § 1232g; 34 CFR 99). While this helps to ensure students' privacy, in some cases the FERPA can be a barrier to health information sharing. Because of school vaccination requirements, school personnel oftentimes have the most up-to-date information regarding a child's vaccination status, but due to the FERPA they are not permitted to enter this information into the state IIS without express written consent from a parent (CDC, 2018a).

Ultimately, there are individual- and community-level benefits to widen use of an IIS; however, the use of an IIS should be balanced with securing individual privacy interests. Policy in these cases can be a lever to develop and maintain an IIS as well as to create a policy framework for optimal use; however, it can also at times pose a barrier to efficient information exchange.

## VACCINE FINANCING AND COVERAGE

### Publicly Insured Children and Adults

Cost varies for vaccines and vaccine administration. Authority to dictate coverage and cost-sharing policies for vaccinations falls to both the federal government and state government depending on how an individual is or is not insured.

The Vaccines for Children Program (VFC) is a federal entitlement program that covers children who qualify for Medicaid and do not have insurance, underinsured children, and American Indian/Alaskan Native children (CDC, 2016a). With funding allocated through the Centers for Medicare & Medicaid Services (CMS), CDC is able to purchase vaccines at a reduced cost for distribution to grantees, such as state health departments (CDC, 2016b). All ACIP-recommended vaccines are covered and provided through the VFC program for children under 19 years of age (CDC, 2016b).

For adults who are insured through Medicaid, which is implemented and operated at the state level, there is more variety in coverage and cost-sharing policies. Most state Medicaid agencies cover at least some adult vaccinations but may not cover all ACIP-recommended vaccines. The Affordable Care Act (ACA) authorized state Medicaid expansion to uninsured adults and children whose incomes are at or below 138% of the federal poverty level (CMS, n.d.-a). Not every state has opted to expand Medicaid. Expansion states are required to cover all ACIP-recommended vaccines with no cost-sharing for adults newly insured under Medicaid expansion. For adults enrolled in Medicaid prior to expansion or in nonexpansion states, vaccine coverage is not guaranteed and cost-sharing may be imposed.

For people like Brenda in Hypothetical Case Study #4 who are 65 or older, Medicare Part B covers annual influenza vaccination and pneumococcal vaccination (CMS, n.d.-b, n.d.-c). Medicare Part B also covers hepatitis B vaccination if the individual is at medium or high risk for hepatitis B; for example, if Medicare recipients have end-stage renal disease, hemophilia, or live in the same household with a hepatitis B carrier (CMS, n.d.-b, n.d.-c). So, it is likely that Brenda's pneumococcal and hepatitis B vaccines will be covered under Medicare. For vaccines covered under Part B, cost-sharing is expressly prohibited (CMS, n.d.-c). Most other vaccines are covered under Medicare Part D if they are commercially available and medically necessary; however, those vaccines are subject to cost-sharing. As such, in Hypothetical Case Study #4, Brenda will probably have to pay out of pocket for the zoster vaccination. Further, if Brenda was not at medium or high risk for hepatitis B, the vaccine would be a Part D benefit and subject to cost-sharing.

Section 317 of the Public Health Service Act is another public funding mechanism for vaccines and programmatic services. Section 317 funds can be used to vaccinate newborns receiving the birth dose of hepatitis B whose bundled insurance plan does not cover it, as well as uninsured or underinsured adults, and fully insured individuals needing vaccines during an outbreak response (CDC, 2016a). Additionally, there are discretionary funds associated with Section 317 that can be used for programmatic services. This funding is meant to serve as a safety net for populations that otherwise could not be vaccinated through other public-financing mechanisms, and as a result is a small funding mechanism compared to others like the VFC entitlement program.

---

**HYPOTHETICAL CASE STUDY #4: VACCINE COVERAGE UNDER MEDICARE**

Brenda is a 68-year-old female who is insured under Medicare. At a routine doctor's visit, her physician recommends the pneumococcal and zoster vaccination. The physician also informs Brenda that, due to her chronic liver disease, hepatitis B vaccination is also recommended. Brenda tells the physician that she is concerned about the out of pocket costs she may have to pay.

1. What is the framework for providing vaccines to publicly insured adults, like Brenda?
2. As Brenda is insured through Medicare, are all of the vaccines that her physician recommended covered?
3. Is it possible that Brenda may still have to pay out of pocket for any of these vaccines? If so, which?

---

## LIFE-COURSE APPROACH TO VACCINATION AND POLICY DEVELOPMENT

This chapter has presented many notable ways in which policy can impact vaccination and demonstrated how these different policies are tailored to specific population groups based on situation and need. Incorporating a life-course approach to vaccination policy development is vital. The life-course approach highlights the importance of access to healthcare services, including vaccination, during critical periods of the life span, as this can impact health trajectories. The United States is currently facing shifting demographics, such as an increasing percentage of an older adult population and a re-emergence of certain VPDs. There has been a shift to prioritize prevention in the healthcare industry (Philip et al., 2018). As a result, prioritizing vaccination efforts through the life course is important. This requires tailoring policies to specific populations based on age, health condition, or lifestyle to ensure that the maximum benefit is derived from vaccination.

For example, one's employment may place a person at higher risk of exposure to a vaccine-preventable disease, such as a healthcare worker or someone who works in a tattoo or piercing establishment. In those cases, there are federal and state laws that require individuals in different places of employment to be vaccinated against specific VPDs, such as flu vaccination requirements at the state level or the OSHA hepatitis B vaccination requirements at the federal level (Bhatti et al., 2017; U.S. Department of Labor, n.d.). Additionally, one can see aspects of the life course approach reflected in the ACIP recommended vaccination schedule that was discussed earlier in the chapter. The vaccination schedule reflects not just which vaccines are recommended from birth to older adulthood, but also different life stages such as pregnancy, high-risk health conditions, employment type, and travel (CDC, 2019b).

## CONCLUSION

Vaccination is considered one of the greatest public health achievements of the 20th century (CDC, 1999). Vaccine initiatives at the federal and state levels work together to support vaccination and vaccination-related services to maximize vaccination rates and ensure safety and efficacy. Law is a critical tool in vaccination, establishing the source and scope of authority for vaccination efforts at the federal and state levels and the limits of this authority when balancing individual liberty against the public's health.

## CHAPTER REVIEW

### Discussion Questions

1. How has the ACA impacted access to vaccines?
2. What is your response to a parent who says, "Why would my unvaccinated child be a threat to others if vaccines work?"
3. Many people still believe that thimerosal, a mercury-containing preservative, causes autism, even though extensive research has found no association. Beginning in 1999 and ending in 2003, the FDA phased out thimerosal from childhood vaccines in the United States (multi-dose influenza vaccines do contain thimerosal). Thimerosal is used in over 120 countries in vaccines protecting against four deadly diseases: diphtheria, tetanus, pertussis, and Hib. Thimerosal helps to stabilize multidose vaccines, which are more efficient and cost-effective than single-dose vaccines when reaching more remote locations or larger numbers of people quickly (World Health Organization [WHO], 2011). While the WHO states that thimerosal is not a concern, some people have questioned the use of vaccines (or any other medical treatments) in developing countries that are not approved in the United States for possible safety reasons. Discuss the ethical implications.
4. What legal recourse exists for potential vaccine injuries? How is this limited?
5. Why do you think the power to regulate interstate commerce and the power to tax and spend are the appropriate legal authority for vaccination efforts at the federal level?
6. What factors do you think should be considered when balancing individual freedoms against the public's health when mandating vaccines? Do you think this should change if there is a threat or current outbreak in the community?
7. A few states (currently WV, MS, CA, NY, ME, and CT) restrict vaccination exemptions only to students with medical contraindications. Discuss whether it is coercive to require vaccination mandates upon school entry with no religious or philosophical exemptions and to exclude unvaccinated students from attending school.
8. What important federal privacy acts limit sharing vaccine information? How?

9.  Should declining to vaccinate a child be considered "neglect" in juvenile dependency (child welfare) cases? Consider both pros and cons.

10. How should courts decide when divorced parents disagree over whether to vaccinate a child?

11. Assume a parent chooses not to vaccinate their otherwise healthy child and their child later contracts a vaccine-preventable disease and spreads it to a child who medically could not be vaccinated and for whom the disease is life-threatening. Should the parent be held civilly, or even criminally, responsible? Consider both pros and cons.

12. Vaccination for human papillomavirus (HPV) prevents against common strains of the virus transmitted through vaginal, anal, or oral sex. While some HPV infections go away on their own, HPV infections can cause cancer, including cancers of the cervix, vagina, and vulva in women, penis in men, and anus and throat in both men and women. Some parents have been resistant to the HPV vaccine. Which states require HPV vaccination for school attendance? Is there a difference between requiring other vaccinations for school attendance and requiring the HPV vaccination? What arguments have been made against requiring HPV for school attendance? How can public health address these concerns?

## Essay Questions

1.  This chapter outlines many different federal and state vaccine policies that work together to maintain herd immunity thresholds and prevent spread of vaccine-preventable disease, such as vaccine development and approval, school vaccination mandates, public or private insurance coverage, and adverse event reporting. Consider the consequences if one of these components were not present. How would vaccination rates and herd immunity thresholds potentially be impacted?

2.  What is the general framework for school vaccination laws (statutes and regulations) in your state? What vaccinations are required and when? All states have medical exemptions. What are the requirements for parents or guardians seeking a medical vaccine exemption for their child? Does your state have religious and/or philosophical exemptions? If yes, what are the requirements for parents or guardians seeking an exemption? Can a child with an exemption be excluded from school during an outbreak? What changes to your state law, if any, would you recommend?

3.  Describe what is meant by "life course vaccination." What is the importance of vaccination throughout an individual's lifetime?

4.  This chapter focuses on vaccination policy generally throughout the life course. Vaccinations may be needed in response to an outbreak, such as COVID-19 pandemic currently occurring at the time of publication of this chapter. Vaccination policies during an emergency may differ. Federal vaccine development and approval may have fast-tracked processes. States may have expanded vaccination authority during an emergency. Questions may be answered differently during an emergency. Who will pay for vaccines? How will vaccines be allocated if there are limited quantities available? What additional liability protections are in place for manufacturers, distributors, and administrators of the vaccine? Who is authorized to administer vaccinations (i.e., doctors, nurses, pharmacists, veterinarians, others)? How shall suspected vaccine injuries be tracked and compensated? Can vaccination be mandated during an emergency, and, if an individual declines, can they be restricted from entering certain places while the outbreak is still occuring? Examine a legal issue related to vaccination and compare/contrast how it may be addressed generally versus in an emergency such as COVID-19. What factors should be considered and which stakeholders would be important to include in the discussion?

## Internet Activities

1. Refer to the current ACIP vaccination recommendations at https://www.cdc.gov/vaccines/schedules/hcp/imz/child-adolescent.html to answer the following:
   a. Baby Gabriella has a 2-month well-visit check with the pediatrician. What vaccinations can her parents expect her to receive?
   b. Toddler Jacob is at his 15-month well-visit at the pediatrician. Assuming his vaccinations are up-to-date, which dosage of DTaP will he be receiving at this visit?
   c. Amari is five and starting kindergarten. His pediatrician says he needs several vaccinations at this well-visit. Assuming he is on-schedule, is rotavirus one of the vaccines he will receive at this appointment?
   d. Fatima is 11 and starting middle school. She has not had all of her vaccines and her new pediatrician plans to use the catch-up schedule. If Fatima receives the first dose of varicella vaccine at this appointment, will she need to return for another dose? If yes, when?
   e. Jaden is 13 and allergic to eggs. He has experienced anaphylaxis. Can he receive the influenza vaccination? If yes, under what circumstances?
2. Why is herd immunity important? Watch this video to better understand this important concept: https://www.vaccinestoday.eu/stories/what-is-herd-immunity
3. Visit your state's health department website. Which of the child/adolescent vaccines recommended by the ACIP are required in your state? Ahead of what grade must a child generally receive these for school attendance?
4. Research what vaccination exemptions are authorized in your state. All states have medical exemptions. What are the requirements for parents or guardians seeking a medical vaccine exemption for their child? Does your state have religious and/or philosophical exemptions? If yes, what are the requirements for parents or guardians seeking an exemption?
5. Using the Vaccine Injury table at https://www.hrsa.gov/sites/default/files/hrsa/vaccine-compensation/vaccine-injury-table.pdf might the following injuries, after review and analysis, if exceeding $1000, be compensated?
   a. Anaphylaxis two hours after MMR vaccination
   b. Shoulder injury one week after Hep B vaccination
   c. Guillain-Barre Syndrome one day after seasonal influenza vaccine
   d. Encephalitis 48 hours after pertussis vaccination
6. Review the data and statistics reported on the VICP at this site: https://www.hrsa.gov/vaccine-compensation/data/index.html. What is wrong with each of the following statements?
   a. "I received an award from the VICP for my injury since the government knows DTaP is dangerous!"
   b. "I never get a seasonal flu shot because the influenza vaccine is the most dangerous of all vaccinations! You can tell because the highest number of claims are filed for the influenza vaccine."
7. Learn more about the history of New York vaccination efforts and the measles outbreak of 2018 to 2019 by reading this article:
   - Paumgarten, N. (2019, August 26). The message of measles. *The New Yorker* https://www.newyorker.com/magazine/2019/09/02/the-message-of-measles

## REFERENCES

29 CFR 1910.1030(f)(2)(i).
29 CFR 1910.1030(f)(1)(ii)(a) and (b).
Bancsi, A., Houle, S., & Grindrod, K. A. (2019). Shoulder injury related to vaccine administration and other injection site events. *Canadian Family Physician*, 65(1), 40–42. https://www.ncbi.nlm.nih.gov/pmc/articles/PMC6347325/

Barraza, L., Schmit, C., & Hoss, A. (2017). The latest in vaccine policies: Selected issues in school vaccinations, healthcare worker vaccinations, and pharmacist vaccination authority laws. *The Journal of Law, Medicine and Ethics, 45*(1_Suppl), 16–19. https://doi.org/10.1177/1073110517 703307

Bhatti, A., Hoss, A., Pepin, D., & Black, J. (2017, October). *Menu of State Hospital influenza vaccination laws.* Centers for Disease Control and Prevention Public Health Law Program. https://www .cdc.gov/phlp/docs/menu-shfluvacclaws.pdf

Blank, N., Caplan, A., & Constable, C. (2013). Exempting schoolchildren from immunizations: States with few barriers had highest rates of NMVEs. *Health Affairs, 32*(7), 1282–1290. https://doi .org/10.1377/hlthaff.2013.0239

Burns, J. F. (2010, May 24). British Medical Council bars doctor who linked vaccine with autism. *New York Times.* https://www.nytimes.com/2010/05/25/health/policy/25autism.html

Centers for Disease Control and Prevention. (1999, April 2). Ten great public health achievements. *Morbidity and Mortality Weekly Report, 48*(12), 241–243. https://www.cdc.gov/mmwr/PDF/wk/ mm4812.pdf

Centers for Disease Control and Prevention. (2000, May 19). Poliomyelitis prevention in the United States: Updated Recommendations of the Advisory Committee on Immunization Practices (ACIP). *Morbidity and Mortality Weekly Report, 49*(RR05), 1–22. https://www.cdc.gov/mmwr/ preview/mmwrhtml/rr4905a1.htm

Centers for Disease Control and Prevention. (2015). Measles. *Epidemiology and Prevention of Vaccine-Preventable Diseases, The Pink Book: Course Textbook – 13th Edition.* https://www.cdc.gov/vaccines/ pubs/pinkbook/meas.html

Centers for Disease Control and Prevention. (2016a, February 17). *Questions on vaccines purchased with 317 funds.* https://www.cdc.gov/vaccines/imz-managers/guides-pubs/qa-317-funds.html

Centers for Disease Control and Prevention. (2016b, February 18). *Vaccines for children program (VFC): About the program.* https://www.cdc.gov/vaccines/programs/vfc/about/index.html

Centers for Disease Control and Prevention. (2017, April 28). *State school and childcare vaccination laws.* https://www.cdc.gov/phlp/publications/topic/vaccinations.html

Centers for Disease Control and Prevention. (2018a, February 14). *Health information & privacy.* https://www.cdc.gov/phlp/publications/topic/healthinformationprivacy.html

Centers for Disease Control and Prevention. (2018b, June 5). *Advisory Committee on Immunization Practices (ACIP) charter.* https://www.cdc.gov/vaccines/acip/committee/charter.html

Centers for Disease Control and Prevention. (2018c, December 10). *ACIP current membership roster.* https://www.cdc.gov/vaccines/acip/members/index.html

Centers for Disease Control and Prevention. (2019a). *Comparison of 20th century annual morbidity and current morbidity: Vaccine preventable diseases.* https://www.cdc.gov/vaccines/ed/surv/ downloads/VPD-morbidity-slide1-mmwr-508.pdf

Centers for Disease Control and Prevention. (2019b). *Immunization schedules.* https://www.cdc.gov /vaccines/schedules/index.html

Centers for Disease Control and Prevention. (2019c). *Measles cases and outbreaks.* https://www.cdc .gov/measles/cases-outbreaks.html

Centers for Disease Control and Prevention. (2019d, June). *Immunization information systems (IIS): About immunization information systems.* https://www.cdc.gov/vaccines/programs/iis/about.html

Centers for Disease Control and Prevention. (2019e, September 17). *Mumps cases and outbreaks.* https://www.cdc.gov/mumps/outbreaks.html

Centers for Disease Control and Prevention. (2019f, September 30). *Widespread person-to-person outbreaks of hepatitis A across the United States.* https://www.cdc.gov/hepatitis/outbreaks/2017March -HepatitisA.htm

Centers for Disease Control and Prevention. (2019g, October). *Vaccinate with confidence.* https://www .cdc.gov/vaccines/partners/vaccinate-with-confidence.html

Centers for Disease Control and Prevention. (2020). *Recommended child and adolescent immunization schedule, United States, 2020.* https://www.cdc.gov/vaccines/schedules/downloads/child/ 0-18yrs-child-combined-schedule.pdf

Centers for Medicare & Medicaid Services. (n.d.-a). *How Medicaid health care expansion affects you.* https://www.healthcare.gov/medicaid-chip/medicaid-expansion-and-you

Centers for Medicare & Medicaid Services. (n.d.-b). *Preventive services.* https://www.medicare.gov/coverage/preventive-screening-services

Centers for Medicare & Medicaid Services. (n.d.-c). *What's Medicare?* https://www.medicare.gov/what-medicare-covers/your-medicare-coverage-choices/whats-medicare

ChangeLab Solutions. (2013). *Preemption and public health advocacy: A frequent concern with far-reaching consequences.* http://www.changelabsolutions.org/sites/default/files/Preemption_PublicHealthAdvocacy_FS_FINAL_20130911.pdf

Dubé, E., Laberge, C., Guay, M., Bramadat, P., Roy, R., & Bettinger, J. (2013). Vaccine hesitancy: An overview. *Human Vaccines and Immunotherapeutics, 9*(8), 1763–1773. https://doi.org/10.4161/hv.24657

Feemster, K. A. (2018). *Vaccines: What everyone needs to know.* Oxford University Press.

Fenner, F., Henderson, D. A., Arita, I., Zdenek, J., & Ivan, L. D. (1988). *Smallpox and its eradication.* World Health Organization. https://apps.who.int/iris/handle/10665/39485

The Food, Drug, and Cosmetic Act of 1938. 21 U.S.C. ch. 9 § 301 et. seq. (1938).

Glatman-Freedman, A., & Nichols, K. (2012). The effect of social determinants on immunization programs. *Human Vaccines and Immunotherapeutics, 8*(7), 916–920. https://doi.org/10.4161/hv.20122

Godlee, F., Smith, J., & Marcovitch, H. (2011). Wakefield's article linking MMR vaccine and autism was fraudulent. *British Medical Journal, 342*(1), c7452–c7452. https://doi.org/10.1136/bmj.c7452

Greenwood, B. (2014). The contribution of vaccination to global health: Past, present and future. *Philosophical Transactions of the Royal Society B: Biological Sciences, 369*(1645), 20130433. https://doi.org/10.1098/rstb.2013.0433

*Jacobson v. Massachusetts,* 197 U.S. 11 (1905).

Health Resources & Services Administration. (2019a, June). *About the national vaccine injury compensation program.* https://www.hrsa.gov/vaccine-compensation/about/index.html

Health Resources & Services Administration. (2019b, June). *National vaccine injury compensation program.* https://www.hrsa.gov/vaccine-compensation/index.html

Health Resources & Services Administration. (2019c, September). *Data & statistics.* https://www.hrsa.gov/sites/default/files/hrsa/vaccine-compensation/data/data-statistics-september-2019.pdf

Heleft, L., & Willingham, E. (2014, September 5). *What is herd immunity?* https://www.pbs.org/wgbh/nova/article/herd-immunity

Institute of Medicine. (2004). *Immunization safety review: Vaccines and autism.* The National Academies Press. https://doi.org/10.17226/10997

Lieu, T. A., Ray, G. T., Klein, N. P., Chung, C., & Kulldorff, M. (2015). Geographic clusters in underimmunization and vaccine refusal. *Pediatrics, 135*(2), 280–289. https://doi.org/10.1542/peds.2014-2715

Malone, K. M., & Hinman, A. R. (2007). Vaccination mandates: The public health imperative and individual rights. In R. A. Goodman, R. E. Hoffman, W. Lopez, G. W. Matthews, M. A. Rothstein, & K. L. Foster (Eds.), *Law in public health practice* (pp. 338–360). Oxford University Press.

Martin, D. W., Lowery, N. E., Brand, B., Gold, R., & Horlick, G. (2015, June). Immunization information systems. *Journal of Public Health Management and Practice, 21*(3), 296–303. https://doi.org/10.1097/phh.0000000000000040

McKee, C., & Bohannon, K. (2016). Exploring the reasons behind parental refusal of vaccines. *The Journal of Pediatric Pharmacology and Therapeutics, 21*(2), 104–109. https://doi.org/10.5863/1551-6776-21.2.104

Metcalf, C., Ferrari, M., Graham, A., & Grenfell, B. (2015). Understanding herd immunity. *Trends in Immunology, 36*(12), 753–755. https://doi.org/10.1016/j.it.2015.10.004

Moulton, A. D., Goodman, R. A., & Parmet, W. E. (2007). Perspective: Law and great public health achievements. In R. A. Goodman, R. E. Hoffman, W. Lopez, G. W. Matthews, M. A. Rothstein, & K. L. Foster (Eds.), *Law in public health practice* (pp. 3–21). Oxford University Press.

National Conference of State Legislatures. (2019, June 14). *States with religious and philosophical exemptions from school immunization requirements.* http://www.ncsl.org/research/health/school-immunization-exemption-state-laws.aspx

National Childhood Vaccine Injury Act of 1986, U.S.C.A.§ §300aa-1 through -34 (1986).

Occupational Safety and Health Administration. (n.d.). *Frequently asked questions.* https://www.osha.gov/dcsp/osp/frequently_asked_questions.html

Office of Infectious Disease and HIV/AIDS Policy (OIDP). Vaccines National Strategic Plan. HHS. Gov, 13 May 2021, www.hhs.gov/vaccines/vaccines-national-strategic-plan/index.html

Omer, S. B., Richards, J. L., Ward, M., & Bednarczyk, R. A. (2012). Vaccination policies and rates of exemption from immunization, 2005–2011. *New England Journal of Medicine, 367*(12), 1170–1171. https://doi.org/10.1056/nejmc1209037

Open Clipart. (n.d.). *Scale.* https://openclipart.org/detail/286612/scale

Orenstein, W. A., & HInman, A. R. (1999). The immunization system in the United States: The role of school immunization laws. *Vaccine, 17*(Suppl. 3), S19–S24. https://doi.org/10.1016/s0264-410x(99)00290-x

Parasidis, E. (2017). Recalibrating vaccination law. *Boston University Law Review, 97*, 2153–2241. http://www.bu.edu/bulawreview/files/2018/01/PARASIDIS.pdf

Philip, R. K., Attwell, K., Breuer, T., Pasquale, A. D., & Lopalco, P. L. (2018). Life-course immunization as a gateway to health. *Expert Review of Vaccines, 17*(10), 851–864. https://doi.org/10.1080/14760584.2018.1527690

*Prince v. Massachusetts,* 321 U.S. 158 (1944).

Public Health Service Act of 1944, 42 U.S.C. §217a (1944).

Ransom, M. M. (2016, April). Public *Health Law Competency Model: Version 1.0.* Centers for Disease Control and Prevention Public Health Law Program. https://www.cdc.gov/phlp/docs/phlcm-v1.pdf

Riedel, S. (2005). Edward Jenner and the history of smallpox and vaccination. *Proceedings (Baylor University Medical Center), 18*(1), 21–25. https://doi.org/10.1080/08998280.2005.11928028

Salmon, D. A., Omer, S. B., Moulton, L. H., Stokley, S., deHart, M. P., Lett, S., Norman, B., Teret, S., & Halsey, N. A. (2005). Exemptions to school immunization requirements: The role of school-level requirements, policies, and procedures. *American Journal of Public Health, 95*(3), 436–440. https://doi.org/10.2105/ajph.2004.046201

Schmit, C. D., & Penn, M. S. (2017). Expanding state laws and a growing role for pharmacists in vaccination services. *Journal of the American Pharmacists Association, 57*(6), 661–669. https://doi.org/10.1016/j.japh.2017.07.001

Thomas, T. L., DiClemente, R., & Snell, S. (2014). Overcoming the triad of rural health disparities: How local culture, lack of economic opportunity, and geographic location instigate health disparities. *Health Education Journal, 73*(3), 285–294. https://doi.org/10.1177/0017896912471049

*U.S. v. Shinnick,* 219 F. Supp. 789 (E.D.N.Y. 1963).

U.S. Court of Federal Claims. (n.d.). *Vaccine claims/Office of Special Masters.* http://www.uscfc.uscourts.gov/vaccine-program-readmore

U.S. Court of Federal Claims, Office of Special Masters. (2010). *The autism proceedings.* https://www.uscfc.uscourts.gov/sites/default/files/vaccine_files/autism.background.2010.pdf

U.S. Department of Health and Human Services. (2010). *2010 National vaccine plan: Protecting the nation's health through immunization.* https://www.hhs.gov/sites/default/files/nvpo/vacc_plan/2010-Plan/nationalvaccineplan.pdf

U.S. Department of Labor. (n.d.). *About OSHA.* https://www.osha.gov/aboutosha

U.S. Food and Drug Association Center for Biologics Evaluation and Research. (2018, January 30). *Vaccines product approval process.* https://www.fda.gov/vaccines-blood-biologics/development-approval-process-cber/vaccine-product-approval-process

Vaccine Adverse Event Reporting System. (n.d.-a). *About VAERS.* https://vaers.hhs.gov/about.html

Vaccine Adverse Event Reporting System. (n.d.-b). *Frequently asked questions.* https://vaers.hhs.gov/faq.html

Vanderbilt, A. A., Dail, M. D., & Jaberi, P. (2015). Reducing health disparities in underserved communities via interprofessional collaboration across health care professions. *Journal of Multidisciplinary Healthcare, 8*, 205–208. https://doi.org/10.2147/JMDH.S74129

World Health Organization. (2011, October). *Thiomersal—Questions and answers.* https://www.who.int/immunization/newsroom/thiomersal_questions_and_answers/en

World Health Organization Regional Office for Europe. (2016, August 4). *Poliomyelitis (polio) and the vaccines used to eradicate it—Questions and answers.* https://www.euro.who.int/en/health-topics/communicable-diseases/poliomyelitis/news/news/2016/04/poliomyelitis-polio-and-the-vaccines-used-to-eradicate-it-questions-and-answers

Yang, Y. T., & Silverman, R. D. (2015). Legislative prescriptions for controlling nonmedical vaccine exemptions. *Journal of the American Medical Association, 313*(3), 247–248. https://doi.org/10.1001/jama.2014.16286

*Zucht v. King,* 43 S.Ct. 24 (1922)

# 7

# Infectious Disease Prevention and Control

## Legal Frameworks

Tina Batra Hershey and Alexandra Bhatti

## Learning Objectives

By the end of this chapter, the reader will be able to:

- Identify the legal authorities enabling and limiting the three major components of infectious disease prevention and control.
- Assess constitutional considerations when making decisions related to isolation and quarantine.

## Key Terminology

**Cordon sanitaire:** the restriction of movement of people into or out of a defined geographic area.

**Disease reporting:** an ongoing and systematic collection of health data specifically related to incidence of infectious diseases; is accomplished by state, Tribal, local, and territorial public health agencies employing mandatory notification requirements when a disease case of public health concern is identified.

**Due process:** fair treatment through the normal judicial system, especially as a citizen's entitlement.

**Equal protection:** refers to the idea that a governmental body may not deny people equal protection of its governing laws; the governing body state must treat an individual in the same manner as others in similar conditions and circumstances.

**Isolation:** separates a person or group of persons known to be contagious with a communicable disease from others who are not sick to prevent disease transmission.

**Nonpharmaceutical interventions (NPIs):** actions, apart from getting vaccinated and taking medicine, people and communities can take to help slow the spread of illnesses like pandemic influenza; also referred to as "community mitigation measures".

**Public health surveillance:** "the ongoing, systematic collection, analysis, and interpretation of health data, essential to the planning, implementation and evaluation of public health practice, closely integrated with the dissemination of these data to those who need to know and linked to prevention and control" (Thacker, 1992).

**Quarantine:** separates and restricts the movement of a person or group of persons who were exposed to a contagious disease to see if they become sick.

**Social distancing measures:** nonpharmaceutical interventions to prevent or slow the spread of communicable disease by restricting when, where, and how people gather together.

## Public Health Law Competencies

This chapter addresses the following competencies from the Public Health Law Competency Model (PHLCM; Ransom, 2016).

1.1  Define basic constitutional concepts and legal principles framing the practice of public health across relevant jurisdictions.

2.2  Identify law-based tools and enforcement procedures available to address day-to-day (nonemergency) public health issues.

---

### Spark Question

How has law been used to protect your community from infectious disease? For example, what laws did your local jurisdiction have in place to address the spread of COVID-19?

---

## INTRODUCTION

**Public health surveillance** is "the ongoing, systematic collection, analysis, and interpretation of health data, essential to the planning, implementation and evaluation of public health practice, closely integrated with the dissemination of these data to those who need to know and linked to prevention and control" (Thacker, 1992). Public health surveillance is a critical tool to support early detection of public health threats, like COVID-19, understand the epidemiology of public health issues, monitor the effectiveness of public health interventions, and inform public health policy and programs (World Health Organization [WHO], n.d.-a). Falling within the principles of public health surveillance, the goals of infectious disease surveillance are "(1) to describe the current burden and epidemiology of disease, (2) to monitor trends, and (3) to identify outbreaks and new pathogens" (Murray & Cohen, 2017 p. 222). Effective surveillance requires a cross-sector approach including healthcare professionals, public and private laboratories, local and state health departments, and public health officials from many governmental agencies and departments.

Primary authority for public health interventions to prevent and control infectious diseases lies with states as a function of their "police powers" provided by the 10th Amendment to the U.S. Constitution (U.S. Const. amend. X). This authority includes the ability to conduct infectious **disease reporting**, investigation, and control activities. "Disease reporting," the collection and appropriate dissemination of data related to the incidence of infectious diseases, occurs as a result of the infectious disease surveillance. Surveillance enables public health agencies to collect and assess data to take necessary action.

State, local, and territorial public health agencies implement mandatory reporting requirements for specific infectious diseases of public health concern such as *Zika* and *E. coli*. Mandatory reporting to public health agencies is essential in facilitating the identification of *clusters* and other indicators of potential disease outbreaks. The term "cluster" means, ". . . an unusual aggregation, real or perceived, of health events that are grouped together in time and space and that are reported to a health agency." Once reported, public health professionals within the

## BOX 7.1  HIPAA'S PUBLIC HEALTH ACTIVITIES EXCEPTION

The Health Insurance Portability and Accountability Act of 1996 (HIPAA) is a federal law that required the creation of national standards to protect sensitive patient health information. As a result, the Department of Health and Human Services (DHHS) issued the Privacy Rule to implement HIPAA requirements. The Privacy Rule sets standards for the use and disclosure of individuals' health information known as "protected health information" (PHI). A covered entity (i.e., healthcare provider, health plan, healthcare clearinghouse) can only use or disclose PHI for limited purposes unless the individual authorizes the use or disclosure (45 CFR § 164.502). PHI disclosure by a covered entity to a public health authority is permitted, however, "for the purpose of **preventing or controlling disease**, injury, or disability, including, but not limited to, the **reporting of disease**, injury, vital events such as birth or death, and the conduct of public health **surveillance**, public health **investigations**, and public health **interventions**." (45 CFR § 164.512). "A 'public health authority' is an agency or authority of the United States government, a State, a territory, a political subdivision of a State or territory, or Indian Tribe that is responsible for public health matters as part of its official mandate, as well as a person or entity acting under a grant of authority from, or under a contract with, a public health agency" (45 CFR § 164.501). State and local laws may still protect the information and limit the amount of information a public health practitioner can access - even if the Privacy Rule does not expressly prohibit or limit it.

public health agency are responsible for determining whether an *investigation* will be conducted to identify the source and determine the scope of any potential outbreak. During the COVID-19 pandemic, states implemented mandatory reporting requirements for positive, negative, and indeterminate COVID-19 laboratory results within 24 hours. For a discussion of public health agencies' disease reporting, investigation, and control activities in relation to the HIPAA Privacy Rule, see Box 7.1.

State authority reserved by the 10th Amendment also includes the ability to use **nonpharmaceutical interventions** like **social distancing measures** to prevent the spread of communicable disease by restricting when, where, and how people travel and gather together to prevent or slow the spread of infectious diseases (Qualls et al., 2017). Such measures can include limiting large groups of people from getting together (e.g., canceling sporting and social events, closing buildings such as shopping malls or churches, imposing curfews). **Isolation** separates a person or group of persons known to be contagious with a communicable disease from others who are not sick to prevent disease transmission (Centers for Disease Control and Prevention [CDC], 2014). **Quarantine** separates and restricts the movement of a person or group of persons who were exposed to a contagious disease to see if they become sick (CDC, 2014). Social distancing measures are used when other interventions are unavailable or ineffective; however, such measures are not without controversy, as they infringe upon individual liberties (i.e., freedom of movement, bodily integrity, the right to assembly, privacy) that are provided under the U.S. Constitution.

## HYPOTHETICAL CASE STUDY #1: DISEASE REPORTING

Lynnette, aged 64 years, visited her healthcare provider as she was experiencing a low-grade fever, cough, and stuffy nose for about a day. Based on her symptoms, the provider orders a COVID-19 test via nasopharyngeal swab. Results confirm the patient has an active COVID-19 infection. The provider checks the list of reportable diseases but does not see COVID specifically listed.

- What is the legal framework for reporting cases of infectious diseases to public health agencies?
- What specific diseases must be reported under state law?
- Can the federal government require states to report incidence of infectious disease to CDC?

## Legal Framework: State and Federal Authority to Require Reporting

State and local health agencies are typically charged with the duty of protecting the public's health. Disease reporting, investigation, control, and prevention are generally included among the list of authorized activities. This is generally authorized through a jurisdiction's enabling statutes and regulations. A jurisdiction's authority to conduct surveillance through required disease reporting is not disputed (Gostin et al., 1999). All 50 states, the District of Columbia, the U.S. Virgin Islands, the Commonwealth of Puerto Rico, the Territory of Guam, and some Tribal jurisdictions have laws that authorize state or local health agencies to collect public health surveillance information and require healthcare providers, facilities, laboratories, and others to report suspected or confirmed cases of specified infectious diseases to the state or local health agency (Roush et al., 1999). There are approximately 3,000 public health departments that gather and report disease data to protect their local communities. Jurisdictional law established the details of reporting requirements, including which diseases and conditions must be reported, timelines and format for reporting, as well as the information that must be reported.

The specific diseases that must be reported vary by jurisdiction. Every jurisdiction has a list of reportable diseases that is updated periodically and provided to the public via statute, regulation, or health department website. Most jurisdictions' lists also contain generalized language intended to impose a reporting requirement for unanticipated or emerging infectious diseases, such as COVID-19, that arise in a population. For example, a state's list may include a requirement to report "any cluster of illnesses" (Georgia Department of Public Health, 2018); "unusual or increased case incidence of any suspect infectious illness" (Minnesota Department of Health, n.d.); or "any case, cluster of cases, outbreak, or exposure to an infectious or non-infectious disease, condition, or agent ... not listed in this rule that is of urgent public health significance" (Florida Administrative Code Ann. r. 64D-3.029).

In addition to these disease-reporting requirements, the CDC established the National Notifiable Diseases Surveillance System, which collects information on over 120 diseases from state and local health departments for national surveillance (CDC, 2018a). Based on the concept of federalism, the federal government cannot require states to report incidence of infectious diseases to CDC; however, all 50 states, five territories, and two local health departments voluntarily notify CDC about the occurrence of diseases that are reportable in their jurisdictions (CDC, 2018b).

## HYPOTHETICAL CASE STUDY #2: DISEASE INVESTIGATION

States nearby the state of *Elsewhere* have been experiencing ongoing hepatitis A (HepA) outbreaks. Through reporting requirements for HepA, Simone, the Elsewhere state epidemiologist, has identified five recent cases of HepA diagnoses at a small local hospital. Patients had similar geographic and other risk factors, indicating a common source. In furtherance of the investigation, the Elsewhere State Health Department requested that the hospital give them access to all patient electronic medical records (EMRs) to look for anyone suspected to be exposed or be a source. After the State of Elsewhere's public health investigators were on site for approximately two months, one of the patients stated he refused to allow the agency's investigators to access his personal health information, citing it was a violation of his privacy.

- What authority does the public health department have to investigate the outbreak?
- What authority does the public health department have to inspect medical records without patient consent?
- Does state or federal law determine a limit or standard for information that must be disclosed to the public health department?

## Legal Framework: State Authority to Investigate

Once a case of a reportable infectious disease is reported to the state or local health department, state laws require the agency investigate to assess and understand the scope of the potential public health threat to the community. Typically, the state's health agency outlines its investigation authorities and procedures in its rules and regulations. The law may authorize a public health investigator to collect information from affected individuals, their close contacts, and others who may have been exposed or who may have information relevant to the investigation (e.g., Alabama Code §420-4-1-.04). The law may also identify activities the department of health may take in conducting the investigation, including activities such as accessing medical records; conducting surveys and interviews of the public, relevant healthcare providers, and infected individuals and their contacts; and collecting biological samples from infected and potentially infected individuals (e.g., New Hampshire Code Admin. R. He-P 301.07). Because such procedures may involve the collection of individually identifiable health information, many jurisdictions' laws include a requirement to keep investigation information confidential (e.g., Alabama Code §420-4-1-.04).

Tensions often arise during public health investigations regarding the need to access records containing individually identifiable health information versus a covered entity's obligation to protect patient information under state and federal law. In addition to the HIPAA Privacy Rule requirements described in Box 7.1, HIPAA also requires covered entities to limit their disclosure of protected information to the minimum necessary amount needed to achieve the public health activity goals (45 CFR § 164.514). The HIPAA does determine a limit or standard for information that must be disclosed to a public health department, and provides that hospitals and other covered entities may reasonably rely on the assurances of the public health authority accessing protected information that the information requested is the minimum necessary to achieve its public health activity goal (45 CFR § 164.514).

---

### HYPOTHETICAL CASE STUDY #3: ISOLATION AND QUARANTINE

Joe, aged 28 and homeless, admitted himself to the hospital, complaining of coughing up blood. After conducting several tests, including a chest x-ray and sputum samples, a hospital physician diagnosed Joe with active tuberculosis (TB). Treatment was immediately started, and Joe received counseling on the nature, treatment, and transmission of TB. Ten days later, before his TB treatment was complete, Joe announced he was leaving the hospital. He also, for the first time, informed the physicians he had been diagnosed with TB five years prior but had refused treatment. As the hospital was concerned that Joe was still contagious and could infect others in the community with TB, the hospital contacted the local health department.

- What is the legal framework for addressing this threat to public health?
- Can Joe be isolated or quarantined?
- If Joe is isolated or quarantined, where should he be detained?
- If Joe is noncompliant, what steps can the health department take to protect the public's health?
- What due process protections are available to Joe?

## Legal Framework: State Authority to Isolate and Quarantine

The authority of states to isolate and quarantine is well-established in the United States (Parmet, 1993; Rothstein, 2015). Indeed, quarantine has been used for centuries to protect public health (Parmet, 1985). Several states passed their first quarantine laws in the 18th century (*Gibbons v. Ogden*, 1824) due to outbreaks from diseases such as smallpox, cholera, typhoid, and bubonic plague (Tyson, 2004). In *Compagnie Francaise de Navigation a Vapeur v. Louisiana State Board of Health* (1902), the U.S. Supreme Court addressed the issue of whether a public health board, with authority delegated from the state, could prohibit a ship from landing in a city or town under quarantine for communicable disease. The Court upheld the power of the state to enact laws delegating its quarantine police power to municipalities to protect public health (*Compagnie Francaise de Navigation a Vapeur v. Louisiana State Board of Health*, 1902).

The states' police powers were tested in the seminal case, *Jacobson v. Massachusetts* (1905). In the early 20th century, smallpox outbreaks were common; to combat this threat, the state of Massachusetts enacted a law allowing municipal health boards to mandate smallpox vaccination for residents if deemed necessary to protect public health. Under this authority, the Cambridge Board of Health adopted a regulation requiring its inhabitants be vaccinated or pay a five dollar fine. The Reverend Henning Jacobson refused to be vaccinated and was convicted by the trial court and ordered to pay the five dollar fine. The conviction was upheld by the appellate court and Jacobson appealed to the U.S. Supreme Court, claiming a violation of his **due process** and **equal protection** rights under the 14th Amendment. The Supreme Court ruled, in this case, public health was more important than individual rights:

> There is, of course, a sphere within which the individual may assert the supremacy of his own will and rightfully dispute the authority of any human government, especially of any free government existing under a written constitution, to interfere with the exercise of that will. But it is equally true that, in every well ordered society charged with the duty of conserving the safety of its members the rights of the individual in respect of his liberty may at times, under the pressure of great dangers, be subjected to such restraint, to be enforced by reasonable regulations, as the safety of the general public may demand (*Jacobson v. Massachusetts*, 1905, p. 29).

While *Jacobson* (1905) is a case about mandatory vaccination, it articulates the principles and authority behind the basic use of state police power and the deference courts will give to such authority (Gostin, 2005; Hershey et al., 2017; Mariner et al., 2005). First, while states may issue and enforce reasonable regulations to protect the health of a community under their police powers, the community must demonstrate a compelling reason to restrain individual liberties to protect public health. Next, courts will defer to the authority given to public health agencies by legislatures so long as such authority is exercised using sound public health evidence, the authority is not exercised in an arbitrary or capricious manner, and due process and equal protection are provided to affected individuals. Finally, the "least restrictive means necessary to protect public health" must be used (e.g., New Jersey Stat. Ann. 26:13–15).

Isolation and quarantine are used routinely across the United States, particularly for airborne infectious diseases like TB and measles. A variety of factors must be considered before isolation or quarantine is implemented, including the following:

- *Infectious disease in question.* What disease is at issue? Deadly diseases like smallpox or a viral hemorrhagic fever such as Ebola are likely to generate a public health response. Diseases like measles, once thought to be eradicated in the United States, are also likely to elicit a response, as are highly communicable diseases like TB.
- *Mode of transmission.* How is the disease transmitted? Through the air, via bodily fluids, and so forth?
- *Incubation and infectious periods.* How long does the disease take to manifest? How long does it take for the disease to be communicated from the affected individual to another person?
- *Location of isolation or quarantine.* Where will the individual be kept while infectious? Home, work, school, healthcare facility are possible locations.
- *Type of treatment.* What type of treatment is needed to cure the disease? Is a hospital or other specialized medical treatment center necessary?

Typically, such measures are not controversial and involve the compliance of the affected individual. Sometimes, however, the affected individual does not comply, and legal challenges ensue (See, e.g., *In re Commitment of J.S.T.*, 2015; *In re Washington*, 2007). An Illinois case illustrates the actions public health authorities may take with respect to a noncompliant individual, as described in Box 7.2.

Every state has the authority to issue and enforce isolation and quarantine statutes under their police powers; these laws vary from state to state (National Conference of State Legislatures, 2014). In some states, an individual may be placed into quarantine or isolation through an administrative order (e.g., an order from the state health department or governor; see, e.g.,

## BOX 7.2 NONCOMPLIANT INDIVIDUALS

In 2014, after repeated documented instances of noncompliance by a 20-year old man diagnosed with active pulmonary TB ("the patient"), the Champaign-Urbana Public Health District (CUPHD) issued an order of isolation in compliance with Illinois law. A hearing was held to enforce the order, but the patient failed to attend. The Illinois court issued an order of isolation that delineated the restrictions on the patient, which included home confinement, directly observed therapy (DOT), a GPS monitoring device, and the provision of sputum samples (*In re Christian Mbemba Ibanda*, 2014). The patient proceeded to violate the isolation order, leaving his home on multiple occasions, refusing to comply with DOT, and failing to charge the batteries of the GPS monitoring device. A petition for indirect criminal contempt was filed by the Champaign County attorney general and the patient was arrested. He served his isolation at a neighboring county's jail, as there was no negative pressure isolation cell at the Champaign County jail, at the cost to Champaign County of $50 per day. While in jail, the patient resumed his TB treatment and was released shortly thereafter, after three negative sputum samples were collected. The isolation order was vacated as the patient was no longer a threat to public health; the indirect criminal contempt charges were dropped several months later (see, e.g., Hershey et al., 2017).

20 Illinois Comp. Stat. 22305/2(b)-(c); Alabama Code §22.12.1–22.12.29; Arkansas Stat. Ann. § 14-262-101-109). Other states require a court order before a person can be placed in isolation or quarantine (see, e.g., Louisiana Rev. Stat. Ann. § 40:17[A]).

There is also variation in the diseases subject to isolation and quarantine (Cole, 2014). Some states specify the diseases in statute or regulation and may have additional laws specific to a disease (e.g., tuberculosis; Cole, 2014). Other states grant the state health department the authority to determine which diseases are subject to isolation and quarantine authority (Cole, 2014). Some states delegate isolation and quarantine authority to local health jurisdictions. For example, under Connecticut law (Conn. Gen. Stat. Ann. § 19a-221),

> Any town, city, borough or district director of health may order any person isolated or quarantined whom such director has reasonable grounds to believe to be infected with a communicable disease or to be contaminated, if such director determines such person poses a substantial threat to the public health and isolation or quarantine is necessary to protect or preserve the public health…

Courts give broad discretion to public health officials who issue isolation and quarantine orders. In *People ex rel. Barmore v. Robertson* (1922), the Supreme Court of Illinois upheld a quarantine order for a typhoid carrier even though she was not contagious:

> One of the most important elements in the administration of health and quarantine regulations is a full measure of common sense. It is not necessary for the health authorities to wait until the person affected with a contagious disease has actually caused others to become sick by contact with him before he is placed under quarantine.

The discretion of health officials, however, is not unlimited. In *Kirk v. Wyman* (1909), the South Carolina Supreme Court struck down an order imposed by local health officials on an older woman with contagious leprosy in part because the quarantine was ordered to be served in a pesthouse rather than a safe and habitable location. "[E]ven temporary isolation in such a place would be a serious affliction and peril to an elderly lady, enfeebled by disease, and accustomed to the comforts of life" (*Kirk v. Wyman*, 1909). Moreover, public health officials must demonstrate that the individual subject to deprivation of personal liberty has a communicable disease in the infectious stage that poses a danger to public health (See, e.g., *State of Arkansas v. Snow*, 1959). Box 7.3 describes a case where the state did not meet its burden to prove restrictions to individual liberty were necessary to protect public health.

## BOX 7.3 MAYHEW v. HICKOX

Kaci Hickox became a household name in the Fall of 2014 after her return from caring for Ebola-infected patients in West Africa and subsequent quarantine in both New Jersey and Maine. On October 24, 2014, Hickox arrived at Newark International Airport, which had recently implemented airport screening measures for individuals returning from West Africa. Hickox registered an elevated temperature and was placed into quarantine in a tent in a hospital parking lot. She was released on October 27, 2014, after testing for Ebola came back negative, and traveled to her home state of Maine. Although she had been asked to contact Maine public health officials, Hickox failed to do so. Upon her arrival in Maine, Maine public health officials immediately requested that Hickox quarantine herself in her home for the 21-day incubation period, receive direct active monitoring from a public health nurse, and restrict her movements to avoid contact with others. While Hickox agreed to participate in direct active monitoring, she refused to quarantine herself or restrict her movements. Under Maine law, ME Rev Stat. Ann. tit 22, § 805, 812,

BOX 7.3 *(continued)*

Maine public health officials are required to request court intervention to effectuate their detention order, and a court will issue a detention order if it finds by clear and convincing evidence that a public health threat exists.

A petition was filed on October 30 by the Maine Attorney General; a temporary order restricting Hickox's activities was also issued by the Maine court. An Order Pending Hearing was issued on October 31, 2014, at which time the Maine court found that, while requiring Hickox to comply with direct active monitoring and other steps was required under Maine law, "[T]he state had not met its burden . . . to prove by clear and convincing evidence that limiting [Hickox's] movements to the degree requested is 'necessary to protect other individuals from the danger of infection,' however. According to the information presented to the court, [Hickox] currently does not show any symptoms of Ebola and is therefore *not* infectious" (emphasis in original). (See, e.g., Hershey et al., 2017.)

The case of Hongkham Souvannarath, a Laotian immigrant residing in the United States who was jailed for 10 months for refusing to take TB medication, illustrates the conundrum facing public health officials regarding where to detain infectious patients (*Souvannarath v. Hadden,* 2002). Souvannarath had limited English proficiency and was ultimately diagnosed with multidrug resistant TB, which required intravenous medication. She was detained in a county jail under an administrative order of isolation after failing to adhere to treatment. The detention order lacked information about the specific reason for detention and failed to inform Souvannarath of her rights under California's TB control laws, such as the right to a hearing and court representation. In addition, the order authorized her confinement in a county jail where she was treated like other inmates. Souvannarath was ultimately released and filed suit against the county and health officials, claiming, among other things, violation of Section 121358(a) of California's TB Control Statute that prohibited detention of noncompliant TB patients in jails (Cal. Health & Safety Code 121358[a]). A California court of appeals affirmed the lower court's ruling that it was legally impermissible to detain nonadherent patients in county prisons (*Souvannarath v. Hadden,* 2002).

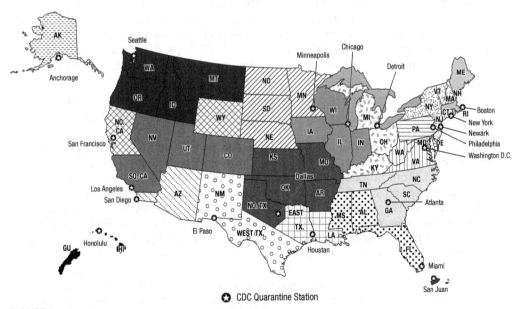

**FIGURE 7.1** CDC quarantine stations by jurisdiction.

*Source*: Centers for Disease Control and Prevention. https://www.cdc.gov/quarantine/images/quarantine -stations-508-map.jpg

## Federal Authority to Isolate and Quarantine

While state and local governments generally exercise the authority to impose isolation and quarantine orders, the federal government also plays a role. The federal government's isolation and quarantine authority is limited to situations involving international or interstate travel (42 USC § 264) or intrastate communicable diseases in the event a state's response is so ineffective that it poses a serious threat to other states (42 CFR § 70.2). Federal isolation and quarantine authority is also limited to certain diseases—including plague, smallpox, and viral hemorrhagic fevers such as Ebola, referred to as quarantinable communicable diseases (42 CFR § 71.1; Executive Order 13295, 2003)—as amended by Executive Order 13375, 2005; Executive Order 13674, 2014). CDC operates 20 quarantine stations across the United States at ports of entry and land border crossings to monitor the arrival of international travel. See Figure 7.1 for a map of CDC quarantine stations. This federal authority is rarely used. Box 7.4 describes one such instance.

In the wake of the 2014–2016 Ebola outbreak, the CDC issued a final rule in January 2017 that clarified and enhanced its disease control powers (Control of Communicable Disease, 2017). Under the new regulations, the CDC may authorize the apprehension, medical examination, quarantine, isolation, or conditional release when there is a "reasonable belief" that an individual is infected with a quarantinable communicable disease and is engaging or about to engage in interstate travel, or a probable source of infection to others who may be engaging in interstate travel (42 C.F.R. § 70.6[a]). The new rules also allow for detention if the CDC has a reasonable belief that a person arriving in the United States from a foreign country is infected with or has been exposed to a quarantinable communicable disease (42 C.F.R. 71.32[a]).

The regulations provide for several due process protections (e.g., specifications regarding detention order contents, mandatory reassessment of federal detention orders within 72 hours; 42 C.F.R. 70.14[a], 42 C.F.R. 70.15[b], 42 C.F.R. 71.37[a], 42 C.F.R. 71.38). However, the reasonable belief standard for detention has been criticized as affording the federal government with too much discretion at the expense of individual liberties (Ulrich & Mariner, 2018).

## Constitutional Considerations

Under the Fifth and Fourteenth Amendments, government must not "deprive any person of life, liberty, or property, without due process of law" (U.S. Const. amend. V, U.S. Const. amend. XIV). There are two types of *due process*: procedural and substantive. "Procedural due process" requires the government provide certain procedural steps (e.g., notice, right to present evidence, right to counsel). The extent of the process provided is dependent upon the scope

### BOX 7.4 THE ANDREW SPEAKER CASE

Andrew Speaker, a Georgia resident, was diagnosed with TB and was asked by Georgia public health officials not to travel to Europe for his honeymoon. Regardless, he left for his trip, and CDC officials determined from lab samples that he may have developed extremely drug-resistant TB (XDR-TB). Speaker was notified and asked to report to Italian health authorities. He refused and returned to the United States by flying into Canada and driving into New York State. At that time, the CDC issued its first federal quarantine order since the 1960s. Speaker finally turned himself in to public health officials and was treated at a Denver hospital with experience treating TB patients. Limited quarantines were ordered for individuals who had been exposed to TB during Speaker's travels. In the end, the CDC determined Speaker had a less serious form of TB rather than XDR-TB. Speaker filed a lawsuit against the CDC, alleging privacy and other violations, which was dismissed (Fidler, 2007; *Speaker v. CDC*, 2012).

and duration of the deprivation of rights (*Matthews v. Eldridge*, 1976). "Substantive due process" requires the government to have an adequate justification for the deprivation of an individual's life, liberty, property interest (*Washington v. Glucksberg*, 1997).

In the context of isolation, quarantine, and other public health measures taken to control the spread of infectious disease, procedural due process requires the state to provide the individual with written notice of the alleged condition and/or behavior that creates a risk to public health; access to legal counsel, including appointed counsel if indigent; a full and impartial hearing, with the ability to be present and to cross-examine and present witnesses; a clear and convincing standard of proof; and the right to obtain a verbatim transcript of the proceeding (*Greene v. Edwards*, 1980). Substantive due process protection with respect to the imposition of social distancing measures includes evidence the individual is either infected with or has been exposed to an individual infected with a communicable disease and is therefore a risk to public health (Fidler et al., 2007). In addition, the public health intervention must be reasonable, effective, and use the least restrictive means (Fidler et al., 2007). In *Newark v. J.S.* (1993), a New Jersey Superior Court stated:

> The parameters of due process require an analysis of both the individual and governmental interests involved and the consequences and avoidability of the risks of error and abuse [citing *Matthews v. Eldridge*, 424 U.S. 319, 335 (1976)]. Here the clash of competing interest is at its peak. Hardly any state interest is higher than protecting its citizenry from disease. Hardly any individual interest is higher than the liberty interest of being free from confinement. The consequences of error and abuse are grave for both the state and the individual.

"Equal protection" is another constitutional concern with respect to disease control and prevention measures. Under this principle, derived from the 14th Amendment, like individuals must be treated similarly. Such principles apply automatically under the 14th Amendment to state and local governments (U.S. Const. amend. XIV). Equal protection principles apply to the federal government through the Fifth Amendment (See, e.g., *Bolling v. Sharpe*, 1954).

*Jew Ho v. Williamson et al* (1900) illustrates the principles of equal protection in the context of disease control and prevention, as well as concerns regarding disease control measures and prejudice, further described in Box 7.5. In early 1900, several cases of bubonic plague were discovered in San Francisco in the city's Chinese quarter. City health officials imposed a **cordon sanitaire** or area quarantine that was specifically applied to a 12-block area predominantly occupied by ethnic Chinese people, rather than target the quarantine to affected areas. A federal appellate court ruled the quarantine could not continue because

> it is unreasonable, unjust, and oppressive, and therefore contrary to the laws limiting the police powers of the state and municipality in such matters; and second, that it is discriminating in is character, and contrary to the provisions of the fourteenth amendment of the constitution of the United States (*Jew Ho v. Williamson et al*, 1900, p. 26).

## The COVID-19 Pandemic: A Legal Timeline

The COVID-19 pandemic provides a timely case study on how law can be used to address and control an infectious disease pandemic. This section offers a timeline of legal issues related to the COVID-19 pandemic, and explores declarations, new laws passed to address COVID-19, and offers examples of how courts have addressed legal issues related to perceived infringement on civil liberties. Box 7.6 offers examples of federal actions to control an infectious disease pandemic.

### Public Health Emergency of International Concern

On December 31, 2019, the WHO was informed of a pneumonia of unknown cause, detected in the city of Wuhan in Hubei province, China. On January 7, 2020, Chinese authorities identified the causative agent to be a novel coronavirus, one not previously identified as causing disease

**BOX 7.5 DISEASE CONTROL MEASURES AND CONCERNS REGARDING PREJUDICE**

In times of disease outbreak and epidemics, the public's fear is heightened and draconian measures that would not occur in "normal times" are seen as necessary to protect the public's health. Oftentimes, such measures are driven by prejudice towards racial and ethnic groups, immigrants, and the LGBTQ community. During yellow fever and plague outbreaks in the 19th and early 20th centuries, prejudice against Asians was rampant, as illustrated in *Jew Ho* (1900). Such prejudice was seen again in 2003 during the SARS outbreak and 2015 during the measles outbreak in California (See, e.g., Bednarczyk et al., 2016; Person et al., 2004). The COVID-19 pandemic saw an increase in anti-Asian attacks (see, e.g., https://www.npr.org/2021/03/10/975722882/the-rise-of-anti-asian-attacks-during-the-covid-19-pandemic). During the 1980s, tremendous fear regarding the emerging disease HIV/AIDS caused extreme reactions against the LGBTQ community, particularly against gay men (see, e.g., Mustich, 2011). And the 2014–2016 Ebola outbreak raised fears about immigrants, particularly those from Africa (see, e.g., Jones, 2014). Thus, it is critical that public health authorities ensure that disease control measures proposed and implemented are not driven by prejudice towards any individual or group.

in humans, which was named SARS-CoV-2. China recorded its first death from SARS-CoV-2 on January 11, 2020. Although believed to be circulating in the United States at the end of 2019, the first case in the U.S. was reported on January 20, 2020 in a 35-year-old man in Snohomish County, Washington, who had recently returned from Wuhan. On January 20, 2020, Wuhan was placed under quarantine, with the entirety of Hubei province under quarantine within a few days. WHO declared a Public Health Emergency (PHE) of International Concern (PHEIC) on January 30, 2020, named the disease caused by the SARS-CoV-2 virus "COVID-19" on February 11, 2020, and declared a pandemic on March 11, 2020 (WHO, n.d.-b). Federal, state, local, Tribal, and territorial governments took varying legal actions to prevent the spread of the SARS-CoV-2 virus and mitigate the impact of the COVID-19 pandemic on the U.S. public health care and healthcare systems.

## Emergency Declarations in the US

On January 31, 2020, United States Secretary of Health and Human Services (HHS Secretary) Azar declared a PHE under section 319 of the Public Health Service Act existed nationwide since January 27, 2020 due to COVID-19. The declaration of PHE was renewed on April 21, 2020 (PHE, 2020a), July 23, 2020 (PHE, 2020b), October 2, 2020 (PHE, 2020c), and January 7, 2021 (PHE, 2021).

President Trump declared dual emergencies, effective March 1, 2020, on March 13, 2020 under the National Emergencies Act and section 501(b) of the Robert T. Stafford Disaster Relief and Emergency Assistance Act (Stafford Act), which allows the federal government to declare an emergency without a governor's request (White House, 2020a, 2020b). All 50 states, the District of Columbia, and four territories were approved for major disaster declarations to assist with additional needs identified under the nationwide emergency declaration for COVID-19 (FEMA, 2021).

On March 10, 2020, HHS Secretary Azar issued a declaration under the Public Readiness and Emergency Preparedness Act (PREP Act) to provide liability immunity for activities related to medical countermeasures against COVID–19. At the writing of this chapter, this declaration has been amended five times (PHE, n.d.).

## New Laws Passed to Address the COVID-19 Infectious Disease Pandemic

In addition to exercising existing statutory authority, new laws were passed to address the pandemic. For example, the Families First Coronavirus Response Act, enacted on March 18, 2020, provided free coronavirus testing and provided paid sick leave and extended family

**BOX 7.6  COVID-19: EXAMPLES OF FEDERAL ACTIONS TO CONTROL AN INFECTIOUS DISEASE PANDEMIC**

Many federal agencies took action in response to the COVID-19 pandemic. For example, under section 1135 of the Social Security Act, the Secretary of the Department of Health and Human Services may temporarily modify or waive certain Medicare, Medicaid, CHIP, or HIPAA requirements through 1135 waivers. The Centers for Medicare and Medicaid Services (CMS) issued numerous waivers under this authority to ensure beneficiaries had access to care and to allow healthcare providers flexibility when providing care (CMS, n.d.). And, the HHS Office for Civil Rights (OCR) issued numerous guidance documents, resources, bulletins, and announcements regarding how patient health information can be used and disclosed in response to the COVID-19 pandemic, as well as enforcement discretion decisions under the HIPAA (U.S. Department of Health & Human Services, n.d.).

leave for workers, and expanded unemployment benefits (H.R.6201 – Families First Coronavirus Response Act, 116th Congress [2019–2020]). The Coronavirus Aid, Relief, and Economic Security (CARES) Act, sprawling legislation enacted on March 27, 2020, included $2.2 trillion in emergency relief to address the crisis and bolster the economy (H.R.748 – CARES Act, 116th Congress (2019–2020)). The CARES Act created the Paycheck Protection Program that provided forgivable loans to small business, provided one-time cash payments to individual Americans up to certain income levels and increased unemployment benefits, provided loans to corporations, and funding to state and local governments. An additional $900 billion in relief was attached to the Consolidated Appropriations Act, 2021, enacted in late December 2020 after the expiration of certain CARES Act programs (H.R.133 – Consolidated Appropriations Act, 2021, 116th Congress [2019–2020]).

Using executive authority, governors, mayors, and state agencies took on the bulk of the pandemic response in 2020 by issuing declarations of emergencies, executive orders, emergency proclamations, and emergency rulemakings to institute social distancing measures, including stay-at-home and shelter-in-place orders, travel restrictions, curfews, mandatory quarantine periods for travelers, face covering requirements, business and school closures, and bans on gatherings of various sizes. States also restricted elective medical procedures and appointments, commandeered medical supplies, expanded access to telehealth, and set vaccine priority populations (KFF, 2021; National League of Cities, 2021). These mitigation measures continued to varying degrees in early 2021.

## COVID-19 in the Courts

The use of disease control measures, however, are not without controversy, as they infringe upon individual liberties provided under the U.S. Constitution, and numerous cases have been filed in both state and federal courts challenging these actions (Ballotpedia, n.d.; Hunton Andrews Kurth, n.d.). Many of these cases raise questions regarding constitutional limits on governmental authority to restrict social and economic activity through social distancing measures, to protect the public's health. They also raise issues regarding separation of powers and governors' authority to impose restrictions.

In one case, a court in the Western District of Pennsylvania held certain restrictions imposed by Pennsylvania Governor Tom Wolf and his administration were unconstitutional. *County of Butler v. Wolf*, 2020 WL 5510690 (W.D. Pa. Sept. 14, 2020). Specifically, the court declared the limits on the number of people who could gather in a space imposed by Governor Wolf in an Executive Order violated the First Amendment's right to free assembly. The Court also found violations of the Fourteenth Amendment's Due Process and Equal Protection clauses in the now lifted stay-at-home and business closure components of certain Executive Orders.

While the Court recognized the Wolf administration "took their actions in a well-intentioned effort to protect Pennsylvanians from the virus ... good intentions toward a laudable goal are not alone enough to uphold governmental action against a constitutional challenge." The Court declined to apply the "extraordinary deference" other courts have shown to *Jacobson*, pointing to that decision's age as well as the U.S. Supreme Court's development of three tiers of constitutional scrutiny since *Jacobson* was decided. *Id.* at *6–10. A panel of judges on the Third Circuit Court of Appeals granted the Governor's request for a stay pending appeal, which restored Pennsylvania's indoor and outdoor gathering limits. *County of Butler. v Governor of Pennsylvania* (3d Cir. Oct. 1, 2020). Previous and subsequent challenges had failed to overturn Governor Wolf's coronavirus orders (see, e.g., *M. Rae, Inc. v. Wolf*, 2020 ; *Wolf v. Scarnati*, 2020).

The U.S. Supreme Court has heard several challenges to limitations on gathering size and the free exercise of religion. In *South Bay United Pentecostal Church v. Newsom* (May 29, 2020), the Supreme Court ruled five to four to reject a California church's attempt to overturn the state's restrictions on in-person religious services. The Court decided a similar case, *Calvary Chapel Dayton Valley v. Sisolak* (July 24, 2020) 2 months later with the same outcome. However, the composition of the court changed after the death of Justice Ruth Bader Ginsberg in September 2020 and the addition of Justice Amy Coney Barrett. In *Roman Catholic Diocese of Brooklyn v. Cuomo* (November 25, 2020), the Court ruled five to four to issue a preliminary injunction, holding New York may not enforce limits on in-person religious worship imposed by New York Governor Andrew Cuomo because the restrictions likely discriminate against religion in violation of the First Amendment. Since this decision, the Court has ordered lower courts to revisit various challenges by religious groups to state restrictions on indoor worship services in light of the *Roman Catholic Diocese of Brooklyn v. Cuomo* decision (see, e.g., *High Plains Harvest Church v. Polis*, December 15, 2020). Indeed, in early 2021, based on the *Roman Catholic Diocese of Brooklyn v. Cuomo* decision, a divided Supreme Court allowed California churches to resume indoor worship services, while still allowing the state to enforce its ban on singing and chanting and limit attendance to 25% of capacity. See *South Bay United Pentecostal Church v. Newsom* (February 5, 2021) and *Harvest Rock Church v. Newsom* (February 5, 2021).

The courts were not the only place challenges to executive authority occurred. State legislatures around the country took steps to curb executive authority exerted during the pandemic. For example, Democratic Kentucky Governor Andy Beshear sued the state's Republican-dominated legislature over limits to his authority (Beshear & Friedlander, 2021). Democratic Wisconsin Governor Tony Evers immediately issued a new mask mandate after the Republican-dominated legislature repealed the previous mandate (The State of Wisconsin, n.d.). Several state legislatures, including New Mexico, Arizona, and New York, have drafted legislation or passed resolutions designed to increase the role of the legislature during public health emergencies (Associated Press, 2021). As the COVID-19 pandemic continued, the tension between the executive, legislative, and judicial branches increased, as state public health emergency laws did not contemplate a protracted emergency.

## CONCLUSION

Surveillance is a fundamental tool in infectious disease prevention and control that enables public health agencies to track pathogen information and monitor trends to detect and respond to outbreaks. It relies on three main components: a) disease reporting; b) disease investigation; and c) disease control and prevention. Disease reporting is accomplished by state and local public health agencies employing mandatory notification requirements when a disease case of public health concern is identified. The agency must determine whether an investigation will be conducted to identify the source and determine the scope of any potential outbreak. The authority of states to isolate sick individuals and quarantine individuals who have been or may have been exposed to infectious disease, as well as take other disease prevention and control measures, is well-established in the United States. As has been seen in the COVID-19 pandemic, however, such disease prevention control measures are not without controversy, as they infringe upon individual liberties provided under the U.S. Constitution. Therefore, such measures are not taken lightly, and many factors must be considered, including due process and equal protection. The federal government also plays a role; however, its isolation and quarantine authority is limited to situations involving international or interstate travel or intrastate communicable disease when a state's response is ineffective and poses a threat to other states.

## CHAPTER REVIEW

### Review Questions

1.  Where in the law do jurisdictions define their list of reportable diseases?
2.  What is the health department's responsibility when notified of the occurrence of a reportable disease?
3.  To what situations is the federal government's isolation and quarantine authority limited?

### Essay Questions

1.  What is the standard for actions a public health agency may take in accessing identifiable information during a public health investigation? How can a public health agency address the tension between accessing pertinent investigation information and protecting patient privacy before an investigation begins?
2.  What factors will public health officials consider before imposing isolation or quarantine?
3.  What due process protections are required before social distancing measures are imposed?
4.  Why might an individual not voluntarily comply with an isolation or quarantine order?

### Internet Activities

1.  Find your state or local health department's disease-reporting website. Does the website provide a list of reportable diseases and indicate who must report those diseases to the health department? Is measles a reportable disease in your jurisdiction?
2.  Can you find a recent example in the news of public health investigators accessing medical records as part of an outbreak investigation? Can you find another example of a local public health investigation involving an outbreak outside of the healthcare facility setting? What information did investigators use to identify the source of each outbreak?

## REFERENCES

20 Ill. Comp. Stat. 22305/2(b)-(c).
42 CFR 70.14(a).
42 CFR 70.15(b).
42 CFR § 70.2.
42 CFR § 70.6(a).
42 CFR § 71.1.
42 CFR 71.32(a).
42 CFR 71.37(a).
42 CFR 71.38.
42 USC § 264.
45 CFR § 164.501.
45 CFR § 164.502.
45 CFR § 164.512.
45 CFR § 164.514.
Alabama Code §22.12.1–22.12.29.

Alabama Code §420-4-1-.04.

Arkansas Stat. Ann. § 14-262-101-109.

Associated Press. (2021, February 3). New Mexico latest legislature to question emergency power. *U.S. News.* https://www.usnews.com/news/best-states/new-mexico/articles/2021-02-03/new -mexico-latest-legislature-to-question-emergency-powers

Ballotpedia. (n.d). *Lawsuits about state actions and policies in response to the coronavirus (COVID-19) pandemic, 2020–2021.* https://ballotpedia.org/Lawsuits_about_state_actions_and_policies_in _response_to_the_coronavirus_(COVID-19)_pandemic,_2020-2021

Bednarczyk, R. V., Rebolledo, P. A., & Omer, S. B. (2016). Assessment of the role of international travel and unauthorized immigration on measles importation to the United States. *Journal of Travel Medicine, 23*(3), 1–6. https://doi.org/10.1093/jtm/taw019

Beshear, A., & Friedlander, E. (2021, February 2). *Commonwealth of Kentucky Franklin circuit court.* https://governor.ky.gov/attachments/202010202_Filed-Pleadings.pdf

*Bolling v. Sharpe,* 347 U.S. 497 (1954).

California Health & Safety Code 121358(a).

Calvary Chapel Dayton Valley v. Sisolak (July 24, 2020)

Centers for Disease Control and Prevention. (2014, August 28). *About quarantine and isolation.* https:// www.cdc.gov/quarantine/quarantineisolation.html

Centers for Disease Control and Prevention. (2018a, March 21) *National notifiable diseases surveillance system (NNDSS): About NNDSS.* https://wwwn.cdc.gov/nndss/infographic-intro.html

Centers for Disease Control and Prevention. (2018b, September 28) *National notifiable diseases surveillance system (NNDSS): Data collection and reporting.* https://wwwn.cdc.gov/nndss/data -collection.html

Centers for Medicare & Medicaid Services. (n.d.). *Coronavirus waivers & flexibilities.* https://www .cms.gov/about-cms/emergency-preparedness-response-operations/current-emergencies/ coronavirus-waivers

*City of Newark v. J.S.,* 652 A.2d 265, 191-192 (New Jersey Super 1993).

Cole, J. (2014). *Federal and state quarantine and isolation authority.* Congressional Research Service. https://fas.org/sgp/crs/homesec/RL33201.pdf

*Compagnie Francaise de Navigation a Vapeur v. Louisiana State Board of Health,* 186 U.S. 380 (1902).

Connecticut Gen. Stat. Ann. § 19a-221.

Control of Communicable Disease, 82 Fed. Reg. 6890 (January 19, 2017).

*County of Butler. v Governor of Pennsylvania,* 2020 WL 5868393 (October 1, 2020).

Executive Order 13295 (April 4, 2003), as amended by Executive Order 13375 (April 1, 2005).

Executive Order 13674 (July 31, 2014).

Federal Emergency Management Administration. (2021). *COVID-19 disaster declarations.* https:// www.fema.gov/disasters/coronavirus/disaster-declarations

Fidler, D. P., Gostin, L. O., & Markel, H. (2007). Through the quarantine looking glass: Drug resistant tuberculosis and public health governance, law, and ethics. *The Journal of Law, Medicine & Ethics, 35,* 612–628. https://doi.org/10.1111/j.1748-720X.2007.00185.x

Florida Admin. Code Ann. r. 64D-3.029.

Georgia Department of Public Health. (2018, July). *Notifiable disease/condition reporting.* https://dph .georgia.gov/sites/dph.georgia.gov/files/GA%20Notifiable%20Disease%20Poster%207-2018.pdf

Gostin, L. O. (2005). *Jacobson v. Massachusetts* at 100 years: Police powers and civil liberties in tension. *American Journal of Public Health, 95*(4), 576–581. https://doi.org/10.2105/AJPH.2004.055152

Gostin, L. O., Burris, S., & Lazzarini, Z. (1999). The law and the public's health: A study of infectious disease law in the United States. *Columbia Law Review, 99*(1), 59–128. https://doi. org/10.2307/1123597

*Greene v. Edwards,* 263 S.E.2d 661 (West Virginia, 1980).

Harvest Rock Church v. Newsom (February 5, 2021)

Hershey, T. B., Pryde, J. A., Mwaungulu, G. S., Phifer, V. I., & Roszak, A. R. (2017). Putting the law into practice: A comparison of isolation and quarantine as tools to control Tuberculosis and Ebola. *Journal of Public Health Management & Practice, 23*(2), e25–e31. https://doi.org/10.1097/ PHH.0000000000000327

High Plains Harvest Church v. Polis, December 15, 2020

H.R.133 - Consolidated Appropriations Act, 2021, 116th Congress (2019–2020). https://www.congress .gov/bill/116th-congress/house-bill/133/text

H.R. 6201 – Families First Coronavirus Response Act, 116th Congress (2019–2020). https://www .congress.gov/bill/116th-congress/house-bill/6201/text

H.R.748 – CARES Act, 116th Congress (2019–2020). https://www.congress.gov/bill/116th-congress/ house-bill/748/text?q=%7B%22search%22%3A%5B%22coronavirus+aid+relief+and+economic %22%5D%7D&r=2&s=1

Hunton Andrews Kurth. (n.d.). *COVID-19 complaint tracker.* https://www.huntonak.com/en/covid -19-tracker.html

In re Commitment of J.S.T., 478 S.W.3d 856 (2015)

In re Washington, 735 N.W.2d 111 (Wisc. 2007).

*Jacobson v. Massachusetts,* 197 U.S. 11 (1905).

*Jew Ho v. Williamson et al,* 103 F.10 (1900).

Jones, A. J. (2014, October 21). Ebola fears turn into an epidemic of racism and hysteria. *The Intercept.* https://theintercept.com/2014/10/21/cant-ebola-become-latest-racist-national-security-issue

Kaiser Family Foundation. (2021, April 6). *State COVID-19 data and policy actions.* https://www.kff .org/coronavirus-covid-19/issue-brief/state-covid-19-data-and-policy-actions

*Kirk v. Wyman,* 83 S.C. 372, 391 (1909).

Louisiana Rev. Stat. Ann. § 40:17(A).

*M. Rae, Inc. v. Wolf,* 2020 WL 7642596 (M.D. Pa, 2020).

Mariner, W. K., Annas, G. J., & Glantz, L. H. (2005). *Jacobson v. Massachusetts*: It's not your great-grandfather's public health law. *American Journal of Public Health, 95*(4), 581–590. https://doi .org/10.2105/AJPH.2004.055160

*Matthews v. Eldridge,* 424 U.S. 319 (1976).

Minnesota Department of Health. (n.d.). *Diseases reportable to the Minnesota Department of Health.* https://www.health.state.mn.us/diseases/reportable/rule/poster.pdf

Murray, J., & Cohen, A. L. (2017). Infectious disease surveillance. *International Encyclopedia of Public Health, 2017,* 222–229. https://doi.org/10.1016/B978-0-12-803678-5.00517-8

Mustich, E. (2011, June 5). *A history of AIDS hysteria.* Salon. https://www.salon.com/2011/06/05/ aids_hysteria/

National Conference of State Legislatures. (2014, October 29). *State quarantine and isolation statutes.* http://www.ncsl.org/research/health/state-quarantine-and-isolation-statutes.aspx

National League of Cities. (2021, March 6). *COVID-19: Local action tracker.* https://covid19.nlc.org/ resources/covid-19-local-action-tracker

New Hampshire Code Admin. R. He-P 301.07.

New Jersey Stat, Ann. 26:13–15.

Parmet, W. E. (1985). AIDS and quarantine: The revival of an archaic doctrine. *Hofstra Law Review, 14*(1). https://scholarlycommons.law.hofstra.edu/hlr/vol14/iss1/4

Parmet, W. E. (1993). Health care and the constitution: Public health and the role of the state in the framing era. *Hastings Constitutional Law Quarterly, 20*(2), 267–335. https://repository.uchastings. edu/hastings_constitutional_law_quaterly/vol20/iss2/1/

*People ex rel. Barmore v. Robertson,* 302 Ill 422, 434 (1922).

Person, B., Sy, F., Holton, K., Govert, B., Liang, A., & the NCID, SARS Community Outreach Team. (2004). Fear and stigma: The epidemic within the SARS outbreak. *Emerging Infectious Diseases, 10*(2), 358–363. http://dx.doi.org/10.3201/eid1002.030750

Public Health Emergency. (2020a, April 21). *Renewal of determination that a public health emergency exists.* https://www.phe.gov/emergency/news/healthactions/phe/Pages/covid19-21apr2020.aspx

Public Health Emergency. (2020b, July 23). *Renewal of determination that a public health emergency exists.* https://www.phe.gov/emergency/news/healthactions/phe/Pages/covid19-23June2020.aspx

Public Health Emergency. (2020c, October 2). *Renewal of determination that a public health emergency exists.* https://www.phe.gov/emergency/news/healthactions/phe/Pages/covid19-2Oct2020.aspx

Public Health Emergency. (2021, January 7). *Renewal of determination that a public health emergency exists.* https://www.phe.gov/emergency/news/healthactions/phe/Pages/covid19-07Jan2021.aspx

Public Health Emergency. (n.d.). *Public readiness and emergency preparedness act.* https://www.phe .gov/Preparedness/legal/prepact/Pages/default.aspx

Qualls, N., Levitt, A., Kanade, N., Wright-Jegede, N., Dopson, S., Biggerstaff, M., Reed, C., & Uzicanin, A. (2017) Community mitigation guidelines to prevent pandemic influenza—United States, 2017. *Morbidity and Mortality Weekly Report Recommendations and Reports, 66*(No. RR-1), 1–34. http://dx.doi .org/10.15585/mmwr.rr6601a1

Ransom, M. M. (Ed.). (2016). *Public health law competency model: Version 1.0.* https://www.cdc.gov/phlp/docs/phlcm-v1.pdf

Roman Catholic Diocese of Brooklyn v. Cuomo (November 25, 2020)

Rothstein, M. A. (2015). From SARS to Ebola: Legal and ethical considerations for modern quarantine. *Indiana Health Law Review, 12*(1), 2–3. https://doi.org/10.18060/18963.

Roush, S., Birkhead, G., Koo, D., Cobb, A., & Fleming, D. (1999). Mandatory reporting of diseases and conditions by health care professionals and laboratories. *Journal of the American Medical Association, 282*(2), 164–170. https://doi.org/10.1001/jama.282.2.164

South Bay United Pentecostal Church v. Newsom (May 29, 2020)

South Bay United Pentecostal Church v. Newsom (February 5, 2021)

*Souvannarath v Hadden*, 95 Calif App 4th 1115 (Calif App 2002).

*Speaker v. Centers for Disease Control and Prevention*, 489 F. App'x 425 (11th Cir. 2012).

*State of Arkansas v. Snow*, 230 Ark. 746 (1959).

*State of Illinois v. Ibanda*, No. 14-MR-296 (Cir. Ct. Champaign County April 11, 2014).

State of Wisconsin. (n.d.). *Emergency order #1: Relating to stopping the spread of COVID-19 by requiring face coverings.* https://content.govdelivery.com/attachments/WIGOV/2021/02/04/file_attachments/1684996/2020_02_04%20FebFaceCovering.pdf

Thacker, S. B., & Berkelman, R. L. (1992). History of public health surveillance. In W. Halperin & E. L. Baker (Eds.), *Public health surveillance.* Van Norstrand Reinhold. https://www.cdc.gov/mmwr/preview/mmwrhtml/su6103a3.htm#:~:text=The%20current%20definition%20is%20%22Public,to%20know%20and%20linked%20to

*Third Circuit County of Butler v. Wolf*, No. 20-2936 (3d Cir. Oct. 1, 2020).

Tyson, P. (2004, October 12). *A short history of quarantine.* http://www.pbs.org/wgbh/nova/body/short-history-of-quarantine.html

Ulrich, M. R., & Mariner, W. K. (2018). Quarantine and the federal role in epidemics. *SMU Law Review, 71*(2), 391. https://scholar.smu.edu/smulr/vol71/iss2/2

U.S. Constitution amend. V.

U.S. Constitution amend. X.

U.S. Constitution amend. XIV.

U.S. Department of Health & Human Services. (n.d.). *HIPAA and COVID-19.* https://www.hhs.gov/hipaa/for-professionals/special-topics/hipaa-covid19/index.html

*Washington v. Glucksberg*, 521 U.S. 702 (1997).

White House. (2020a, March 13). *Letter from President Donald J. Trump on emergency determination under the Stafford act.* https://trumpwhitehouse.archives.gov/briefings-statements/letter-president-donald-j-trump-emergency-determination-stafford-act

White House. (2020b, March 13). *Proclamation on declaring a national emergency concerning the novel coronavirus disease (COVID-19) outbreak.* https://trumpwhitehouse.archives.gov/presidential-actions/proclamation-declaring-national-emergency-concerning-novel-coronavirus-disease-covid-19-outbreak/

*Wolf v. Scarnati*, 233 A.3d 679 (Sup. Ct. Pa 2020).

World Health Organization. (n.d.-a). *Public health surveillance.* https://www.who.int/immunization/monitoring_surveillance/burden/vpd/en

World Health Organization. (n.d.-b). *Timeline: WHO's COVID-19 response.* https://www.who.int/emergencies/diseases/novel-coronavirus-2019/interactive-timeline#

## Additional Resources

- **Principles of Epidemiology in Public Health Practice—Lesson 5: Public Health Surveillance**
  https://www.cdc.gov/csels/dsepd/ss1978/lesson5/section1.html
- **Principles of Epidemiology in Public Health Practice—Lesson 6: Investigating an Outbreak**
  https://www.cdc.gov/csels/dsepd/ss1978/lesson6/section1.html
- **Legal Authorities for Isolation and Quarantine**
  https://www.cdc.gov/quarantine/aboutlawsregulationsquarantineisolation.html
- **Legal Authority for Infectious Disease Reporting in the United States: Case Study of the 2009 H1N1 Influenza Pandemic**
  https://www.ncbi.nlm.nih.gov/pmc/articles/PMC4265911

# 8

# Public Health Law in Chronic Disease Prevention and Management

Ashley Wennerstrom, Sharada Shantharam, Floribella Redondo, and Siobhan Gilchrist*

## Learning Objectives

By the end of this chapter, the reader will be able to:

- Illustrate the application of law to promote health equity and encourage healthy lifestyles.
- Analyze the role of law in defining scope of practice for chronic disease prevention and health equity.
- Appraise the importance of healthcare financing to promote health equity.

## Key Terminology

**Chronic Disease:** Conditions that last one year or more and require ongoing medical attention and/or limit activities of daily living.

**Collaborative Practice Agreements:** Formal, written relationships between healthcare providers that allow for certain expanded services for patients and the healthcare team.

**Community-Clinical Linkages:** Connections between community and clinical sectors to improve population health.

**Community Health Worker:** A trusted member of and/or someone who has an unusually close understanding of the community served, who serves as a link between health/social services and the community to facilitate access to services and improve the quality and cultural competence of service delivery.

**Health Equity:** The idea that everyone should have an equal opportunity to reach their maximum potential in terms of health. Achieving health equity requires removing barriers to achieving good health, especially for underserved and marginalized communities (Braveman et al., 2017).

**Medicaid:** A federal healthcare program jointly financed by state governments established in 1965 through an amendment to the Social Security Act of 1935 (Title XIX of the Social Security Amendments of 1965, 42 U.S.C. § 1396 et seq) to provide health insurance coverage for low-income people.

---

* The views expressed are the author's own and do not reflect the views of the United States Government or the U.S. Department of Health and Human Services.

**Scope of Practice:** Roles and responsibilities that a healthcare provider is allowed to undertake within the scope of their professional license.

**Team-based care:** A strategy that can be implemented at the health system level to enhance patient care by having two or more healthcare providers working collaboratively with each patient.

**The Patient Protection and Affordable Care Act, 42 U.S.C. § 18001 et seq Acronym for this term is provided on page 121, 2nd para.** A federal healthcare law enacted in 2010, and amended by the Health Care and Education Reconciliation Act in 2010, to ensure affordable health insurance coverage, expand the Medicaid program, and support innovative healthcare delivery models.

## Public Health Law Competencies

This chapter addresses the following competencies from the Legal Epidemiology Competency Model (LECM; Ransom, Ramanathan, & Yassine, 2018) and Public Health Law Competency Model (PHLCM; Ransom, 2016).

1.1 LECM 3.1: Identify opportunities for a legal evaluation study to address existing legal, health, or other issues.

1.2 PHLCM 2.2: Identify law-based tools and enforcement procedures available to address day-to-day (nonemergency) public health issues.

> ### Spark Question
> How has law been used to prevent and manage chronic diseases like cardiovascular disease, diabetes, and so on?

## INTRODUCTION

Six out of 10 individuals in the United States live with at least one **chronic disease** (Centers for Disease Control and Prevention [CDC], 2019a). Chronic diseases, like cardiovascular disease (CVD) and diabetes, can be prevented by eating well, being physically active, avoiding tobacco and excessive drinking, and getting regular health screenings. Barriers to health and **health equity** associated with racism, education, income, location, and other social factors increase the burden of chronic disease on certain subpopulations. Public health law can serve an integral role in advancing health equity, improving environments to make healthy choices easier, enhancing community linkages to clinical services, and strengthening healthcare systems.

Applying a Socio-Ecological Model (SEM) provides an understanding of the factors that can lead to or prevent chronic disease. Considering how individual, interpersonal, institutional, community, and policy factors influence health equity provides a comprehensive model to assess barriers and opportunities to health. For example:

- Individual factors, such as personal knowledge, attitudes, skills, and behaviors, influence food choices, physical activity, and smoking. Individual factors also shape a healthcare provider's cultural humility.
- Interpersonal factors, including formal and informal social networks and social support systems, affect care given by family and friends.
- Institutional factors, such as organizational structures, characteristics, and rules, impact whether patients have access to high-quality healthcare services and ongoing treatment for chronic disease.
- Community factors involve community structures, characteristics, and environments that play an important role in making healthy choices easier for people. This may include affordable, easy access to healthy foods, safe transportation, infrastructure that promotes physical activity, and smoke-free environments.
- Policy factors include local, state, and national laws and policies that drive the distribution of health-related opportunities and economic resources. These may allow us to solve

---

**BOX 8.1  LEGAL PRINCIPLES**

**Medicaid**, an example of "cooperative federalism" (also defined in Chapter 2), is a joint initiative by the federal government and states to provide health coverage to individuals in need—particularly those of low-income. Each state develops and pays for a plan to provide health coverage to Medicaid recipients that satisfies minimum federal requirements. In turn, the Centers for Medicare and Medicaid Services (CMS), the federal agency that administers the Medicaid program, reimburses the state for some portion of its spending based on the "Federal Medical Assistance Percentage" (FMAP) calculation.

States have some flexibility in implementing Medicaid as long as they meet federal approval, and some states provide more comprehensive coverage than others. States can propose changes to their Medicaid plans by submitting amendments or waivers to the CMS.

---

public health problems or to create conditions for those public health problems to be resolved (e.g., improved transportation, education, housing; Jones, 2000).

This chapter provides examples of how law can be used to promote health equity, influence the provision and availability of healthcare services, and enhance **community-clinical linkages** necessary to prevent and manage chronic disease.

---

### HYPOTHETICAL CASE STUDY #1: COMMUNITY HEALTH WORKERS AND MEDICAID

Amal is a recent public health graduate who has just moved to a Northwest state to work as a Lead Program Coordinator for a new Community-Clinical Linkages (CCLs) initiative housed within the state health department's Cardiovascular Disease Prevention and Control office. She has learned CCLs are connections between community and clinical sectors to improve population health (CDC, 2016). Her role is to develop and implement a statewide program to improve upon these connections, with overarching goals of improving outcomes for CVD and type 2 diabetes among priority populations and to reduce disparities. Amal realizes that because **community health workers** (CHWs) are a critical professional workforce who address social determinants of health at multiple levels of the socioecological model (e.g., limited transportation, poor housing, poverty, discrimination, unemployment, and inaccessible healthcare) among priority populations, public health laws and policies that provide a supportive and sustainable environment for CHWs to work are instrumental in advancing health equity. She reaches the conclusion that CHWs would be an appropriate workforce to engage and include in the program because they serve as a bridge between underserved communities and clinical and social service sectors. Accordingly, she proposes and receives her supervisors' approval to implement a statewide CCL program with the following objectives:

1. Recruit and sustainably employ in the public health department several CHWs from communities experiencing inequities related to CVD and give them a central role in the implementation of the CCL initiative to connect community-based organizations to clinical sectors.
2. Engage these CHWs in activities focused on changing individuals' behavior and addressing social determinants of health, including activities demonstrating one's health is impacted by more than individual behaviors and decisions.

> **3.** Facilitate collaboration with other CHWs who are employed by other agencies in both the clinical (e.g., Medicaid Managed Care Organizations [MCO]) and community (e.g., social services, public housing) sectors to ensure there is coordination and no duplication of services.

To begin the implementation process, the first step Amal takes is to learn about the CHW workforce in her state, including its history and any existing laws or policies that may influence CHW inclusion in healthcare settings (e.g., core competencies, **scope of practice**, financing, access to client health data). To better understand the potential need for CHW services, she researches existing state data from qualitative (e.g., focus groups) and quantitative (e.g., state's public health database) sources in order to learn about health inequities across the state, identify priority populations, and gain an understanding about the underlying root causes of the disparities. Amal finds, as a whole, the state is relatively healthy. However, public health data stratified by socioeconomic status and demographic groups (e.g., race and/or ethnicity, socioeconomic position, new immigrants, insurance status) and by census-tract level show large health disparities in chronic disease conditions, with highest rates of diabetes, hypertension, stroke, and heart attack among non-White Medicaid members with low socioeconomic status (SES) in several geographic areas of the state. The data also indicate these population groups contend with challenging social determinants of health. She finds studies that describe how these social determinants of health are shaped largely by current and historical policies.

- What public health framework could Amal apply to plan for how a statewide CCL initiative engaging CHWs could be implemented?
- What federal and state laws does Amal need to learn about in her search for sources of sustainable financing for employing CHWs in the CCL initiative?
- What federal law could impact the provision of CHW services to populations experiencing inequities in CVD and type 2 diabetes in this CCL initiative?

## Public Health Framework

The SEM can also be applied to initiatives employing CHWs. Understanding the laws and policies impacting the CHW workforce is essential to promoting changes to advance their inclusion in healthcare and social service delivery systems and teams. Practitioners should also be aware of current and historical policies and laws, particularly those related to social determinants of health that impact the populations CHWs serve. CHWs also help facilitate collaborations with organizations in community, public health, and clinical sectors whose structures and policies are well-poised to support health equity through improved service access and through promoting community development. For example, community organizations such as food pantries improve access to nutrition; community development organizations can increase neighborhood walkability; and clinical organizations such as federally qualified health centers facilitate access to healthcare. As described previously, CHWs focus on communities (as defined by groups of people who are affiliated or connected by race and/or ethnicity and geography) that are experiencing inequities related to CVD, type 2 diabetes, and other chronic conditions, as well as activities focused on changing individuals' behaviors such as education and health coaching.

## Federal and State Legal Framework

The increasing evidence of CHWs' contributions to attaining positive health outcomes in CVD and type 2 diabetes provides a strong argument for the value of incorporating CHWs into chronic disease prevention strategies. CHWs have historically been funded by short-term grants, so there is a need to develop sustainable CHW workforce–financing models, particularly through Medicaid payment. Under Medicaid, the federal government calculates and pays the Federal Medical Assistance Percentage to match state expenses. Most states also enter into written contracts with MCOs to deliver health services to Medicaid members. MCOs are increasingly including population health improvement strategies, social determinants of health, and CHWs (Center for Health Care Strategies, 2018). Medicaid managed care provides for the delivery of Medicaid health benefits and additional services through contracted arrangements between state Medicaid agencies and MCOs that accept a set per-member–per-month (capitation) payment for these services (Medicaid.gov, n.d.). Medicaid managed care typically provides more flexibility than traditional Medicaid to cover additional services, and this flexibility has been leveraged to support CHWs (Albritton, 2016).

Additionally, Section 1332 of the Affordable Care Act (ACA) permits a state to apply for a "state innovation waiver" (now also referred to as a "state relief and empowerment waiver") to pursue innovative strategies for providing their residents with access to high-quality, affordable health insurance while retaining the basic protections of the ACA (Centers for Medicare & Medicaid Services, n.d.). These waivers are used by many states to test alternate benefit designs or new models for delivering care. Additionally, some states have used these waivers to fund engaging CHWs in models that focus on specific populations (Albritton, 2016). Medicaid can also support CHWs for delivering a broader set of services if states choose to expand their list of services. Another model the Center for Medicare and Medicaid Innovation is authorized to implement under Section 3021 of the ACA (Section 1115A of the Social Security Act) is the Accountable Health Communities Model that focuses on the CCLs in health-delivery reform, and states are beginning to include CHWs in implementation of this model as well (Institute for Public Health Innovation, 2018).

State laws and policies addressing CHW definitions, scope of practice, financing, certification, and training differ by state (CDC, 2016). In some cases, states have implemented rules around CHW certification, in efforts to develop a sustainable financing mechanism (e.g., via Medicaid) for the workforce. There is sparse evidence on whether such certification affects health outcomes at all, creating a need to gather data in partnership with CHWs to determine whether CHW certification can be linked to improvements in health outcomes.

## Selected Concepts for Discussion

1.  How do state policies pertaining to Medicaid impact a program's capacity to sustainably employ CHWs in providing CCLs and addressing social determinants of health?
2.  How could proposed changes to federal healthcare law impact the inclusion of CHWs in care teams and health delivery systems?

### BOX 8.2 LEGAL PRINCIPLES

The practice of medicine is typically described in a state's "Medical Practice Act," often through a provision that defines the "unlawful" practice of medicine and is enforceable under the state's criminal act. In general, it pertains to physicians and includes attempting to or performing the acts of prescribing drugs, diagnosing and treating illness, disease, or injuries, or performing surgery on humans. For this reason, it is important to understand that simple acts such as a pharmacist taking a person's blood pressure in the context of chronic disease diagnosis could be considered an unlawful medical practice unless otherwise authorized by law.

## HYPOTHETICAL CASE STUDY #2: COLLABORATIVE PRACTICE AGREEMENT— PHARMACIST SCOPE OF PRACTICE

Jessie R. was diagnosed with hypertension 5 years ago and had been prescribed an antihypertensive medication. Last year, he was diagnosed with high cholesterol and was also prescribed a statin drug to lower his cholesterol level. He lives in a small, rural community in the upper Midwest. Although he tries to visit his nurse practitioner (NP) regularly, a recent job change and transportation challenges have made it difficult for him to get to follow-up office appointments. He has experienced what he believes are side effects from taking both medications and let his hypertensive medication refill lapse a few months ago. Dr. K, a community pharmacist, is aware of the transportation and other barriers Jessie and other community members face in staying adherent to medications for chronic disease management. Also, she understands many drivers of health inequities are influenced by organizational and structural policies and practices that impact how local healthcare services are accessed and delivered. When Jessie stops by the community pharmacy to pick up an antibiotic, Dr. K notes that Jessie had not filled his antihypertensive medication as scheduled. She tells him she has a **collaborative practice agreement** (CPA) with his NP for several patients. Dr. K explains she could draft a CPA with his NP that would allow her to help manage his hypertension and high cholesterol by changing his medications to reduce side effects as needed without him having to go back to the NP for a new prescription. She asks him whether she has his consent to speak directly with the NP about a CPA for his care. Happy to save time and avoid additional unpaid leave hours, Jessie says "Yes."

- What is the federal and state legal framework regarding the practice of medicine?
- How do states use the law to define scope of practice for healthcare providers?
- By what authority can the NP delegate medical functions to a pharmacist?

## Public Health Framework

Applying a combination of interventions across multiple levels of the SEM provides a more effective approach to chronic disease prevention. Scope of practice laws that allow each provider to practice at the top of their license, education, and training can be leveraged to enhance the healthcare services available to the community and allow for organizational polices to support **team-based care**. Such laws can help to facilitate interpersonal interactions between patients and healthcare providers which may prompt individual-level changes in knowledge, behaviors, and self-efficacy necessary to improve medication adherence.

## Federal and State Legal Framework

As explained in Chapter 2, under the 10th Amendment, states have the inherent authority to promote the public health, safety, and well-being of their populations (*Gibbons v. Ogden*, 1824; *Smith v. Turner*, 1849), and this power extends to the practice of medicine. State governments have a compelling interest in ensuring that the public is safe from the "incompetent, fraudulent or deceptive practice of medicine" (Richards, 1999). States accomplish this by regulating the practice of medicine through state practice acts and regulations promulgated by state Boards of Medicine, Nursing, Pharmacy, and other health professions that specify the requisite training, education, qualifications, and other factors necessary for professional licensure. The federal government has a larger role in ensuring medications and medical devices are safe and effective largely through the Federal Food, Drug, and Cosmetic Act of 2007, which authorizes the U.S. Food and Drug Administration (FDA) to regulate market access to safe drugs, medical devices, and other products (Federal Food, Drug, and Cosmetic Act, 2018). In addition, as authorized by the federal Controlled Substances Act of 1970, the U.S. Drug Enforcement Agency (DEA) places some limits on health providers' prescribing practices (Comprehensive Drug Abuse Prevention and Control Act of 1970, 21 U.S.C. 801 et seq). Other federal and state statutes and regulations also affect health professional practices. However, the laws just mentioned directly affect their scope of practice.

## State Scope of Practice Laws

All states and Washington, D.C. have enacted legislation and promulgated regulations that set forth the parameters for the practices of healthcare providers. NP scope of practice varies by state, with some states licensing qualified NPs as independent practitioners with full practice authority to "evaluate patients, diagnose, order and interpret diagnostic tests, prescribe medications, and treat patients," and other states requiring licensed NPs to practice in collaboration with or under the supervision of a licensed practicing physician (CDC, 2019b; American Association of Nurse Practitioners, 2018). In these states, the physician delegates certain medical practices to the NP either through a written collaborative agreement or oversight of the NPs patient care services. The scope of practice for licensed pharmacists also varies by state, with some states authorizing pharmacists with advanced training and certification to perform clinical services outside of their normal scope of practice either independently as clinical pharmacists or through a CPA with another healthcare practitioner (e.g., physician, NP) with prescribing authority (National Alliance of State Pharmacy Associations, n.d.).

## CONCLUSION

Public health law can be used to advance health equity, improve environments to make it easier for people to make healthy choices, enhance community linkages to clinical services, and strengthen healthcare systems. CHWs, pharmacists, and NPs are valued members of the healthcare workforce who can impact population health at multiple levels. Federal financing models and participatory involvement in developing state laws and policies addressing definitions, scope of practice, financing, certification, and training continue to shape these healthcare workforces. Scope of practice laws can help to facilitate interpersonal interactions between patients and healthcare providers, which can improve patient knowledge, behaviors, and self-efficacy.

## CHAPTER REVIEW

### Review Questions

1. What are two ways in which CHWs can impact chronic disease according to the SEM?
2. Which of the following public health law competencies are covered in this chapter?
   a. Implement the use of relevant legal information, tools, procedures, and remedies, including injunctions, closing orders, and abatement orders.
   b. Identify opportunities for a legal evaluation study to address existing legal, health, or other issues.

   c.  Collect and analyze qualitative and quantitative data using generally accepted research methodologies.

   d.  Integrate legal information into the exercise of professional public health judgment within the larger public health response.

   e.  Describe the protocol for contacting and best practices for engaging with legal and/or ethical advisors and other key public health law resources.

## Essay Questions

1. Compare and contrast state and federal legal frameworks in the role of healthcare providers in preventing chronic disease.
2. Discuss three ways law is used to promote health equity in chronic disease prevention and control.

## Internet Activities

1. Law and the Social Ecological Model
   - Research your state legislative website. Find one chronic disease-related bill that may impact one or more levels of the SEM.
2. Collaborative Practice
   - Find the Minnesota Pharmacy Practice Act and Board of Pharmacy Regulations to see if collaborative practice between pharmacists and nurse practitioners is authorized and under what circumstances.
3. CHW Policy and Community-Clinical Linkages
   - Conduct a literature review on CHW-based policy interventions for improving community-clinical linkages.

## REFERENCES

Albritton, E. (2016). *How states can fund community health workers through Medicaid to improve people's health, decrease costs, and reduce disparities.* Families USA.

American Association of Nurse Practitioners. (2018). *State practice environment.* https://www.aanp.org/advocacy/state/state-practice-environment

Braveman, P., Arkin, E., Orleans, T., Proctor, D., & Plough, A. (2017). *What is health equity?* https://www.rwjf.org/en/library/research/2017/05/what-is-health-equity-.html

Center for Health Care Strategies. (2018). *Addressing social determinants of health via Medicaid managed care contracts and section 1115 demonstrations.* https://www.chcs.org/media/Addressing-SDOH-Medicaid-Contracts-1115-Demonstrations-121118.pdf

Centers for Disease Control and Prevention. (2016). *State law fact sheet: A summary of state community health worker laws.* https://www.cdc.gov/dhdsp/pubs/docs/chw_state_laws.pdf

Centers for Disease Control and Prevention. (2019a). *National Center for Chronic Disease Prevention and Health Promotion.* https://www.cdc.gov/chronicdisease/index.htm

Centers for Disease Control and Prevention. (2019b). *Practical implications of state law amendments granting nurse practitioner full practice authority.* https://www.cdc.gov/dhdsp/pubs/docs/Nurses_Case_Study-508.pdf

Centers for Medicare & Medicaid Services. (n.d.). *Section 1332: State innovation waivers.* 42 U.S.C. 1315a (2018). https://www.cms.gov/cciio/programs-and-initiatives/state-innovation-waivers/section_1332_state_innovation_waivers-.html

Federal Comprehensive Drug Abuse Prevention and Control Act of 1970, 21 U.S.C. § 801 et seq.

Federal Food, Drug, and Cosmetic Act of 2007, 21 U.S.C. § 301 et seq.

*Gibbons v. Ogden,* 22 U.S. 1 (1824).

Institute for Public Health Innovation. (2018). *Community health worker—Accountable health communities.* (2018). https://www.institutephi.org/careers/chw02-05-2018

Jones, C. P. (2000). Levels of racism: A theoretic framework and a gardener's tale. *American Journal of Public Health, 90*(8), 1212–1215. https://doi.org/10.2105/ajph.90.8.1212

Medicaid.gov. (n.d.). *Managed care.* https://www.medicaid.gov/medicaid/managed-care/index.html

National Alliance of State Pharmacy Associations. (n.d.). *Pharmacist prescribing: Statewide protocols and more.* https://naspa.us/resource/swp

Patient Protection and Affordable Care Act, 42 U.S.C. § 18001 et seq.

Ransom, M. M. (Ed.). (2016). *Public health law competency model: Version 1.0.* https://www.cdc.gov/phlp/docs/phlcm-v1.pdf

Ransom, M. M., Ramanathan, T., & Yassine, B. (Eds.). (2018). *The legal epidemiology competency model: Version 1.0.* https://www.cdc.gov/phlp/publications/topic/resources/legalepimodel/ index.html

Richards, E. P. (1999). The police power and the regulation of medical practice: A historical review and guide for medical licensing board regulation of physicians in ERISA-qualified managed care organizations. *Annals of Health Law, 8*(1), 1–37. (PMID: 10622904).

*Smith v. Turner,* 48 U.S. 283 (1849).

Title XIX of the Social Security Amendments of 1965, 42 U.S.C. § 1396 et seq.

## Additional Resources

- About Chronic Diseases (CDC) https://www.cdc.gov/chronicdisease/about/index.htm
- Addressing Health Disparities in Diabetes (CDC) https://www.cdc.gov/diabetes/disparities.html
- Public Health Grand Rounds (CDC) http://www.cdc.gov/cdcgrandrounds/archives/2014/oct2014.htm
- Affordable Care Act (CMS) https://www.healthcare.gov/glossary/affordable-care-act/
- Public Health Law Academy (CDC) https://www.cdc.gov/phlp/publications/topic/phlacademy.html
- Medicaid Program History (CMS) https://www.medicaid.gov/about-us/program-history/index.html

### Hypothetical Case Study #1

- Community Health Workers Community Member Section (APHA) https://www.apha.org/apha-communities/member-sections/community-health-workers
- Community Health Worker Toolkit (CDC) https://www.cdc.gov/dhdsp/pubs/toolkits/chw-toolkit.htm

### Hypothetical Case Study #2

- A Guide for Public Health: Partnering with Pharmacists in the Prevention and A Guide for Public Health: Partnering with Pharmacists in the Prevention and Control of Chronic Diseases (CDC) http://www.cdc.gov/dhdsp/programs/spha/docs/pharmacist_guide.pdf
- Collaborative Practice Agreements and Pharmacists' Patient Care Process: A Resource for Pharmacists (CDC) https://www.cdc.gov/dhdsp/pubs/docs/Translational_Tools_Pharmacists.pdf
- Pharmacy Resources Toolkit (CDC) https://www.cdc.gov/dhdsp/pubs/toolkits/pharmacy.htm
- Collaborative Drug Therapy Management: Case Studies of Three Community-Based Models of Care (PCD) https://www.cdc.gov/pcd/issues/2015/14_0504.htm
- Pharmacist Collaborative Practice Agreements: Public Health Law Academy training (Changelab Solutions) https://www.changelabsolutions.org/product/pharmacist-collaborative-practice-agreements

# 9

# Intentional Injury Prevention and Control

## Adolescent Sexual Violence and the Law

Keri McDonald Hill, LeKara Simmons, and Daniella Thorne

## Learning Objectives

By the end of this chapter, the reader will be able to:

- Explain sexual violence.
- Discuss varying state legal approaches to preventing adolescent sexual violence.
- Characterize sexual consent laws for minors.
- Analyze the major provisions of Erin's law and its intent.

## Key Terminology

**Consent:** All partners freely choose, with clear understanding, to engage in a specific activity, at the moment the activity will take place (Sexual Trauma Services of the Midlands, 2016).

**Erin's Law:** Public schools in each state where Erin's Law has been adopted are required to implement child sexual abuse prevention programming.

**Mandated reporter:** A person who, because of their profession, is legally required to report any suspicion of child abuse or neglect to the relevant authorities ("What is a mandated reporter?" n.d.).

**Rape:** Penetration, no matter how slight, of the vagina or anus with any body part or object, or oral penetration by a sex organ of another person, without the consent of the victim.

**Sexting:** Sending sexually explicit digital images, videos, text, and/or emails, usually sent through a mobile device.

**Sexual assault:** A nonconsensual sexual act proscribed by federal, Tribal, or state law, including when the victim lacks capacity to consent.

**Sexual battery:** An unwanted form of contact with an intimate part of the body that is made for purposes of sexual arousal, sexual gratification, or sexual abuse.

---

The authors graciously thank colleagues from the Georgia Campaign for Adolescent Power and Potential who provided support, insight, and expertise that greatly assisted bringing this chapter to fruition.

**Sexual violence:** Use of force or manipulation into unwanted sexual activity without consent.

**Statutory rape:** Sexual intercourse with a person under the age of lawful consent.

## Public Health Law Competencies

This chapter addresses the following competencies from the Public Health Law Competency Model (PHLCM; Ransom, 2016).

**1.2** Identify and apply public health laws pertinent to practitioner's jurisdiction, agency, program, and profession.

**2.2** Identify law-based tools and enforcement procedures to address day-to-day (nonemergency) public health issues.

**2.3** Recognize the legal authority and limits of critical system partners and others who influence health outcomes.

---

### Spark Question

What is one law you would recommend to address adolescent sexual violence in your community? Why do you believe such a law is necessary?

---

## INTRODUCTION

Violence can affect everyone at all stages of life, regardless of age, gender identity, race, or economic status. Both unintentional injuries and those caused by acts of violence, referred to as "intentional injuries," are among the top 15 killers for Americans of all ages. They are the leading cause of death and disability worldwide, and specifically a leading cause of premature death. In the first half of life, more Americans die from violence and injuries than from any other cause, including cancer, HIV, or the flu (Centers for Disease Control and Prevention [CDC], n.d.).

Beyond their immediate health consequences, injuries and violence have a significant impact on public health and well-being and exact enormous psychological, social, and economic costs. Studies show the effect of injuries and violence contribute to premature death, years of potential life lost, disability, poor mental health, high medical costs, and loss of productivity (*Healthy People*, n.d.).

This chapter focuses on the role of law in addressing an emerging issue in violence and injury prevention and control as identified by the Department of Health and Human Services' (DHHS) *Healthy People* 2020 initiative: sexual violence among youth. This chapter explores varying state legal approaches to prevent adolescent sexual violence and characterizes sexual consent laws for minors. Sexual violence is considered an intentional injury, that is widespread in the United States, and many survivors are under the age of 18 when they first experience it. According to the National Intimate Partner and Sexual Violence Survey (NISVS), sexual violence is common among youth and is usually committed by someone the victim knows. Violence in youth, without appropriate trauma-informed interventions, can result in immediate and lifelong consequences, including physical, emotional, behavioral, and social challenges, as well as suffering future abuse or continuing the cycle in adulthood by abusing others.

## SEXUAL VIOLENCE

**Sexual violence** is the use of force or manipulation into unwanted sexual activity without consent. **Consent** is best defined as "all partners freely choose, with a clear understanding, to

## BOX 9.1  SEXUAL VIOLENCE HEALTH DISPARITIES

"More than one in three women and nearly one in four men have experienced sexual violence involving physical contact at some point in their lives. Nearly one in five women and one in 38 men have experienced completed or attempted rape in their lifetimes" (Smith et al., 2019).

Moreover, there is higher risk of sexual violence for the LGBTQ community, individuals with disabilities, individuals who are experiencing homelessness, individuals who are incarcerated, and previous survivors of sexual violence.

engage in a specific activity, at the moment the activity will take place" (Sexual Trauma Services of the Midlands, 2016). Consent cannot be given if any party is under the state's legal age of consent, or the influence of alcohol and/or drugs. Forms of sexual violence include forced penetration, incest, unwanted sexual contact/touching, sexual harassment, sexual exploitation, showing one's genitals or naked body to other(s) without consent, masturbating in public, and watching someone in a private act without their knowledge or permission (National Sexual Violence Resource Center, 2010).

Sexual violence has plagued institutions, communities, and nations since the beginning of time. As discussed in Boxes 9.1 and 9.2, some populations, including the LGBTQ community and women of color, have historically been disproportionately impacted. During the last decade, national attention has been given to sexual violence prevention in the wake of the #MeToo movement and **Erin's Law** legislation. Survivors have spoken their truth and state laws have been strengthened to penalize offenders and bolster prevention education in school settings.

## VARIABILITY OF SEXUAL VIOLENCE LAWS

Although the current definition of **rape** applies nationally, it is important for public health practitioners to know that states have varied definitions, categories, and penalties for sexual

## BOX 9.2  RAPE: RACE AND GENDER

"The violation of a woman forcibly and against her will" was the definition of rape Colonial Americans primarily relied on. Later, the definition changed to include only free women or exclusively White women capable of being raped, with the exclusion of enslaved women from legal protection (Barnes, 2018).

The 1865 to 1870 Reconstruction Amendments granted Black women the protection under the law and the right to bring rape charges against White men. White supremacist groups refused to accept these changes and continued sexual violence attacks, and resistance continued into the Civil Rights era (Barnes, 2018).

The 2012 "Rape is Rape" campaign demanded the definition be changed. At the time, **sexual assault** was based on the definition "carnal knowledge of a female, forcibly and against her will." The definition included only "the slightest penetration of a female (vagina) by the sexual organ of the male (penis)" (Federal Bureau of Investigation [FBI], 2004, p. 19). The definition excluded sexual assault of male victims by female offenders, and other acts of sexual assault, and contributed to the underreporting of sexual assault cases (Barnes, 2018).

The U.S. Department of Justice's definition of "rape" ultimately changed to "the penetration, no matter how slight, of the vagina or anus, with any body part or object, or oral penetration by a sex organ of another person, without the consent of the victim" (U.S. Department of Justice, 2012, p. 1).

violence. These variations contribute to the complexities associated with addressing sexual violence, as described here:

- **California**: "Rape" falls under sexual assault, which includes offenses such as groping and other unwanted sexual contact (California Rape Laws, n.d.).
- **Florida**: "Rape" is currently an offense under sexual battery and there is no longer a separate legal definition of rape.
- **Montana**: Montana categorizes "rape" as sexual intercourse without consent and states that a person who knowingly has sexual intercourse without consent with another person commits the offense of sexual intercourse without consent. The penalty for sexual assault without consent shall be punished by life imprisonment or by imprisonment in the state prison for a term of not less than 2 years or more than 100 years ("Sexual Intercourse Without Consent," n.d.).
- **Kansas**: "Rape" is defined as knowingly engaging in sexual intercourse with a victim who does not consent to the sexual intercourse. The penalty in Kansas for rape is considered a severity level 1, person felony (Sex Offenses, 2012).

## Sexual Battery

**Sexual battery** may occur whether the victim is clothed or not ("Sexual Battery Law and Legal Definition," n.d.). Like rape, the laws will vary from state to state. In Georgia, sexual battery is defined as physical contact with the intimate parts of the body without consent, which is considered a misdemeanor. In Indiana, sexual battery is defined as a victim who is "compelled to submit to the touching" by use of threat of force or a victim who is mentally disabled and cannot consent ("Sexual Assault Statutes in the United States Chart," 2016).

## Sexting

**Sexting** is defined as "the sending or receiving of sexually explicit text messages including the digital recording of naked, semi-naked, sexually suggestive or explicit images and their distribution via mobile phone messaging, email or social network sites" (Arthur, 2019). Some states include laws that criminalize sexting due to specific circumstances. These laws vary per state.

According to most state laws, if sexually explicit material is sent to a person under the age of 18 years, it is considered child pornography ("Sexting Legal Consequences," n.d.). Depending on the state, the penalty for this offense may be up to 5 years in prison with a potential $1,000 to $10,000 in fines for first offenses ("Sexting Legal Consequences," n.d.). However, there are some states who have adopted sexting laws that indicate specifically targeted images sent between or among youth. For example, Connecticut's sexting law targets teens (anyone between 13 and 17 years) who either send or possess nude or obscene photos of either themselves or another teenager. The Connecticut law also makes distinctions between the ages of the sender and the recipient, penalizing senders between the ages of 13 and 15 who send pictures of themselves, and recipients between the ages of 13 and 17 who receive any images. Nonetheless, state laws differ significantly. Louisiana, for example, prohibits anyone under the age of 17 from sending or keeping explicit photographs, while Texas allows an exception for sexting if a minor sexts with another minor who is no more than two years older or younger and the two are dating (Theoharis, n.d.). Consequently, unlike other sexual assault offenses, with sexting, consent of receiving or sending a video is not a valid defense ("Sexting Legal Consequences," n.d.).

## Internet & Sex Trafficking

Most youth use the internet daily (U.S. Department of Education [US DoE], 2019). Youth between the ages of three to 18 reported a higher percentage of access to internet use at home in

2017 than in 2010 (64% versus 58%; U.S. Department of Commerce 2018). This access allows children and youth to access vast amounts of information and forms of entertainment. Children and youth often use the internet to complete schoolwork, play online games, and watch films, but many also use it to maintain relationships and meet new people for friendship.

"Sex trafficking" of a minor is when a sexual act is performed by someone under the age of 18 years in exchange for an item of value. Sex trafficking criminals use coercive measures and sexually exploitive practices such as violence, threats, lies, and offering money and drugs to compel or force youth to engage in sexual acts that are unwanted and against their will (The Child Advocacy Center, n.d.; www.caclapeer.org/lapeercacblog). It is more common for children to become victims of sex trafficking by being tricked by traffickers who present themselves as a friend, boyfriend, or protective employer. Others become child sex trafficking victims by being kidnapped or sold by their parents (de Chesnay, 2013). The emergence of social media networks and other online communities have increased access to youth making it easier for traffickers to find victims (The Child Advocacy Center, n.d.). For example, children may encounter online predators who use the internet to lure victims through online chat rooms, social networking sites, and unsolicited emails. These channels allow individuals to sexually abuse victims of sex trafficking without direct physical contact, such as by coercing, directing a child to perform sexual acts through a webcam, or witnessing sexual activity by adults (U.S. Department of Justice , 2009).

There are federal laws that address sex trafficking. For example, The Trafficking Victims Protection Act of 2000 and its subsequent reauthorizations define human trafficking as sex trafficking in which a commercial sex act is induced by force, fraud, or coercion, or in which the person induced to perform such act has not attained 18 years of age. State laws also exist, but vary across states in terms of definitions, penalties, and enforcement priorities. (University of Southern California, n.d.).

## SEXUAL VIOLENCE PREVENTION EDUCATION

According to the CDC, the public health approach to addressing sexual violence includes (a) promoting social norms that protect against violence, (b) teaching skills to prevent sexual violence, (c) providing opportunities to empower and support girls and women, (d) creating protective environments, and (e) supporting victims/survivors to lessen harms (CDC, 2019).

Like sexual violence laws and definitions, requirements for sexual violence prevention education vary throughout the United States. However, sexual violence education and prevention has been bolstered with the introduction of *Erin's Law*. Legislators named the law after Erin Merryn, a child abuse survivor who continues to advocate for sexual abuse education in schools. In each state where it has been adopted, Erin's Law requires all public schools in that state implement an age-appropriate, prevention-oriented child sexual abuse program (Erin's Law, 2020). Erin's Law is limited to sexual abuse education but does not include other sexual violence prevention topics such as boundary setting, sexting, online safety, healthy relationships, human trafficking, effective communication, sexualization in the media, and gender stereotypes. Additional sexual violence and life-skills topics can be often found embedded in sex education and HIV-related laws and policies. Table 9.1 highlights additional topics required by state sex education and HIV education mandates.

### HYPOTHETICAL CASE STUDY #1: THE ROMEO AND JULIET CLAUSE

David is a health educator at a local health department. The county runs a teen clinic every Tuesday and Thursday evening to increase access to clinical services after school hours. Haley, age 15, comes in requesting information on the various forms of hormonal birth control. During the discussion, Haley shares that she has been engaging in sexual intercourse with her partner, Jordan. David provides Haley the requested information and continues in casual conversation about her plans for the upcoming weekend. Haley informs David she is going to the movies to celebrate Jordan's 18th birthday.

The legal age of consent in David's state is 16. However, there is a *Romeo and Juliet* clause in the state statutory rape law.

1. Is it possible for Haley to legally engage in *consensual* sex? Why or why not?
2. What is a Romeo and Juliet clause? How might it impact the situation described in Case Study #1?
3. Are you mandated by law to report the Haley and Jordan's age difference to your supervisor?

## Age of Consent, Statutory Rape, and Romeo & Juliet Clause

All states have an established minimum age for an individual to legally consent to sex (Bierie & Budd, 2018). The legal age of consent varies from state to state for persons aged 16 to 18 years old nationwide (U.S. Age of Consent Map, 2020). Understanding that the age of consent varies from state to state, the laws related to **statutory rape** will as a result vary. Table 9.2 shows a chart listing each state's age of consent.

Age of consent laws prohibit sexual intercourse with persons under a particular age, stating that no individual can agree to engage in sex until they are of the legal age of consent (Kern, 2013). Violations to age of consent statutes are referred to as "statutory rape," which is "the carnal knowledge of a person who is deemed underage as proscribed by statute and who is therefore presumed to be incapable of consenting to sexual activity" (Catherine, 2003). Statutory rape laws prohibit sexual intercourse with an individual who is below the age of consent defined by statute regardless of whether or not the activity is against the victim's will (Flynn, 2013). As discussed in Box 9.3, these laws are gender-neutral, and are designed to protect minors from

### TABLE 9.1 Topics Mandated by Law to Be Included in School-Based Sex and HIV Education

| TOPICS | NUMBER OF STATES |
|---|---|
| Prevention of teen dating violence and sexual violence | 38 + D.C. |
| Require provision of information on preventing, recognizing, and responding to teen dating violence and sexual violence | 37 + D.C. |
| Skills for healthy romantic and sexual relationships | 35 + D.C. |
| Information on healthy relationships | 31 + D.C. |
| Instruction on self-control and decision-making about sexuality | 26 + D.C. |
| Provision of information on asserting personal boundaries and refusing unwanted sexual advances | 24 + D.C. |
| The importance of consent to sexual activity to be covered | 8 |

*Source:* Guttmacher Institute. (2020). *Sex and HIV education.* https://www.guttmacher.org/print/state-policy/explore/sex-and-hiv-education

## TABLE 9.2  United States: Age of Consent

| STATE | AGE OF CONSENT |
|---|---|
| Alabama, Alaska, Arkansas, Connecticut, District of Columbia, Georgia, Hawaii, Indiana, Iowa, Kansas, Kentucky, Maine, Maryland, Massachusetts, Michigan, Minnesota, Mississippi, Montana, Nebraska, Nevada, New Hampshire, New Jersey, New Mexico, North Carolina, Ohio, Oklahoma, Pennsylvania, Rhode Island, South Carolina, South Dakota, Vermont, Washington, West Virginia, Wyoming | 16 |
| Colorado, Illinois, Louisiana, Missouri, New York, Texas | 17 |
| Arizona, California, Delaware, Florida, Idaho, North Dakota, Oregon, Tennessee, Utah, Virginia, Wisconsin | 18 |

*Source:* United States Age of Consent Map. (2020). https://www.ageofconsent.net/states

---

### BOX 9.3  STATUTORY RAPE: GENDER & AGE

Traditionally, society viewed statutory rape through a gender-specific lens, allowing for an offense to be considered as statutory rape only when an adult male victimized a minor female, in response to concerns such as teenage pregnancy and vulnerability of young girls. Additionally, the discussion was only around younger adolescents (ages 10 to 12 years) and excluded older teens.

The crime is now prosecuted as a gender-neutral, strict liability offense given the minor's incapability to consent to sexual activity with an adult (Klein & Cooper, 2017; Tenzer, 2019).

---

coercive and involuntary sexual activity perpetrated by adults or by peers (Kern, 2013). The main premise is that, based on their neurological development, minors lack the cognitive capacity to effectively guard themselves from manipulation by adults, and this issue is particularly pronounced with the increase in age differences between sexual partners (Bierie & Budd, 2018).

Adolescence is a period of exploration, which includes sexual exploration and experimentation on varying levels. Although some forms of exploring can be healthy, the regulation of sexual activity among adolescents can be difficult to oversee (Klein & Cooper, 2017). In 2017, the percentage of high school students who reported ever having sexual intercourse was 39.5% (CDC, 2017). National statistics also demonstrate a vast majority of these sexual encounters to be deemed by teens as consensual. The reality that sexual behaviors between adolescents are common and most teens believe these actions to be consensual does not mean that these acts are lacking in exploitation or that these behaviors are healthy, but the public is skeptical that sexual encounters between youth of similar ages should all be considered criminal (Bierie & Budd, 2018). The sexual behavior may not involve physical force, but due to the minor status of the younger party, consent cannot legally be given, which allows for prosecution of the older party for sexual offense against a minor (Klein & Cooper, 2017). The disconnect between public opinion, the law, and the reality of trends in adolescent sexual activity places some teens in jeopardy of being charged with statutory rape and being labeled as sex offenders (Kern, 2013). To prevent unfair persecution, most states have age-gap provisions that provide legal protections through exceptions to statutory rape (Flynn, 2013). These laws are often referred to as "Romeo and Juliet clauses" (Kern, 2013).

## BOX 9.4 JUDICIAL DISCRETION: ROMEO AND JULIET CLAUSES

Many jurisdictions have been thought to be highly selective in reviewing the large number of potential cases from which to "pick and choose" to pursue. In some states it is found to be more common for only males to be prosecuted, though both minors are both victims and offenders. Disproportionate convictions of minority men have also been cited (Kern, 2013).

A 17-year-old engaging in sexual activity with their 16-year-old partner may be legally permitted, but once the person turns 18, sexual encounters with their partner may be considered illegal under the definition above. This means that in Case Study #1, Haley, age 15, is not able to *legally* consent to sexual intercourse with her partner, Jordan.

Romeo and Juliet clauses mitigate penalties associated with teens who engage in sexual activity when one is below the age of consent. Many states use a version of a Romeo and Juliet clause associated with their statutory rape law. The term "Romeo and Juliet" is often used interchangeably with "age-gap provision" (Kern, 2013). For instance, if Haley were 16, the age of consent in her respective state, she would be able to *legally* consent to sexual intercourse with Jordan. Since there is a Romeo and Juliet clause in their state, 16-year-old Haley and 17-year-old Jordan's sexual encounters would be *legally* consensual and prevent Jordan from statutory rape violations after his 18th birthday.

## Mandatory Reporting Laws

A **mandated reporter** is a person who, because of their profession, is legally required to report any suspicion of child abuse or neglect to the relevant authorities ("What Is a Mandated Reporter?", n.d.). Mandatory reporting laws are crucial toward the protection of young people in such cases. Mandated reporting procedures vary not only by state, but also by institutions. Many institutions have internal policies and procedures for handling reports of abuse, and these usually require the person who suspects abuse to notify the head of the institution that abuse or neglect has been discovered or is suspected and needs to be reported to child protective services or other appropriate authorities (Child Welfare Information Gateway, 2019).

Statutes in 32 States, the District of Columbia, and the Virgin Islands provide procedures that must be followed in those cases. In 18 States, the District of Columbia, and the Virgin Islands, any staff member who suspects abuse must notify the head of the institution when the staff member feels abuse or possible abuse should be reported to an appropriate authority. In nine States, the District of Columbia, and the Virgin Islands, the staff member who suspects abuse notifies the head of the institution first, and then the head or their designee is required to make the report. In nine States, the individual reporter must make the report to the appropriate child protection authority first and then notify the institution that a report has been made. Laws in 17 States, the District of Columbia, and the Virgin Islands make clear that, regardless of any policies within the organization, the mandatory reporter is not relieved (Child Welfare Information Gateway, 2019). Moreover, in most cases where sexual abuse may be present or possible, mandated reporters must be able to recognize the signs of minor sexual abuse. Some signs of sexual abuse of a minor may include recurring pain during urination or bowel movements, sexually transmitted diseases, anxiety and depression, rebellion or withdrawal, and poor self-esteem ("Identifying Child Sexual Abuse," n.d.).

Based on the mandated reporter definition, David is not required to report Jordan and Hailey's relationship. Mandated reporting is applicable only when there is suspicion of child abuse or neglect. Hailey did not disclose any act of sexual violence while discussing birth control methods with David. If she did, David would follow his organization's mandated reporting protocol. As a youth-serving public health professional, it is necessary to be well informed of your organization's mandating reporting protocol.

## CONCLUSION

Every young person possesses tremendous potential to grow into their own and impact the communities around them. But all too often their potential goes unrecognized, untapped, or gets lost in all the challenges they face, like fragile family situations, anxiety, academic pressure, unhealthy and risky behavior, and complicated relationships with their peers and adults. As discussed in this chapter, one emerging challenge for public health and public health law is ensuring we are using law as a tool to help protect our youth from sexual violence. Varying laws, decades of stereotypes, and political influences make legal responses to sexual violence a complicated issue. It is promising that the legal definitions associated with sexual violence continue to become more inclusive. However, highly publicized cases such as Hollywood's Harvey Weinstein, Bill Cosby, and Jeffrey Epstein remind us there is work still to be done. Legislation to address sexual violence topics and issues, such as Erin's Law, is one step to ensure that youth and young adults have the knowledge and skills to create a society that is free of sexual violence.

## CHAPTER REVIEW

### Review Questions

1. According to the CDC, the public health approach to addressing sexual violence includes opportunities to empower and support girls and women.
   True/False

2. When it comes to sexting, all state laws make a distinction between the age of the sender and the recipient.
   True/False

3. In the states that have adopted it, what does Erin's Law require? (short answer)

### Essay Questions

1. Using the public health approach outlined by CDC, develop a description of a law or policy that you might implement to address adolescent sexual violence in your community. Be sure to include language describing the intent of the new law and the specific population the law is meant to benefit.

2. Discuss how adolescent sexual violence laws are like adolescent sexual reproductive rights. How are they different?

## Internet Activities

1.  Did you know the #MeToo movement was "founded in 2006 to help survivors of sexual violence, particularly Black women and girls, and other young women of color from low wealth communities, find pathways to healing?" (Me too, 2018). How has the movement changed over time? Find out more information at https://metoomvmt.org
2.  Use the following site to help you find the statutory rape laws and clauses in your home state: https://legaldictionary.net/romeo-and-juliet-laws
3.  Is your state one of the 37 states where Erin's Law is mandated for age-appropriate sexual abuse awareness education in public schools? Visit http://www.erinslaw.org to find out.

## REFERENCES

Arthur, R. (2019). Regulating youth sexuality, agency and citizenship: Developing a coherent criminal justice response to youth sexting. *King's Law Journal, 30*(3), 377–395. https://doi.org/10.1080/09615768.2019.1686229

Barnes, E. (2018). Justice at what cost? As today, accusations of rape in 19th-Century America inevitably, and repeatedly, met with harsh backlashes against the victims. *History Today, 68*(12), 8–11. https://www.historytoday.com/history-matters/justice-what-cost

Bierie, D., & Budd, K. (2018). Romeo, Juliet, and statutory rape. *Sexual Abuse, 30*(3), 296–321. https://doi.org/10.1177/1079063216658451

California Rape Laws. (n.d.). https://statelaws.findlaw.com/california-law/california-rape-laws.html

Catherine, L. C. (2003). On statutory rape, strict liability, and the public welfare offense model. *American University Law Review, 53*(2). https://ssrn.com/abstract=907682

Centers for Disease Control and Prevention. (2017). *Youth risk behavior survey.* https://www.cdc.gov/healthyyouth/data/yrbs/index.htm

Centers for Disease Control and Prevention. (2019). *Sexual violence.* https://www.cdc.gov/violenceprevention/sexualviolence/index.html

Centers for Disease Control and Prevention. (n.d.). *Injury prevention & control.* https://www.cdc.gov/injury/wisqars/overview/key_data.html

The Child Advocacy Center. (n.d.). *Human trafficking and the internet.* https://www.caclapeer.org/lapeercacblog/human-trafficking-the-internet

Child Welfare Information Gateway. (2019). *Mandatory reporters of child abuse and neglect.* https://www.childwelfare.gov/pubPDFs/manda.pdf#page=5&view=Summaries%20of%20State%20laws

Darkness to Light. (n.d.). *Identifying child sexual abuse.* https://www.d2l.org/get-help/identifying-abuse

De Chesnay, M. (2013). *Sex trafficking: A clinical guide for nurses.* Springer Publishing Company.

Erin's Law. (2020). *What is Erin's Law.* http://www.erinslaw.org/erins-law

Federal Bureau of Investigation. (2014). *Frequently asked questions about the change in the UCR definition of rape.* https://ucr.fbi.gov/recent-program-updates/new-rape-definition-frequently-asked-questions

Flynn, D. (2013). All the kids are doing it: The unconstitutionality of enforcing statutory rape laws against children and teenagers. *New England Law Review, 47*(3), 681–713. https://heinonline.org/HOL/LandingPage?handle=hein.journals/newlr47&div=37&id=&page=

Georgia Coalition for Adolescent Power and Potential. (n.d.). https://www.gcapp.org/sites/default/files/images/GCAPP%202018%20Annual%20Report.pdf

Guttmacher Institute. (2020). *Sex and HIV education.* https://www.guttmacher.org/print/state-policy/explore/sex-and-hiv-education

HealthyPeople. (n.d.). *Injury and violence prevention.* https://www.healthypeople.gov/2020/topics-objectives/topic/injury-and-violence-prevention

Identifying Child Sexual Abuse. (n.d.). https://www.d2l.org/get-help/identifying-abuse

Kern, J. (2013). Trends in teen sex are changing, but are Minnesota's Romeo and Juliet laws? *William Mitchell Law Review, 39*(5), 1606–1622. https://open.mitchellhamline.edu/cgi/viewcontent.cgi?article=1530&context=wmlr

Klein, J. L., & Cooper, D. T. (2017). Do perceptions of statutory rape vary based on offender and victim pairings? Testing the effects of race and gender. *Applied Psychology in Criminal Justice, 13*(1), 33–50. http://www.apcj.org/journal/index.php?mode=view&item=122

Me Too. (2018). *History and vision.* https://metoomvmt.org/about/#history

National Sexual Violence Resource Center. (2010). *Fact sheet.* https://www.nsvrc.org/sites/default/files/Publications_NSVRC_Factsheet_What-is-sexual-violence_1.pdf

Ransom, M. M. (2016, April). *Public health law competency model: Version 1.0.* CDC. https://www.cdc.gov/phlp/docs/phlcm-v1.pdf

Sex Offenses, Kansas. Stat. § 21-5503 (2012). http://www.kslegislature.org/li_2012/b2011_12/statute/021_000_0000_chapter/021_055_0000_article/021_055_0003_section/021_055_0003_k

Sexting Legal Consequences. (n.d.). https://www.hg.org/legal-articles/sexting-legal-consequences-39370

Sexual Assault Statutes in the United States Chart. (2016). https://ndaa.org/wp-content/uploads/sexual-assault-chart.pdf

Sexual Battery Law and Legal Definition. (n.d.). https://definitions.uslegal.com/s/sexual-battery

Sexual Intercourse Without Consent. (n.d.). https://leg.mt.gov/bills/mca/45/5/45-5-503.htm

Sexual Trauma Services of the Midlands. (2016). *Building healthier communities.* https://www.stsm.org/

Smith, S. G., Zhang, X., Basile, K. C., Merrick, M. T., Wang, J., Kresnow, M., & Chen, J. (2019). *The national intimate partner and sexual violence survey: 2015 data brief—Updated release.* https://www.cdc.gov/violenceprevention/pdf/2015data-brief508.pdf

Tenzer, L. Y. (2019). #METOO, statutory rape laws, and the persistence of gender stereotypes. *Utah Law Review, 1,* 117–157. https://dc.law.utah.edu/cgi/viewcontent.cgi?article=1200&context=ulr

Theoharis, M. (n.d.). *Teen sexting: Learn the details about teen sexting laws and penalties and get specific information about your state's laws.* https://www.criminaldefenselawyer.com/crime-penalties/juvenile/sexting.htm

University of Southern California. (n.d.). *Technology and human trafficking.* https://technologyandtrafficking.usc.edu

U.S. Age of Consent Map. (2020). https://www.ageofconsent.net/states

U.S. Bureau of Labor and Statistics. (2015). *Average hours per weekday spent by high school students in various activities.* http://www.bls.gov/tus/charts/students.htm

U.S. Department of Commerce. (2018). *Census Bureau, Current Population Survey, October 2010 & November 2017. Digest of Education Statistics 2018, Table 702.35.* https://www.census.gov/programs-surveys/cps.html

U.S. Department of Education. (2019). *The Condition of Education 2019 (NCES 2019-144).* National Center for Education Statistics. https://nces.ed.gov/programs/coe/pdf/coe_cch.pdf

U.S. Department of Justice. (2009). Criminal Division. Global symposium for examining the relationship between online and offline offenses and preventing the sexual exploitation of children. https://www.justice.gov/sites/default/files/criminal-ceos/legacy/2012/03/19/SymposiumReport20090519.pdf

U.S. Department of Justice. (2012). Attorney General Eric Holder announces revisions to the uniform crime report's definition of rape. *Justice News.* https://www.justice.gov/opa/pr/attorney-general-eric-holder-announces-revisions-uniform-crime-report-s-definition-rape

What Is a Mandated Reporter? (n.d.). https://www.socialworkdegreeguide.com/faq/what-is-a-mandated-reporter

## Additional Resources

- **Society for Adolescent Health and Medicine**
  https://www.adolescenthealth.org/Resources/Clinical-Care-Resources/Sexual-Reproductive-Health/Clinical-Care-Guidelines/Sexual-Violence.aspx
- **The Georgia Coalition for Adolescent Power and Potential**
  https://www.gcapp.org
- **Preventing Sexual Violence (CDC)**
  https://www.cdc.gov/violenceprevention/sexualviolence/fastfact.html
  https://grassrootschange.net

# 10

# Unintentional Injury Prevention and Control

## Opioid Use Disorder

Mara Howard-Williams, Corey Davis, and Harry Nelson

## Learning Objectives

By the end of this chapter, the reader will be able to:

- Describe the impact of public health law as both a barrier to and facilitator of evidence-based responses to reducing opioid-related harm.
- Identify the legal concepts of nondiscrimination in access to treatment for chronic pain and substance use disorder.
- Recognize selected legal frameworks for regulating prescribing, overdose prevention, and substance use disorder treatment.

## Key Terminology

**Americans With Disability Act (ADA):** A federal law, passed in 1990, that prohibits discrimination against people with certain disabilities.

**Medications for opioid use disorder:** Prescription medications that have been shown to reduce the negative impacts of opioid use disorder. There are currently three such medications approved by the Food and Drug Administration (FDA): buprenorphine, methadone, and naltrexone (Substance Abuse and Mental Health Services Administration [SAMHSA], n.d.-a).

**Naloxone:** A medication that reverses the respiratory depression and other physical symptoms associated with opioid overdose (Chamberlain & Klein, 1994).

**Overdose Good Samaritan Laws:** This term refers to laws that shield someone from being arrested or prosecuted for certain charges if they summon emergency assistance for a suspected overdose. In many cases, these protections also apply to the person who overdosed.

## Public Health Law Competencies

This chapter addresses the following competencies from the Public Health Law Competency Model (PHLCM; Ransom, 2016).

**1.2** Identify and apply public health laws pertinent to practitioner's jurisdiction, agency, program, and profession.

**2.2** Identify law-based tools and enforcement procedures to address day-to-day (nonemergency) public health issues.

**2.3** Recognize the legal authority and limits of critical system partners and others who influence health outcomes.

---

**Spark Questions**

1. What are some of the public health legal responses to the crisis of opioid-related harm?
2. To what extent does the response to the crisis of opioid-related harm reflect a shift in attitudes toward harm reduction?
3. How does public health law interact with other areas of law in the context of drug-related harm?
4. Do you think opioid use disorder should be a disability?

---

## INTRODUCTION

Injuries that are unplanned and generally preventable are known as "unintentional injuries." According to the Centers for Disease Control and Prevention (CDC), an unintentional injury is "the physical damage that results when a human body is suddenly subjected to energy in amounts that exceed the threshold of physiologic tolerance—or else the result of a lack of one or more vital elements, such as oxygen" (CDC, 2012, p. 15). While drowning, motor vehicle crashes, falls, fires, and poisonings are all common forms of unintentional injury, the leading cause of such injuries in the United States today is drug overdose (CDC, n.d.). This is being driven largely by overdose related to the use of opioids and underscores the importance of exploring ways that law and policy can address the increasingly destructive toll that opioid use disorder (OUD) has catalyzed.

Beginning in the late 1990s, rates of opioid-related morbidity and mortality have risen steadily. By 2018, opioids, either alone or in combination, were involved in nearly 48,000 deaths in the United States, a nearly sixfold increase over two decades (Scholl et al., 2018). Opioid-related harms increased in three related but somewhat distinct waves. First, a rise in the prescription of opioids for pain led to both increases in opioid painkiller use as well as OUD. Beginning in approximately 2010, as concerns mounted over the overprescribing of opioids for pain management, states and other actors began to decrease access to some prescription opioids (Piper et al., 2018). Some individuals who found it harder to access prescribed opioids reacted by shifting to the illicit opioid market.

Partially as a result of this shift, heroin-involved overdose deaths approximately tripled between 2010 and 2015 (Hedegaard et al., 2015). Beginning in 2013, the third wave of opioid-related harm was caused by an influx of illicitly manufactured fentanyl and its analogs into the illicit drug supply (Ciccarone, 2019). These drugs are much more potent than other street opioids and are often indistinguishable from them to the naked eye. As of 2015, OUDs affected 2 million people aged 12 and over, with 600,000 people aged 12 or over meeting the criteria for heroin use disorder (Wu et al., 2016).

This chapter describes the impact of public health law as both a barrier to and facilitator of evidence-based responses to reducing opioid-related harm. Through the lens of a hypothetical case study, this chapter explores the legal concepts of nondiscrimination in access to treatment for chronic pain and substance use disorder and offers a discussion of selected legal frameworks for regulating prescribing, overdose prevention, and substance use disorder treatment.

## LEGAL BARRIERS AND FACILITATORS

States and the federal government have passed a variety of laws designed to mitigate opioid-related harms and, in some cases, used existing law to attempt to increase access to evidence-based interventions to reverse opioid overdose and mitigate the harms associated with OUD. However, in some cases, existing laws that predate the current crisis reduce access to both proven treatment and the overdose reversal medication **naloxone**.

### Naloxone Access

Naloxone is a medication that quickly and effectively reduces the respiratory depression that characterizes opioid overdose (Chamberlain & Klein, 1994). Although it is not a controlled substance and has no misuse potential, it is a prescription medication in the United States (Davis & Carr, 2015). This status reduces access to the medication, as many people at highest risk of overdose face barriers accessing the traditional medical system (Paquette et al., 2018).

As the overdose crisis deepened, states passed a variety of laws to increase access to naloxone. Although only the federal government can remove the prescription requirement, states have broad latitude to set the standards for the prescribing and dispensing of prescription medicines. In the case of naloxone, states have used that flexibility to increase access to naloxone in a number of ways. First, nearly all states permit naloxone to be prescribed to people that the prescriber has not personally examined (referred to as "third-party" prescribing), and most permit it to be dispensed to any person who meets criteria specified by the prescriber (referred to as "non-patient-specific" or "standing order" prescribing; Davis & Carr, 2017b). Some have also given pharmacists the authority to prescribe naloxone without the patient seeing another provider (Davis & Carr, 2017b). Finally, most states provide immunity from potential civil and criminal penalties for providers who act according to the law (Davis & Carr, 2017b; Table 10.1).

These legal changes have been associated with an increase in the amount of naloxone dispensed from pharmacies as well as the number of community organizations distributing naloxone (Xu et al., 2018). They have also been associated with decreases in overdose deaths (McClellan et al., 2018). However, since law still acts as a barrier to naloxone access, further

## TABLE 10.1 Number of States That Have Expanded Naloxone Access (as of 2017)

| | |
|---|---|
| Any law expanding access to naloxone? | 50 states + D.C. |
| Pharmacist can dispense/distribute without patient-specific prescription from another medical professional | 49 states + D.C. |
| Pharmacists can dispense/distribute under a standing order | 42 states + D.C. |
| Pharmacists can dispense/distribute under pharmacist prescriptive authority | 6 states + D.C. |
| Naloxone prescription authorization to third parties | 45 states + D.C. |

Source: Prescription Drug Abuse Policy System. http://pdaps.org/datasets/laws-regulating-administration-of-naloxone-1501695139

interventions, such as mandating insurance cover the medication and removing the prescription requirement entirely, should be considered (Davis & Carr, 2020).

## Buprenorphine and Methadone for Opioid Use Disorder Treatment

Law and policy can facilitate reductions in OUD-related harm, as in laws designed to increase access to naloxone. However, they can also act as a significant barrier to evidence-based treatment interventions. One of the most pressing examples of such legal barriers is laws and regulations that limit access to **medications for opioid use disorder** (MOUD), particularly methadone and buprenorphine. Both medications adhere to the brain receptors to which opioids attach, fully or partially blocking their effects (Connery, 2015). Extensive research shows that MOUD treatment provides many positive effects, including reducing the risk of relapse and risk of contracting bloodborne diseases such as HIV and hepatitis C (Connock et al., 2007). More importantly, it reduces the risk of opioid overdose among people with OUD by as much as 50% (Sordo et al., 2017).

However, restrictive federal, state, and local laws and policies, in addition to structural and systemic factors such as stigma and insufficient funding, significantly impede access to MOUD. This is one of the many reasons that fewer than half of all drug treatment facilities provide any type of medication for OUD (SAMHSA, 2018). Methadone for MOUD is one of the most restricted medications in the country. It can be dispensed only from specially licensed clinics, and only to patients who meet certain requirements. Further, patients must generally come to the methadone clinic every day to receive their medication (take-home doses are permitted under limited circumstances) and initial dosage amounts are limited (Davis & Carr, 2019). There is no evidence that these restrictions improve outcomes; rather, they serve as a barrier to treatment (Amiri et al., 2018). States often further limit methadone access by placing restrictions on new clinics and permitting localities to restrict where they can be sited.

There are also significant limitations on buprenorphine access. The most important of these is a federal requirement that prescribers obtain a special certification (typically referred to as a "waiver") before prescribing buprenorphine for OUD, even though no such restrictions exist when the same medication is prescribed for treatment of pain (21 U.S.C. § 823(g)). Physicians must attend 8 hours of additional training to become waivered; the mid-level practitioners who are able to obtain a waiver are required to attend a full 24 hours of training (21 U.S.C. § 823[g][2][G]). Federal law also limits the number of patients most providers can treat at a time to 30 in the first year after receiving a waiver and 100 patients thereafter (SAMHSA, n.d.-b). These restrictions are widely viewed as unnecessary limitations on the ability of medical providers to effectively treat OUD (Fiscella et al., 2019).

Some changes have been made to increase access to buprenorphine. In 2016, the Comprehensive Addiction and Recovery Act (Public Law No. 114-198, 114th Congress Public Law 198) temporarily permitted specially trained physician assistants and nurse practitioners to become waivered, and later that year the Department of Health and Human Services increased the number of concurrent patients a waivered provider could treat from 100 to 275 (Davis & Carr, 2017a). In 2018, the SUPPORT Act (Public Law No. 115-271 115th Congress) made permanent the provision permitting nurse practitioners and physician assistants to prescribe buprenorphine for OUD; temporarily permitted clinical nurse specialists, certified registered nurse anesthetists, and certified nurse midwives to become waivered; and permitted some providers to treat 100 patients in the first year instead of the previously permitted 30 (Davis, 2019). However, access still remains well below the level of need. Indeed, only approximately 4% of American physicians were waivered to prescribe buprenorphine in 2016, leaving nearly half of America's 3,100 counties, including over 60% of rural counties, without a single physician authorized to prescribe the medication (Andrilla et al., 2017).

## BOX 10.1 OUD, HEALTH DISPARITIES, AND HEALTH EQUITY

- Data demonstrates that White non-Hispanic people experience the highest rates of opioid overdose deaths in nearly every state. (https://www.cdc.gov/mmwr/volumes/69/wr/mm6911a4.htm). American Indian and Alaskan Natives experience the second-highest rate of overdose deaths, followed closely by non-Hispanic Black people. (https://www.ihs.gov/opioids/data)
- Probably because previous laws disproportionately impacted people of color, laws designed to increase access to overdose treatment appear to disproportionately benefit people of color. One nationwide study found that naloxone access and Good Samaritan laws were associated with 14% and 15% reductions in overall opioid overdose deaths. These decreases were much more pronounced among African Americans, where the laws were associated with 23% and 26% declines (Mcclellan et al., infra.).
- Evidence shows that people on Medicaid as well as people who identify as Hispanic are less likely than people with commercial insurance and White people to begin MOUD treatment. (https://www.jabfm.org/content/32/5/724.long)

---

### HYPOTHETICAL CASE STUDY #1: OPIOID USE DISORDER AND THE ADA

Darien works as an intake specialist at a local public health clinic. Mr. Brown is a new patient who is at the clinic to treat his chronic pain. While filling out the intake paperwork, Mr. Brown lists Suboxone as a current medication. When the clinic reviews his paperwork, Darien tells Mr. Brown that unfortunately the clinic has a policy that does not allow them to accept new patients who take buprenorphine (which is a component of Suboxone). The clinic created the policy because Suboxone is a common form of medication-assisted treatment (MAT), and as such is often indicative of an OUD. Because Suboxone combines buprenorphine, a partial opioid antagonist, and naloxone, an opioid antagonist, it is often prescribed to patients who were dependent on prescription or illicitly manufactured opioids to avoid withdrawal symptoms and reduce cravings.

Upset about the clinic's policy, Mr. Brown tells Darien that he is going to complain to the Office of Civil Rights of the U.S. Department of Justice and tell them that the clinic is violating the **Americans With Disabilities Act**.

1. Do you think Darien and the clinic have discriminated against Mr. Brown under the ADA?
2. What public health issue is implicated here?
3. How do you think the Department of Justice should respond to Mr. Brown's discrimination claim?

---

## Americans With Disabilities Act

The **ADA**, signed into law in 1990, protects individuals with certain disabilities from certain types of discrimination. Some parts of the act prevent discrimination in employment practices while others ensure equal access to public and private entities and services. People often remember the ADA as the law that requires installing ramps or elevators at places that have stairs to ensure those with disabilities can navigate the building.

**TABLE 10.2  Overdose Good Samaritan Laws (as of July 2018)**

| | |
|---|---|
| Any Overdose Good Samaritan Protection | 45 + D.C. |
| In relation to possession of a controlled substance, the Good Samaritan law protects against: | |
| Arrest | 21 + D.C. |
| Charge | 29 + D.C. |
| In relation to drug paraphernalia, the Good Samaritan law protects against: | |
| Arrest | 16 + D.C. |
| Charge | 21 + D.C. |
| Protection against probation/parole violations | 23 |

*Source:* Prescription Drug Abuse Policy System. http://pdaps.org/datasets/good-samaritan-overdose-laws-1501695153

Defining "disability" under the ADA can be tricky. The law defines disability as "[a] physical or mental impairment that substantially limits one or more of the major life activities of such an individual," and adds that the term "shall be construed broadly in favor of expansive coverage" (28 C.F.R. § 36.105). Specifically, the ADA includes drug addiction as a physical or mental impairment, but specifically *excludes* "psychoactive substance use disorders resulting from current illegal use of drugs." So, drug use disorders like OUD are considered disabilities under the ADA so long as the individual is in a recovery phase and is not presently using illegal drugs.

---

### BOX 10.2 OVERDOSE GOOD SAMARITAN LAWS

Good Samaritan laws protect people from lawsuits, or sometimes criminal penalties, for acting to help someone else. In the overdose context, **overdose Good Samaritan laws** protect someone from being arrested for or charged with certain crimes if they call for help during an overdose. Most laws provide protections for the person who overdosed as well.

Often, someone witnessing an overdose is afraid to call 911. Sometimes, the witness has illegal opioids or drug paraphernalia on them, or they may be afraid the person experiencing the overdose may be arrested.

As of 2018, 46 states had an overdose Good Samaritan law that protected certain people from criminal penalties for calling for help if they suspected an opioid overdose (Table 10.2). These laws vary widely by state. A small number of states have a "one free pass" approach, so a 911 caller is protected only for the first time they call. If they call in a subsequent overdose, they are no longer protected by the Good Samaritan law. A few states provide expansive protection under Good Samaritan laws that protect against all drug offenses, including possession and sale.

Good Samaritan laws show initial promise to reduce drug overdose deaths, but they must be expansive enough and publicized enough for those who would report overdoses to understand and use the protection these laws provide.

Title III of the ADA prohibits public accommodations, commercial facilities, and private entities from discriminating against individuals on the basis of disability. Places like doctors' offices fall under the category of places required to allow equal access to those with disabilities.

The ADA has become an important tool to help people with OUD access treatment. In several instances, the Department of Justice has brought suit, alleging that failure to provide MOUD violates the ADA. In one example, the U.S. Attorney for the District of Massachusetts reached a settlement with a skilled nursing facility that refused to take a patient who was receiving buprenorphine (U.S. Department of Justice, 2018). Several courts have now ruled that jails violate the ADA if they do not continue MOUD for individuals who are receiving them when they become incarcerated (Fuller, 2019; U.S. Court of Appeals, 2019). In another case, the U.S. Department of Justice sued an outpatient medical clinic for a violation of the ADA based on a policy of declining to treat patients for pain based solely on the patients' prescribed use of buprenorphine.

Ensuring nondiscrimination in the primary care setting for those with a history of OUD is an important public health issue because discrimination impacts access to care. While denial at one clinic may not prevent someone from receiving primary care, if increasingly more clinics refuse to see patients with a history of OUD, these individuals may become completely unable to access primary care. While general access to primary care is important in and of itself, studies demonstrate that primary care is an important component of treatment for OUD, with or without specifically using buprenorphine (Fiscella et al., 2019; Wakeman & Barnett, 2018).

Additional public health considerations are invoked in the previous example. Discrimination—both social and structural—based on health status implicitly occurs when a clinic uses preexisting health conditions as a basis to deny treatment. From a broader policy perspective, it is important to make sure that individuals who want treatment for OUD have access to that treatment. Denying access to primary care can severely limit access to any treatment for someone with OUD.

## United States v. Selma Medical Associates

The previous hypothetical case study is based on a recent case in which a patient was turned away from a family medicine clinic for having a history of OUD. The patient sought treatment for chronic pain from a family practice medical clinic. In his initial intake conversation with the clinic, the patient disclosed that he had previously been prescribed and was taking Suboxone, a common form of MAT approved by the FDA. Suboxone combines buprenorphine, a partial opioid agonist, and naltrexone, an opioid antagonist, and is commonly prescribed to patients who were previously dependent on prescription or illicitly manufactured opioids, avoiding withdrawal symptoms that would otherwise be experienced and reducing cravings.

Similar to Darien in Case Study #1, upon learning that the patient was taking Suboxone, the medical clinic staff declined to schedule a new patient appointment on the grounds that it had a policy to decline treating pain in patients on buprenorphine. Suboxone is sometimes stigmatized as a "substitute" or "replacement" medication that avoids the "work" of "true" recovery from addiction and does not represent abstinence and sobriety, which are primary goals of many in the addiction recovery community. Some providers also regard treatment of pain as more complex in patients who have experienced an OUD, given that the patients may be at higher risk of dependency or relapse if prescribed analgesic medication.

In hypothetical Case Study #1, Mr. Brown threatened to complain to the Office of Civil Rights of the U.S. Department of Justice. In the actual case, the patient actually did file a complaint, and the Office of Civil Rights of the U.S. Department of Justice found enough merit in it that they filed a legal complaint against Selma Medical Associates. In its complaint, the

Department of Justice argued that the clinic's refusal to treat the patient constituted a violation of Title III of the Americans With Disabilities Act.

In January 2019, the Department of Justice and Selma Medical Associates reached a settlement of the matter. The settlement specifically describes that a person who has OUD and has not engaged in the "illegal use of drugs" and has "participated in a supervised rehabilitation program" has a qualifying disability under the ADA (Settlement Agreement between the United States of America and Selma Medical Associates, 2019). Additionally, the settlement describes that Selma Medical's policy is discriminatory against those with OUD since the clinic "screened out or tended to screen out individuals with OUD" and did not provide any other reasonable modifications to its policies to accommodate those with OUD (Settlement Agreement between the United States of America and Selma Medical Associates, 2019).

The settlement required the clinic agree to pay damages and create a nondiscrimination policy to ensure all patients have access to the clinic's services without discriminating against those with OUD (Settlement Agreement between the United States of America and Selma Medical Associates, 2019). The clinic must also train its management and patient-facing employees in the ADA (Settlement Agreement between the United States of America and Selma Medical Associates, 2019).

## CONCLUSION

Law is an important tool in preventing opioid-related injuries and fostering recovery from OUD. In recent years, the law has expanded to provide more people with access to naloxone, which has saved many lives. Additionally, law has increased access to MOUD by allowing more practitioners to prescribe MOUD and to increase the number of patients who can receive a MOUD prescription from a practitioner. The law has also evolved to prevent discrimination against individuals with OUD, which increases access to treatment for individuals with OUD and recognizes OUD as a disability.

Although the law has made important improvements in addressing opioid injuries, there is still more the law can do to reduce opioid injuries. Greater access to MOUD and naloxone can remove barriers to treatment for people with OUD. Overdose Good Samaritan laws can be expanded to provide broader and more comprehensive protections for individuals who report overdoses to encourage more reporting and ultimately save lives. The wide variations of these laws state to state can make it difficult to summarize the landscape of opioid-related legislation, but it provides important information to understand which laws can have the greatest impact on public health.

## CHAPTER REVIEW

### Review Questions

1. It is illegal for a doctor to prescribe methadone.
   True/False
2. Medication-assisted therapy can be helpful to treat opioid use disorder.
   True/False
3. There is no way to reverse an opioid overdose.
   True/False
4. Under what circumstances does the ADA consider opioid use disorder a disability?
5. What health problems can medications like methadone help to prevent?
6. Does your state have an overdose Good Samaritan law? What does the law cover? Look for things like arrest, prosecution, and probation violations in the law.

## Essay Question

1. Has your state changed its law on who can access naloxone and how they can access it? Why or why not? Can you come up with arguments both for and against expanding naloxone access?
2. What are the potential consequences of categorizing opioid use disorder as a "disability"? For example, do you think what was previously identified as addiction to other drugs (heroin, cocaine, etc.) will now qualify as a disability under this legal categorization?
3. What barriers does federal law impose on access to medications for opioid use disorder?
4. How do laws intended to reduce discrimination such as the Americans With Disabilities Act apply in the context of opioid use disorder?

## Internet Activities

1. Network for Public Health Law: Legal interventions to reduce overdose mortality: Naloxone access and overdose Good Samaritan laws. Visit this resource, which catalogs state laws designed to increase access to naloxone. What differences do you notice? What might explain these differences? https://www.networkforphl.org/wp-content/uploads/2021/04/NAL-FINAL-4-12.pdf
2. Good Samaritan Overdose Prevention Laws: Use this interactive tool to see which states have passed overdose Good Samaritan laws and the types of protection they offer: http://pdaps.org/datasets/good-samaritan-overdose-laws-1501695153

## REFERENCES

21 U.S.C. § 823(g).
21 U.S.C. § 823(g)(2)(G).
Amiri, S., Lutz, R., Socias, M. E., McDonell, M. G., Roll, J. M., & Amram, O. (2018). Increased distance was associated with lower daily attendance to an opioid treatment program in Spokane County Washington. *Journal of Substance Abuse Treatment, 93*, 26–30. https://doi.org/10.1016/j.jsat.2018.07.006
Andrilla, C. H. A., Coulthard, C., & Larson, E. H. (2017). *Changes in the supply of physicians with a DEA DATA waiver to prescribe buprenorphine for opioid use disorder, Data Brief #162.* University of Washington.
Centers for Disease Control and Prevention. (2012). *National action plan for child injury prevention.* https://www.cdc.gov/safechild/pdf/National_Action_Plan_for_Child_Injury_Prevention-a.pdf
Centers for Disease Control and Prevention. (n.d.). *Opioid overdose.* https://www.cdc.gov/drugoverdose/index.html
Chamberlain, J. M., & Klein, B. L. (1994). A comprehensive review of naloxone for the emergency physician. *American Journal of Emergency Medicine, 12*, 650–660. https://doi.org/10.1016/0735-6757(94)90033-7
Ciccarone, D. H. (2019). The triple wave epidemic: Supply and demand drivers of the US opioid overdose crisis. *International Journal of Drug Policy, 71*, 183–188. https://doi.org/10.1016/j.drugpo.2019.01.010
Connery, H. S. (2015). Medication-assisted treatment of opioid use disorder: Review of the evidence and future directions. *Harvard Review of Psychiatry, 23*, 63–75. https://doi.org/10.1097/HRP.0000000000000075
Connock, M., Juarez-Garcia, A., Jowett, S., Frew, E., Liu, Z., Taylor, R. J., Fry-Smith, A., Day, E., Lintzeris, N., Roberts, T., Burls, A., & Taylor, R. S. (2007). Methadone and buprenorphine for

the management of opioid dependence: A systematic review and economic evaluation. *Health Technology Assessment, 11*, 1–171. https://doi.org/10.3310/hta11090

Davis, C. S. (2019). The SUPPORT for Patients and Communities Act—What will it mean for the opioid-overdose crisis? *New England Journal of Medicine, 380*, 3–5. http://doi.org/10.1056/NEJMp1813961

Davis, C. S., & Carr, D. (2015). Legal changes to increase access to naloxone for opioid overdose reversal in the United States. *Drug and Alcohol Dependence, 157*, 112–120. http://doi.org/10.1016/j.drugalcdep.2015.10.013

Davis, C. S., & Carr, D. (2017a). The law and policy of opioids for pain management, Addiction treatment, and overdose reversal. *Indiana Health Law Review, 14*(1), 1–39. https://doi.org/10.18060/3911.0027

Davis, C. S., & Carr, D. (2017b). State legal innovations to encourage naloxone dispensing. *Journal of the American Pharmacists Association, 57*(2), S180–S184. https://doi.org/10.1016/j.japh.2016.11.007

Davis, C. S., & Carr, D. (2019). Legal and policy changes urgently needed to increase access to opioid agonist therapy in the United States. *International Journal of Drug Policy, 73*, 42–48. https://doi.org/10.1016/j.drugpo.2019.07.006

Davis, C. S., & Carr, D. (2020). Over the counter naloxone needed to save lives in the United States. *Preventive Medicine, 130*, 105932. https://doi.org/10.1016/j.ypmed.2019.105932

Fiscella, K., Wakeman, S. E., Beletsky, L. (2019). Buprenorphine deregulation and mainstreaming treatment for opioid use disorder: X the X Waiver. *JAMA Psychiatry, 76*(3), 229–230. https://www.ncbi.nlm.nih.gov/pubmed/30586140

Fuller, A. (2019). Shifting Tides: District of Massachusetts Orders Correctional Facility to Provide Opioid Treatment. *Boston Bar Journal.* https://bostonbarjournal.com/2019/06/06/shifting-tides-district-of-massachusetts-orders-correctional-facility-to-provide-opioid-treatment

Hedegaard, H., Chen, L.-H., & Warner, M. (2015). *Drug-poisoning deaths involving heroin: United States, 2000-2013, NCHS Data Brief (heroin deaths nearly quadrupled from 2010 to 2013).* https://www.cdc.gov/nchs/products/databriefs/db190.htm

Lambdin, B., Davis, C. S., Wheeler, E., Tueller, S., & Kral, A. (2018). Naloxone laws facilitate the establishment of overdose education and naloxone distribution programs in the United States. *Drug and Alcohol Dependence, 188*, 370–376. https://doi.org/10.1016/j.drugalcdep.2018.04.004

Mannelli, P., & Wu, L.-T. (2016). Primary care for opioid use disorder. *Substance Abuse and Rehabilitation, 7*, 107–109. https://www.ncbi.nlm.nih.gov/pmc/articles/PMC4993411/

McClellan, C., Lambdin, B., Ali, M., Mutter, R., Davis, C. S., Wheeler, E., Pemberton, M., & Kral, A. (2018). Opioid overdose laws association with opioid use and overdose mortality. *Addictive Behaviors, 86*, 90–95. https://doi.org/10.1016/j.addbeh.2018.03.014

Paquette, C. E., Syvertsen, J. L., & Pollini, R. A. (2018). Stigma at every turn: Health services experiences among people who inject drugs. *International Journal of Drug Policy, 57*, 104–110. https://doi.org/10.1016/j.drugpo.2018.04.004

Piper, B. J., Shah, D. T., Simoyan, O. M., McCall, K. L., & Nichols, S. D. (2018). Trends in medical use of opioids in the U.S., 2006–2016. *American Journal of Preventive Medicine, 54*(5), 652–660. https://doi.org/10.1016/j.amepre.2018.01.034

Public Law No. 114-198, 114th Congress Public Law 198. https://www.congress.gov/bill/114th-congress/senate-bill/524/text

Public Law No. 115-271 115th Congress. https://www.congress.gov/bill/115th-congress/house-bill/6

Scholl, L., Seth, P., Kariisa, M., Wilson, N., & Baldwin, G. (2018). Drug and opioid-involved overdose deaths—United States, 2013–2017. *MMWR Morbidity and Mortality Weekly Report, 67*, 1419–1427. https://www.cdc.gov/mmwr/volumes/67/wr/mm675152e1.htm

Settlement Agreement between the United States of America and Selma Medical Associates, Inc. (2019). *Under the Americans with Disabilities Act.* https://www.ada.gov/selma_medical_sa.html

Sordo, L., Barrio, G., Bravo, M. J., Indave, B. I., Degenhardt, L., Wiessing, L., et al. (2017). Mortality risk during and after opioid substitution treatment: Systematic review and meta-analysis of cohort studies. *British Medical Journal, 357*, j1550. https://doi.org/10.1136/bmj.j1550

Substance Abuse and Mental Health Services Administration. (2018). *National Survey of Substance Abuse Treatment Services (N-SSATS).* https://wwwdasis.samhsa.gov/dasis2/nssats/NSSATS-2018-R.pdf

Substance Abuse and Mental Health Services Administration. (n.d.-a). https://store.samhsa.gov/system/files/tip63_fulldoc_052919_508.pdf

Substance Abuse and Mental Health Services Administration. (n.d.-b). *Apply for a practitioner waiver.* https://www.samhsa.gov/medication-assisted-treatment/training-materials-resources/apply-for-practitioner-waiver

U.S. Court of Appeals. (2019). Brenda Smith vs. Aroostook County, Shawn D. Gillen. http://media.ca1.uscourts.gov/pdf.opinions/19-1340P-01A.pdf

U.S. Department of Justice. (2018, May 10). *U.S. Attorney's Office settles disability discrimination allegations at skilled nursing facility.* https://www.justice.gov/usao-ma/pr/us-attorney-s-office-settles-disability-discrimination-allegations-skilled-nursing

Wakeman, S. E., & Barnett, M. L. (2018). Primary care and the opioid-overdose crisis: Buprenorphine myths and realities. *The New England Journal of Medicine, 379,* 1–4. https://doi.org/10.1056/NEJMp1802741

Wu, L.-T., Zhu, H., & Swartz, M. S. (2016). Treatment utilization among persons with opioid use disorder in the United States. *Drug and Alcohol Dependence, 169,* 117–127. https://doi.org/10.1016/j.drugalcdep.2016.10.015

Xu, J., Davis, C. S., Cruz, M., & Lurie, P. (2018). State naloxone access laws are associated with an increase in the number of naloxone prescriptions dispensed in retail pharmacies. *Drug and Alcohol Dependence, 189,* 37–41. https://doi.org/10.1016/j.drugalcdep.2018.04.020

## Additional Resources

- **Legal and Policy Approaches to Reducing Prescription Drug Overdose; Public Health Law Academy Training**
  https://www.changelabsolutions.org/product/reducing-prescription-drug-overdose
- **Full settlement of United States vs. Selma Medical Associates**
  https://www.ada.gov/selma_medical_sa.html

# 11

# Public Health Emergency Law

Jennifer L. Piatt, Sarah Wetter, and James G. Hodge, Jr.

## Learning Objectives

By the end of this chapter, the reader will be able to:

- Provide a detailed account of the evolution of public health emergencies and the role of various public health actors in addressing emergency scenarios.
- Understand the importance of developing and utilizing public health emergency (PHE) powers.
- Explain the framework of legal options available to governmental and private sector actors during a PHE, as well as limitations on those powers.
- Illustrate real-time legal and policy challenges presented during a PHE.

## Key Terminology

**Emergency declaration:** A legal designation vested in federal, state, Tribal, local, or territorial executive branch officials authorizing the use of optional and expedited public health powers relating to individuals, groups, or property during exigencies.

**Emergency liability protection:** A limitation on exposure to civil or criminal liability or penalties for actions taken during or in response to a PHE.

**Federalist system:** A system of government in which power is distributed between national and regional governmental bodies with differing responsibilities; in the United States, the federalist system encompasses the distribution of power between the federal government and state governments.

**Isolation:** The physical confinement and separation of an individual/groups who are reasonably believed or known to be infected with a contagious/possibly contagious disease from nonisolated individuals/groups, to limit transmission of the disease.

**Model State Emergency Health Powers Act:** A model act drafted with national input by the Centers for Law and the Public's Health at Georgetown and Johns Hopkins Universities in 2001 that provides a menu of model emergency powers and authorities that adopting states or other governments can use to define, declare, and respond to public health emergencies.

**Quarantine:** The physical separation and confinement of an individual/groups who have/may have been exposed to a contagious/possibly contagious disease and who do not show symptoms or other signs of a contagious disease from nonquarantined individuals/groups, to limit transmission of the disease.

The contents of this chapter are solely the responsibility of the authors and do not necessarily represent the positions of the Network for Public Health Law, Arizona State University, or Georgetown University.

## Public Health Law Competencies

This chapter addresses the following competencies from the Public Health Emergency Law Competency Model Version 1.0 (PHELCM; Centers for Disease Control and Prevention [CDC], 2014).

**1.1**  Act within the scope of federal, state, Tribal, and local statutory and regulatory authority during emergency situations, and through state and/or federal declarations of emergency.

**1.4**  Integrate legal information into the exercise of professional public health judgment within the larger public health response.

**3.1**  Implement the use of relevant legal information, tools, procedures, and remedies related to social distancing including evacuation, quarantine and isolation orders, closure of public places, and curfews.

**3.2**  Recognize the sources of potential civil and criminal liability of public health personnel and consider due process issues before taking legal action.

---

### Spark Questions

1.  During a public health emergency (PHE), why might a fluid and flexible approach underlying response efforts be preferable to more rigid laws or policies applicable in normal circumstances?
2.  When might it be ethically appropriate and legally defensible for PHE powers to encroach on individual/group rights?

---

## INTRODUCTION

PHE law refers to how public and private sectors wield laws, policies, and ethics to plan for, prevent, and respond to emerging infectious diseases (e.g., H1N1, Ebola, and COVID-19), catastrophic events (e.g., hurricanes, tornados, fires, and earthquakes), and other exigencies (e.g., bioterrorism, drug addiction, and mental health crises) that may directly affect the public's health (Hodge, 2017). The potential for these and other conditions to simultaneously impact thousands or millions of persons sustains real-time **emergency declarations** (Sunshine et al., 2019). Some PHEs, alternatively, entail risks to human health on a more granular level, including localized chemical spills, limited food contaminations, or outbreaks of diseases in specific settings (e.g., long-term care facilities, schools, or hospitals). As discussed in Box 11.1, there are also health equity considerations at play.

No matter the source or cause of exigencies, preventing excess morbidity and mortality during or after PHEs requires advance planning and preparedness activities coupled with rapid governmental responses in partnership with private sector actors and entities. Societal capacities to effectively plan, assess, and respond to PHEs necessitate sufficient legal authorities that

---

### BOX 11.1 HEALTH EQUITY AND DISASTER RESPONSE

"Reviewing, updating, and creating plans that engage and include vulnerable populations helps to ensure that our preparedness plans serve the diverse needs of our communities. It also makes these plans more universally applicable[,] meaning they will do more than sit on a shelf—they will be actionable roadmaps that serve entire communities when the next disaster strikes."

Kertanis, J. C. (2020). *Developing emergency preparedness plans with a health equity focus.* https://www.naccho.org/blog/articles/developing-emergency-preparedness-plans-with-a-health-equity-focus

(a) directly authorize or support an array of essential activities, (b) facilitate critical response efforts designed to save lives or lessen morbidity, and (c) adequately balance communal interests and individual rights.

As seen during the COVID-19 pandemic in 2020, appropriately balancing these factors is not easy when people's lives and livelihoods are at stake. PHE legal preparedness and response efforts can be politically volatile, economically damaging, and subject to substantial variations across borders.

Emergency legal preparedness and response efforts are often mired in interjurisdictional disputes and discord. What is legally permissible or required in declared emergencies varies extensively depending on perceived and actual threats, available information, and changing circumstances. Even when legal powers are well-defined, what is ethically or politically viable may be unclear or run counter to legal interventions. During the COVID-19 pandemic, for example, the availability of vaccines in late 2020 raised immediate questions over who may be legally or ethically required to receive them (e.g., healthcare workers [HCWs]). In real-time emergencies, delays or confusion over critical decisions or practical applications can contribute to excess injuries or deaths. Yet, so can ill-advised or uninformed actions that drain resources or lack proof of efficacy, which can be difficult to measure when available empirical data are elusive in the throes of substantial health threats like COVID-19.

Protecting the public's health in emergencies is precarious, but it starts with core knowledge and practice skills grounded in an understanding of the underpinnings of modern PHE laws since 2001. Preparedness and response activities are authorized largely through legal classifications and declarations of varied emergencies triggering an expansive series of public health powers (nearly all of which were used during the COVID-19 pandemic).

Extensive and long-term uses of PHE powers raise unique legal and ethical challenges. Interwoven principles of PHE ethics contribute to a dynamic "legal triage" environment where real-time decisions impact peoples' lives (Hodge & Anderson, 2009, pp. 249, 250). Effectuating sound decisions involving administration of healthcare or public health services requires affirmative legal support to (a) coordinate roles and responsibilities of diverse entities and personnel, (b) allocate scarce resources, (c) shift standards of care, (d) alter scopes of practice among licensed HCWS, and (e) assess liability risks and protections for workers, volunteers, and entities.

## EVOLVING CONCEPTS REGARDING THE SCOPE OF PUBLIC HEALTH EMERGENCIES

Like public health threats, PHE laws are always evolving. For decades, public health exigencies in the United States were legally classified under broad conceptions of "emergencies" or "disasters" (Sunshine, 2017, pp. 397, 400). Under an "all hazards" approach reflected in general emergency laws and policies, public health response efforts typically fell under the direction of federal, state, Tribal, or local emergency management agencies (EMAs). Consequently, approaches and powers that EMAs might deploy to respond to natural disasters like hurricanes were similarly used to address rapidly emerging infectious diseases or other distinct health threats. The concept of PHEs as a distinct legal classification was largely nonexistent.

Following the terrorist acts on September 11, 2001 and the ensuing anthrax attacks that same Fall, combatting acts of terrorism, specifically bioterrorism, became national priorities. Policymakers at all levels of government sought reforms of generalized emergency laws to better prepare for, and respond to, PHEs. A series of legislative and regulatory reforms were initiated to (a) define PHEs, (b) clarify public and private sector response capabilities, and (c) coordinate efforts across jurisdictions.

As noted in what follows, crafting modern legal principles guiding PHE preparedness and response did not come easy. Harsh critics framed model PHE law efforts as sensational, draconian, or contrary to individual freedoms (Annas, 2010). Despite these concerns, modern PHE laws arose and dominated responses to national and regional emergencies over the next two decades. Although major events like Hurricane Katrina (2005) and the H1N1 pandemic (2009) were followed with major legal reforms, the premier test for revamped PHE laws came with the inception of the COVID-19 pandemic in 2020.

## Interjurisdictional Coordination and Response

Effective PHE preparedness and response rely on interjurisdictional coordination among public and private sectors (Obama, 2011). Consequently, enhancing coordination across jurisdictions was a lynchpin to significant federal and state PHE legal reforms. For much of the 20th century, frontline preparedness and response efforts were reserved largely to states tasked with protecting and promoting the public's health within the **federalist system**. States (and localities pursuant to delegated state authority) wield traditional "police powers" to protect the health, safety, and general welfare of populations (Gostin, 2002). Federal agencies including the Federal Emergency Management Agency (FEMA), the U.S. Department of Health and Human Services (DHHS), and its subsidiaries, the Centers for Disease Control and Prevention (CDC) and the Food and Drug Administration (FDA), provided substantial guidance, expertise, and resources. Yet, they often lacked direct legal authority or manpower to address public health exigencies, with the exception of national security events where federal responses are dominant. While clarifying interjurisdictional roles of governments has been a central policy objective since 9/11, it remains elusive as seen through fragmented efforts in response to COVID-19.

## Federal Emergency Powers and Roles

Congress has vested considerable federal emergency powers in the president, the DHHS, and other federal agencies primarily through the (a) Robert T. Stafford Disaster Relief and Emergency Assistance Act (Stafford Act; Stafford Disaster Relief and Emergency Assistance Act. 42 U.S.C.A § 5121 et seq.), (b) National Emergencies Act (NEA; National Emergencies Act. 50 U.S.C.A. §§ 1601, 1621, 1622, 1631, 1641, 1651), (c) Public Health Service Act (PHSA; Public Health Service Act. 42 U.S.C.A. § 201 et seq.), and (d) Pandemic and All-Hazards Preparedness Act (PAHPA; Pandemic and All-Hazards Preparedness Act, Pub. L. No. 109-417, 120 Stat. 2831, renewed in 2013; Hodge, 2018).

Collectively, these laws authorize the federal government to declare states of "emergency", "disaster", and "PHE". Declarations of emergency or disaster are made by the president via the Stafford Act or the NEA. A Stafford Act emergency can be declared generally only after a state governor requests federal assistance "to save lives and to protect property and public health and safety, or to lessen or avert the threat of a catastrophe" (42 U.S.C.A. §§ 5170, 5122[1]). The president declares states of disaster usually in response to natural calamities (e.g., tornadoes, earthquakes, snowstorms, or droughts). However, these same declarations are also used to coordinate and mobilize federal powers and responses to public health crises. On March 13, 2020, President Trump declared dual states of emergency via the Stafford Act and National Emergencies Act in response to escalating impacts of the COVID-19 pandemic.

National emergency or disaster powers, however, are not necessarily well-tailored to PHEs involving direct and immediate disease threats to the health of populations. Consequently, the PHSA authorizes the secretary of the DHHS to declare a federal PHE whenever "a disease or disorder presents a [PHE]" or in response to "significant outbreaks of infectious diseases or bioterrorist attacks" (42 U.S.C.A. § 247d[a]). Pursuant to these declarations (which last 90 days subject to reauthorization), the DHHS can rapidly execute grants or contracts, cover expenses, conduct and support disease investigations, and access emergency funds. Certain Medicare and Medicaid requirements can be temporarily waived. The DHHS can also initiate emergency use authorizations (EUAs) of yet-to-be approved drugs, vaccines, tests, or devices through FDA (2017). Over the last two decades, federal PHE declarations have been issued in response to manifold events, including Hurricane Katrina (2005), the H1N1 pandemic (2009–2010), the opioid epidemic (2017), and the COVID-19 pandemic (2020).

Multiple other federal laws guide national emergency preparedness and response efforts. The Homeland Security Act of 2002 creates and sets responsibilities of the Department of Homeland Security (DHS), which plays prominent roles in emergency coordination and management nationally (Homeland Security Act of 2002. Pub. L. No. 107-296, 116 Stat. 2135). The Public Health Security and Bioterrorism Preparedness and Response Act of 2002 authorizes the implementation of the National Disaster Medical System (NDMS) to coordinate rapid deployment of specialized response teams (Public Health Security and Bioterrorism Preparedness Response Act, Pub. L. No. 107-188, 116 Stat. 594). The Project BioShield Act of 2004 establishes the Strategic National Stockpile (SNS) to expedite distribution of essential medicines and supplies nationally. Amendments to the Social Security Act allow emergency waivers of select emergency medical screening and stabilization provisions of the Emergency Medical Treatment and Active Labor Act (EMTALA. 42 U.S.C.A. § 1320b-5; Project BioShield Act of 2004, Pub. L. No. 108-276, 118 Stat. 835).

The Public Readiness and Emergency Preparedness (PREP) Act authorizes rapid distribution and implementation of federally approved medical countermeasures (MCMs; e.g., medicines, vaccines, or supplies; 42 U.S.C. § 247d–6d). Subject to a PREP Act declaration by the secretary of the DHHS, immunity from liability claims may be extended to officials, manufacturers, drug distributors, pharmacies, HCWs, and others in the pipeline of development, distribution, and administration of MCMs. A compensation fund sets aside money for claims of individuals injured by the administration or use of MCMs. The PREP Act declarations may be retroactive, contemporaneous, or proactive. For example, on March 10, 2020, DHHS Secretary Azar issued a PREP Act declaration in response to COVID-19 (which was subsequently amended multiple times to address real-time issues throughout the year; DHHS, 2020a). On December 2, 2020, during the zenith of the COVID pandemic, he also issued a separate PREP Act declaration to address potential, future impacts of the deadly Marburg virus despite no known cases in the United States (DHHS, 2020c).

## State, Tribal, and Local Emergency Powers and Roles

Substantial transformations of state/territorial, Tribal, and local public health authorities post 9/11 center on how to prevent and respond to bioterrorism incidents and other threats with the potential for systemic, long-term, and widespread disability and death in the population. Many legal reforms are derived from the **Model State Emergency Health Powers Act** (MSEHPA) drafted by the Centers for Law and the Public's Health at Georgetown and Johns Hopkins Universities with CDC (and other) support between October to December 2001 (Gostin et al., 2002).

The MSEHPA introduced a structured and cohesive series of model provisions for governments considering how to respond to public health crises. As discussed further in what follows, it provides a menu of existing, expedited public health powers for consideration and use in a PHE, defined as:

> an occurrence or imminent threat of an illness or health condition that: (1) is believed to be caused by … bioterrorism; the appearance of a novel or previously controlled or eradicated infectious agent or biological toxin [*or other causes*]; … and (2) poses a high probability of … a large number of deaths … or serious or long-term disabilities in the affected population; or widespread exposure to an infectious or toxic agent that poses a significant risk of substantial future harm to a large number of people in the affected population (MSEHPA § 104[m]).

Some critics viewed this definition as overly broad and a potential source for unwarranted infringements of individual rights in favor of communal objectives. In reality, this definition of PHE was far more precise and limiting on governmental powers than existing all-hazards approaches. State-based declarations of "emergency" or "disaster" could typically be issued almost completely at the discretion of state governors, Tribal leaders, local mayors, or county executives. Pursuant to MSEHPA, a PHE can be declared by a governor (with recommended input from the state health commissioner) only when a public health threat poses a "high probability" of a large number of deaths, disabilities, or exposures to harmful agents in an affected population. Declarations are limited in their duration (subject to renewal) and expedited public health powers are framed within constitutional limits (e.g., respect for autonomy, liberty, due process, and equal protection).

State and local uptake of key provisions of the MSEHPA was extensive. By 2006, 39 states' legislatures had passed bills related to the Act (The Center for Law and the Public's Health at Georgetown and Johns Hopkins Universities, 2006). By 2015, the Network for Public Health Law determined that 34 states and the District of Columbia had legislatively crafted explicit definitions of PHEs (or like terms) into their laws (The Network for Public Health Law, 2015). The MSEHPA provisions regarding public health powers, licensure reciprocity, and liability protections were included in other model acts, including the Turning Point Model State Public Health Act of 2003 and the Uniform Emergency Volunteer Health Practitioners Act (UEVHPA) of 2007.

## Shifting Scope of Public Health Emergencies

Legal boundaries crafted around PHEs were intended to confine declarations to instances where quickly developing factors militate rapid, effective, and balanced public health responses. Consistent with these purposes, many national or regional PHE declarations are warranted, including in response to (a) contagious diseases like H1N1 (2009), Ebola virus (2014), and Zika virus (2016); (b) natural disasters impacting human lives such as hurricanes Katrina (2005), Sandy (2012), and Harvey (2017); and (c) emerging health conditions like opioid misuse (2017), Alzheimer's and other mental health conditions (2018), and antibiotic resistance (2019).

Yet PHEs have also been formally declared to address an array of differing events and conditions (e.g., water contamination, domestic violence, food insecurity, homelessness, vaping, and medical cannabis) that stretch the concept beyond its core foundations. In addition, policymakers, scholars, media, and others have classified multifarious public health threats as "crises," "tragedies," "catastrophes," or "epidemics." These tags have been applied to a range of conditions (e.g., microaggression [2015], decreased sperm counts [2017], video game addiction [2018], skin bleaching [2018], and pornography [2019]). Framing these and other conditions as emergencies and the like confuses and diminishes the legal meaning and appropriate uses of PHEs (Hodge et al., 2019).

The COVID-19 pandemic recalibrated the concept of a true PHE in 2020 based in large part on original conceptions noted in the MSEHPA and subsequent legal reforms. Unprecedented PHE legal responses to the pandemic included: (a) federal invocation of emergency and PHE declarations; (b) simultaneous emergency declarations across all 50 states and thousands of Tribal/local governments; and (c) implementation of crisis standards of care (CSC) plans in multiple jurisdictions. As deaths exceeded hundreds of thousands, virtually all PHE powers and responses were exercised against the backdrop of an epidemiologically-complex infectious disease that swept across populations in multiple waves.

To the extent COVID-19 presented the first major test of modern PHE legal preparedness to respond to a significant, sustained, and largely preventable threat, many may suggest the U.S. public health system failed. Law- and policy-makers scrambled to issue emergency declarations, legislate quick fixes (including actions to address enormous economic impacts of long-standing social distancing orders), and address substantial judicial challenges to efficacious public health response efforts. The aftermath of the pandemic will unquestionably lead to additional reforms of PHE laws at all levels of government. The Uniform Law Commission has proposed multiple model law projects to address perceived or actual gaps in legal preparedness and response.

However, as compared with other industrialized countries, multifactorial causes of excess morbidity and mortality due to COVID-19 in the United States may be tied more to politics than extant legal gaps in a federalist system of government. Despite historic and contemporaneous proof of efficacy of significant PHE legal interventions (e.g., social distancing, closures, face masks, hygiene, and testing), political factors severely limited their use in response to the pandemic. As federal authorities concentrated on rapid development of vaccines, states, Tribes, and localities were left largely to combat the virus on the frontlines while pleading for greater federal assistance. Interjurisdictional variations across states and localities grounded in politics, instead of science or law, contributed substantially to deleterious public health and economic impacts of the pandemic.

## EMERGENCY LEGAL PLANNING, PREPAREDNESS, AND RESPONSE

Against this backdrop of PHEs, shifting legal landscapes, and resulting health impacts, effective emergency planning, preparedness, and response are critical. Public health actors must carefully consider advance emergency planning, the scope of available PHE powers, and limitations on PHE powers to optimize health outcomes during an emergency.

### Advance Emergency Planning

Advance emergency planning is a legal and ethical imperative in ensuring effective PHE response and management. Prompt implementation of emergency plans can reduce morbidity and mortality (Binder, 2002, pp. 791, 793; Kanu et al., 2020). As discussed previously, after 9/11 substantial additional resources were allocated into advance emergency planning largely at national and state levels. From 2002 to 2010, the federal government provided roughly $7.6 billion to states and territories to strengthen emergency preparedness (Lister, 2011).

In addition, state, Tribal, and federal laws may provide for and require advance emergency planning. California's Emergency Services Act, for example, requires the governor to coordinate state- and local-level emergency plans (Fla. Stat. § 252.35). The Code of the Snoqualmie Tribe (WA) requires its Emergency Management Department to develop a "Tribal Comprehensive Emergency Management Plan" (Snoqualmie Tribal Code 10.1, §§ 4.0, 6.0). In addition to governmental requirements, private actors may be obligated contractually or otherwise to implement emergency planning. The Joint Commission, which sets national health facility accreditation standards, requires hospitals to demonstrate emergency preparedness through planning (The Joint Commission, 2016). The federal Centers for Medicare and Medicaid Services (CMS) requires entities receiving federal funds to include certain standards in their emergency plans (42 C.F.R. § 482.15).

PHE planning is undergirded by ethical duties. Core public health ethics principles support the moral obligation of public and private actors/entities to provide for the public's health (Thomas et al., 2002). Investing in planning proactively reflects the utilitarian goal of maximizing population health outcomes (Hick et al., 2020). Preparing to act in an ethical manner helps avoid hasty actions that may exacerbate existing health inequities or create new ones.

Certain populations face heightened risks during PHEs, including the elderly, pregnant women, children, individuals with disabilities, prisoners, vulnerable ethnic groups, those facing language barriers, persons experiencing homelessness, and other impoverished groups (Hoffman, 2009). During Hurricane Katrina (2005), emergency plan failures impacted populations who were unable to self-evacuate, including impoverished persons, the elderly, or individuals with disabilities. These vulnerable persons were most likely to perish; more than 75% of those who died in the aftermath of the hurricane were over the age of 60 (U.S. Army Corps of Engineers, 2006). Swift political backlash led Congress to pass the Post-Katrina Emergency Reform Act of 2006, which established a "Disability Coordinator" within FEMA (Post-Katrina Emergency Reform Act of 2006, Pub. L. 109-295, § 513). Some states have taken similar legislative actions. Florida's Emergency Management Act, for example, requires state agencies contracting with care providers for persons with disabilities to include emergency- and disaster-planning provisions in provider contracts (Fla. Stat. § 252.356).

Inadequate planning for vulnerable populations may lead to liability claims. After Hurricanes Irene (2011) and Sandy (2012) swept across New York City, a class action lawsuit filed on behalf of all persons with disabilities against the City and then-Mayor Michael Bloomberg alleged failures of the City's emergency response program. The court concluded that the City had violated the Americans with Disabilities Act, the federal Rehabilitation Act, and New York City Human Rights law by failing to (a) accommodate evacuation needs of individuals with disabilities living in multistory buildings; (b) provide accessible shelters; and (c) inform persons with disabilities about accessible services during emergencies, among other failures (*Brooklyn Ctr. for Indep. of Disabled v. Bloomberg*, 2013). A comprehensive settlement agreement addressed multiple failings identified in the order.

## HYPOTHETICAL CASE STUDY: PANDEMIC HEALTH EMERGENCY

The outbreak of a highly infectious and deadly viral disease begins with a few isolated cases that worried physicians and epidemiologists in Southeast Asia. Attempts at testing, screening, contact tracing, and containment are employed quickly, but the contagion is difficult to quell. Within weeks, additional cases are identified in Rome, Paris, London, and then in large U.S. cities including Seattle, Chicago, and Miami. Cases escalate in urban environments as intrastate movement through air, train, and vehicular transportation results in rapid continental spread.

Governors and public health officials across the United States declare PHEs and consider additional orders to promote social distancing and prevent further devastation, but they are unsure how long they can sustain emergency responses. Hospitals in major urban areas are reaching maximum capacity in intensive care units (ICUs) and are in short supply of personal protective equipment (PPE). Hospitals' staff-infected rates climb exponentially. Several hospitals cannot maintain effective care for infected and noninfected patients without greater assistance, despite triage efforts. Workers on the front lines feel they are inadequately protected from infection. They worry about their potential liability given real-time risks of screening and treating surging numbers of patients.

Scientists are working hard to develop effective countermeasures. Several vaccines are in early development, but a safe and effective vaccine may take 6 months to complete initial trials and another 6–12 months to vaccinate sufficient numbers of Americans beginning with select categories of frontline HCWs. Thousands of Americans are dying each week. Hundreds of thousands more may expire absent significant utilization of effective public health powers and response efforts.

- What legal powers affecting individuals or their property can public health officials and emergency managers exercise in response to the pandemic?
- How can hospitals legally respond to staff shortages under existing declared states of PHE?
- What legal options pursuant to PHE declarations and waivers of existing laws or policies may help improve the availability of HCWs and volunteers to screen, treat, or later vaccinate individuals?
- What liability protections may insulate HCWs and entities from unwarranted claims in the throes of the PHE?

## Public Health Emergency Powers

PHE declarations at every level of government rapidly reshape the legal landscape by authorizing a series of expedited and optional public health powers to respond to the emergency. These include powers (a) affecting individuals or groups, (b) governing uses of property, and (c) waiving existing statutes or regulations that inhibit effective responses.

Many PHE powers directly affect individuals or groups. During pandemics, where disease often spreads easily between individuals absent interventions, PHE actions may seek to promote or require social distancing as a means of reducing transmission. During disasters, terroristic threats or attacks, pandemics, and other emergencies, affected areas may require assistance from additional HCWs facilitated via PHE powers. Additionally, in any emergency, public health actors must disseminate transparent and accurate information to the public to obtain and maintain public trust. The aforementioned MSEHPA addresses these and other issues through a menu of PHE powers affecting individuals or groups, including the following:

- Real-time testing, screening, vaccinating, and treating persons exposed or infected with a communicable condition
- Implementing mass evacuations to prevent further loss of life (especially in cases of natural disasters)
- Collecting laboratory specimens from living or deceased persons or animals
- Separating exposed or infected individuals from others via **isolation** or **quarantine** measures to reduce transmission
- Obtaining assistance from out-of-state HCWs or volunteers through licensure reciprocity
- Informing populations via effective, culturally-appropriate public communications.

PHE powers also target the control and management of property. Government actors can destroy or abate hazardous materials or nuisances threatening the public's health. Pandemic or disaster emergencies can implicate seizure and use of private property (with just compensation) to (a) provide additional space for separating and treating patients or (b) free-up greater resources for use by HCWs or emergency responders. Additional powers governing property management set forth in the MSEHPA include the following:

- Gathering specimens and using safe handling procedures for the disposal of human remains or infectious waste, including syringes and bodily secretions
- Controlling healthcare supplies via procurement, rationing, prioritization, and distribution
- Limiting price gouging of essential needs
- Closing roads or businesses to limit disease spread or exposure to dangerous conditions.

Of course, not all of these optional PHE powers may be executed simultaneously in an emergency. Rather, PHE powers should be tailored and used only as warranted to protect the public's health. Judicious, flexible uses of vast and varied powers enable public and private actors to address ever-changing and unprecedented circumstances.

Emergency legal interventions may also necessitate moving beyond routine laws and policies that inhibit responses. Consequently, the MSEHPA and similar state laws typically allow state governors or public health officials to waive existing laws and regulations to effectuate response efforts. For example, under a declared state of disaster emergency in Pennsylvania, state agency rules may be suspended if strict compliance would hinder emergency response (35 Pa. Cons. Stat. § 7301[f][1]). During the COVID-19 emergency, Pennsylvania Governor Tom Wolf and the Department of State expedited temporary licensure to out-of-state practitioners and licensure reactivation for retired HCWs or those with inactive or lapsed licenses (Pennsylvania Department of State, 2020a, 2020b).

## Limits on Use of Public Health Emergency Powers

Despite the breadth and flexibility of PHE powers, public health actors must consider several important limitations when engaging in emergency response. PHE powers are limited through: (a) appropriate balancing with individual rights; (b) durational restrictions; (c) proof of efficacy; and (d) political accountability.

First, public health interventions must always be balanced against potential or actual unjustified intrusions on individual rights. Public health actors are ethically and often legally required to utilize only the least restrictive interventions available to ensure due consideration of individual liberty (Kass, 2001, pp. 1776, 1780). For example, to the extent that isolation and quarantine powers directly implicate individual freedoms of movement and rights to travel, they must be utilized only when needed to attain substantial public health objectives and must be consistent with procedural due process. Express language regarding implementation of quarantine and isolation powers in the MSEHPA sets forth extensive due process protections, including specific notice and hearing requirements for affected individuals or groups (MSEHPA § 605[b], 2019).

As a second limitation on PHE powers, durational restrictions may be written into federal or state statutes/regulations or imposed by courts via case-based challenges. During the COVID-19 pandemic, Michigan Governor Gretchen Whitmer's statutory PHE powers were curtailed by the Michigan Supreme Court when it determined that state statutes required the Michigan legislature's consent to extend the emergency declaration beyond its initial issuance (*In re Certified Questions from U.S. Dist. Ct.*, 2020). Durational limitations also ensure continual review of the necessity of PHE powers. The MSEHPA provides for automatic termination of a declaration after 30 days unless renewed under the same standards guiding the initial issuance. For months throughout the COVID-19 pandemic, multiple governors consistently reissued PHE declarations based on continued warranted needs.

A third limitation on exercising PHE powers relates to proof of efficacy. Public health interventions should not be implemented without known or reasonably believed efficacy that PHE actions will directly benefit individual or communal health, and proof of efficacy is doubly necessary when political motivations cut against interventions (Hensel & Wolf, 2011). PHE powers lacking efficacy may be questioned judicially or ethically. Actions impacting individuals (e.g., vaccine mandates) without concomitant public health benefits (e.g., significant reductions in transmissibility and assurances of safety) erode public trust (Hodge et al., 2015).

Finally, use of PHE powers must meet political accountability. In PHEs, the public trusts that political actors will focus their responses on reducing morbidity and mortality. Failures to achieve these objectives may be measured at the ballot box. In a 2011 study, researchers concluded that voters who experience a severe weather event tend to "punish politicians who do not take action" (Gasper & Reeves, 2011, pp. 1, 14). Abject failures to control COVID-19 infections nationally in 2020 impacted national and regional elections. Just as ineffective, real-time emergency responses carry political repercussions, overly excessive reactions restricting individuals or groups may be deemed arbitrary or unjustified.

## REAL-TIME LEGAL CHALLENGES IN EMERGENCY PREPAREDNESS AND RESPONSE

As the legal landscape at all levels of government changes dramatically and instantaneously in declared PHEs, rapid emergency response implementation raises major challenges. Supported by interwoven ethics principles, carefully crafted emergency laws can provide a foundation for altered scopes of practice, licensure reciprocity, CSC, and liability protections to help public health actors address evolving emergency circumstances.

## Practicing Legal Triage

Hospitals or other providers experiencing patient surges during PHEs must prioritize patient care based on urgency of need. Similarly, legal practitioners must "triage"—or prioritize and resolve—legal issues arising during PHEs to effectuate appropriate public health responses (Hodge, 2006). Practitioners must assess the public health needs of affected populations using evidence-based information from the field to identify legal opportunities or barriers that either facilitate or impede effective responses. Working with public- and private-sector decision-makers, lawyers must craft legal tools and solutions to overcome these barriers and further public health responses through communications that are translatable on the frontlines of responses as well as to the general public.

Throughout the duration of a declared PHE, competing individual and communal interests must be weighed and balanced in legally and ethically sound ways. Under changing emergency circumstances, constitutional, statutory, and regulatory norms may be adjusted as necessary to facilitate emergency responses. Many HCWs or other essential frontline responders may be unable to assess the legality of their actions during emergencies—potentially exposing them to legal risk or dissuading them from acting due to fear of liability. Conflicts may arise between governmental and private actors, especially where public health and economic interests are seemingly at odds. Individuals subject to governmental restrictions (e.g., quarantine or contact tracing) may assert their rights (e.g., religious freedom, due process, or privacy). While there is no blueprint for managing every legal issue that may arise during PHEs, practitioners adept in legal triage can help assure that individual and communal interests are consistently, appropriately, and regularly balanced as emergency circumstances change.

## Interwoven Principles of Public Health Emergency Ethics

In practice, legal triage entails rapid decision-making against a backdrop of unfolding health threats, incomplete information, and evolving political, economic, and social instability. Inevitable questions arise as to whether a public health response is not only legal, but also ethical. Those engaged in legal triage should be guided by ethics principles including: (a) harm reduction and benefits promotion (i.e., reducing morbidity and mortality), (b) liberty and human rights (i.e., promoting human dignity and autonomy), (c) distributive and social justice (i.e., equitable sharing of benefits and burdens of emergency circumstances), and (d) public accountability and transparent deliberations (i.e., building public trust through sound decision-making processes; Jennings & Arras, 2008).

Embedding PHE ethics into legal triage promotes community values and reinforces public trust and legitimacy in governmental responses. As discussed previously, emergency restrictions on individuals' liberty, autonomy, or property may be ethically justified if tailored to achieve public health and safety objectives. These same measures are ethically suspect, however, if grounded in discrimination and stigmatization. During the COVID-19 pandemic in April 2020, for example, San Diego police officers cleared homeless encampments under the state's stay-home order, contrary to CDC guidance (Halverstadt, 2020). In New York City, minorities were disproportionately cited for social distancing violations under vague enforcement provisions (Bellware, n.d.). Sound emergency laws must clearly and comprehensively address potential ethical pitfalls underlying public health preparedness and response.

## Crisis Standards of Care

Ethics concerns also arise in PHE responses related to distributions of scarce resources (e.g., food, vaccines, beds, and PPE) and the responsibilities of healthcare and other essential workers. In declared emergencies, a shift to CSC enables a substantial change in usual health-care operations and the level of patient care that can be delivered due to a pervasive or catastrophic emergency or disaster. The Institute of Medicine (now known as the National Academy of Medicine [NAM]) conceptualized CSC initially in 2009, updated it in 2012, and revisited it in a November 2019 workshop just prior to the COVID-19 outbreak (Institute of Medicine, 2009). In March 2020, the NAM issued guidance on pertinent issues related to medical triage decisions involving COVID-19 patients (National Academies of Sciences, Engineering, and Medicine, 2020).

Standards for patient care during emergencies fall along a continuum from "conventional" to "contingency" to "crisis" (Gostin & Hanfling, 2009). Conventional standards of care reflect professional norms and expectations outside of emergency circumstances where healthcare resources and personnel may be strained. Contingency standards entail new strains on healthcare systems extending from temporary exigencies (e.g., a hospital facing a surge of patients due to a multivehicle collision in a snowstorm).

During declared emergencies, however, HCWs and entities may experience extensive, long-term shortages of essential resources that necessitate a shift to CSC centered on population-level needs. Under CSC, scarce resources may be prioritized for affected persons with (a) the most urgent health needs or risks and (b) the highest likelihood of benefitting from prioritized care. Shifting medical standards in emergencies requires extensive, advance planning among public and private sectors (Cleveland Manchanda et al., 2020). During the COVID-19 pandemic, many entities activated their CSC plans or released specific CSC guidance for impacted patients (Hodge, 2020).

Allocation decisions involving the lives of individuals and populations are fraught with legal and ethical controversies, including liability claims. During the COVID-19 pandemic, for example, several states' CSC plans were heavily criticized for deprioritizing persons with chronic conditions from receiving ventilators—foreseeably disadvantaging persons with disabilities, minorities, the elderly, and other vulnerable populations. In March 2020, DHHS' Office of Civil Rights opined that several states' CSC plans incorporated unlawful, discriminatory criteria for making triage decisions, leading to immediate adjustments by states (Office of Civil Rights, 2020).

## Altered Scopes of Practice

Another legal mechanism bolstering PHE responses involves expanding the "scope of practice" of the healthcare workforce, which may be overwhelmed by patient surges. Professional scope of practice parameters define and limit the extent and location of specific activities that HCWs and volunteers are authorized to perform based on statutes, regulations, licensure requirements, and professional rules (Hodge et al., 2005). To meet healthcare demands and ensure robust PHE responses, states can legally temporarily expand professional scope of practice parameters provided patient-level care is of sufficient quality. For example, scope of practice may be expanded to allow a greater array of HCWs to administer vaccines or distribute MCMs during a pandemic emergency.

Various legal avenues facilitate expansions of scope of practice during PHEs. As of 2016, laws in 14 states contained built-in exceptions to vaccination authority restrictions for pharmacists during epidemics or emergencies (Schmit & Reddick, 2016). As discussed previously, some state laws authorize waivers or suspensions of statutes or regulations impeding responses. During the COVID-19 pandemic, New York Governor Andrew Cuomo used broad waiver powers to authorize nurse practitioners and others to perform services appropriate to their education and training without typically required physician supervision (Cuomo, 2020). In other cases, professional scopes of practice may be altered via licensing boards, temporary emergency rules or regulations, or legislative amendments. Federal and state emergency rules and regulatory waivers helped increase the types of providers and circumstances permissible for telehealth services during the COVID-19 pandemic (CMS, 2020). Yet, scope of practice expansions must include considerations for protecting patients' health, safety, and privacy, such as adequate training and accountability measures for HCWs.

## Licensure Reciprocity

Similar to scope of practice, professional licensure or certifications of HCWs are grounded in state laws and regulations that differ across jurisdictions. Governments set licensure requirements for practicing HCWs within each state, including minimum education and training requirements, circumstances for practicing a profession, and scope of practice limitations. Outside of routine or emergency provisions, health professionals cannot lawfully practice in a state where they are not licensed. Licensure requirements can impair health professionals' abilities to practice across state lines, either physically or through telemedicine, during PHEs when outside personnel are needed to meet patient surges.

Several established legal mechanisms address these barriers by providing out-of-state licensure reciprocity through routine agreements, emergency provisions, and emergency waivers. Outside of declared emergencies, some states allow HCWs licensed and in good standing in other states to receive licensure reciprocity. As of 2020, 33 states have adopted the Nurse Licensure Compact (NLC), which allows nurses to practice in any other NLC state under an expedited application process (National Council of State Boards of Nursing, n.d.). In declared emergencies, some state laws automatically allow for licensure reciprocity for out-of-state professionals. For example, in Wyoming, "physicians, dentists, veterinarians, nurses or other professional personnel" are eligible for "reciprocity … to practice their professional talents without the normal admissions to practice in this state during the period of the emergency" (Wyoming Stat. Ann. § 19-13-115).

States may also enter mutual aid agreements to share resources or personnel during emergencies, such as the Emergency Management Assistance Compact (EMAC) adopted by all 50 U.S. states. The EMAC expressly recognizes the licensure of out-of-state HCWs in good standing. Provisions of the aforementioned UEVHPA also recognize the license of registered HCWs in declared emergencies (American College of Surgeons, 2014). In other cases, governors may utilize their broad emergency waiver or suspension authorities to temporarily eliminate licensure requirements.

## Liability Protections for Healthcare Workers, Volunteers, and Entities

A principal concern among HCWs called to the frontlines of PHE responses is the potential for unwarranted liability claims amidst CSC, altered scopes of practice, and licensure reciprocity. Some HCWs and entities may limit health services out of fear of liability. Others may choose not to participate at all to avoid the specter of claims of negligence. While there is no universal mechanism to defend against all claims, numerous routine and emergency laws protect HCWs, volunteers, and entities from specific liability claims (The Network for Public Health Law, 2017). These protections may immunize or indemnify persons or entities for acts of ordinary negligence, but generally not for gross negligence or willful, wanton and willful misconduct, or criminal misconduct.

Sovereign immunity principles protect governmental entities and personnel from civil liability claims related to official functions, which may include a government's response to a PHE. Some states' laws authorize nongovernmental personnel to be classified as governmental actors for the limited purposes of emergency response, extending sovereign immunity protections. Other states' laws immunize private sector HCWs, volunteers, and entities in emergencies. For example, in Arizona, a HCW engaged in emergency management activities is immune from claims except in cases of bad faith, willful misconduct, or gross negligence (Arizona Rev. Stat. Ann. § 26-314).

Other laws like the federal Volunteer Protection Act and federal Coronavirus Aid, Relief, and Economic Security Act address liability specifically for emergency volunteers. Under the federal PREP Act, noted previously, HCWs and entities are immune from liability concerning their use of covered countermeasures under an DHHS-declared emergency. Countermeasures can include infectious disease treatments, security countermeasures, and drugs, products, and devices allowed via an FDA EUA. During the COVID-19 pandemic, DHHS Secretary Azar intimated that PREP Act liability coverage extended even to omissions or failures to act (DHHS, 2020b). Thus, a justified decision to choose one person for vaccine over another could not result in a liability claim by the person who did not initially receive the vaccine. The EMAC and other mutual aid agreements offer additional liability protections. Governors may also extend immunities via emergency orders through their waiver and suspension powers.

## CONCLUSION

Legal and ethical public health preparedness fundamentally evolved post-9/11 as public and private sector actors aligned to define, coordinate, and plan for PHEs. Consequently, public health actors are armed with a wide array of optional and expedited PHE powers subject to limits and balancing of individual and community interests. Despite advancements in emergency legal preparedness in the 21st century, the COVID-19 pandemic and prior events exposed significant legal and political challenges subverting effective implementation and response efforts. Wielding legal authorities in real-time consistent with best practices, available data, emerging science, and ethical norms is key to maximizing positive health outcomes when legal responses are needed most.

## CHAPTER REVIEW

### Review Questions

1. How did the legal landscape of PHE powers change post-9/11?
2. What interventions can public health actors utilize to address PHEs?
3. What are some of the primary limitations on PHE powers?
4. How can PHE laws be wielded in real-time to effectuate improved health outcomes for individuals and populations?

### Essay Questions

1. You have been asked to develop a pandemic emergency response training exercise for state health officials in your jurisdiction. What issues will you include to ensure that the training is comprehensive? What legal and ethical issues would you want officials to discuss and address?
2. You have just been assigned the task of presenting on natural disaster legal and ethical preparedness to a group of attorneys who act as advisors to public health officials in your jurisdiction. Using historical and current information from your jurisdiction along with this chapter, develop a natural disaster scenario as a tool to explain the emergency declarations and options that can be taken in response.

## Internet Activities

1.  Take CDC's Public Health Emergency Law Online Training: https://www.cdc.gov/phlp/publications/topic/trainings/ph-emergencylaw.html
2.  Download and review NACCHO and the Network for Public Health Law's Local Public Health Emergency Legal Preparedness Module, available here: https://client.bluesky broadcast.com/naccho/2013/pdf/cd/TrainingCurriculum.ppt

## REFERENCES

35 PA. Cons. Stat. § 7301(f)(1).

42 C.F.R. § 482.15.

42 U.S.C. § 247d–6d (2012).

42 U.S.C.A. § 247d(a) (West 2020).

42 U.S.C.A. §§ 5170, 5122(1) (West 2020).

American College of Surgeons. (2014). *Uniform emergency volunteer health practitioners act* [Organization]. American College of Surgeons. https://www.facs.org/Advocacy/state/UEVHPA

Annas, G. J. (2010). *Worst case bioethics: Death, disaster, and public health.* Oxford University Press.

Arizona Rev. Stat. Ann. § 26-314.

Bellware, K. (n.d.). Violent arrest in New York raises questions about police enforcement of social distancing orders. *Washington Post.* https://www.washingtonpost.com/nation/2020/05/05/donni-wright-nyc-arrest

Binder, D. (2002). *Emergency action plans: A legal and practical blueprint failing to plan is planning to fail* (SSRN Scholarly Paper ID 844428). Social Science Research Network. https://papers.ssrn.com/abstract=844428

*Brooklyn Ctr. for Indep. of Disabled v. Bloomberg,* 1:11-cv-06690-JMF (S.D.N.Y. September 26, 2011). https://www.clearinghouse.net/detail.php?id=13015

Centers for Disease Control and Prevention. (2014, March 7). The Public Health Emergency Law (PHEL) Competency Model Version 1.0 [Government]. Centers for Disease Control and Prevention. https://www.cdc.gov/phlp/docs/compentency-modelv1.pdf

Centers for Medicare and Medicaid Services. (2020, March 17). *Medicare telemedicine health care provider fact sheet* [Government]. Centers for Medicare and Medicaid Services. https://www.cms.gov/newsroom/fact-sheets/medicare-telemedicine-health-care-provider-fact-sheet

Cleveland-Manchanda, E. C., Sanky, C., & Appel, J. M. (2020). Crisis standards of care in the USA: A systematic review and implications for equity amidst COVID-19. *Journal of Racial and Ethnic Health Disparities.* https://doi.org/10.1007/s40615-020-00840-5

Cuomo, A. (2020, March 23). *Executive Order No. 202.10: Continuing temporary suspension and modification of laws relating to the disaster emergency* [Government]. New York State Governor. https://www.governor.ny.gov/news/no-20210-continuing-temporary-suspension-and-modification-laws-relating-disaster-emergency

Emergency Medical Treatment and Active Labor Act. 42 U.S.C.A. § 1320b-5 (West 2019).

Florida Stat. § 252.35.

Florida Stat. § 252.356.

Food and Drug Administration. (2017). *Emergency use authorization of medical products and related authorities: Guidance for industry and other stakeholders* (Guidance HHS-0910-2017-F-1308). U.S. Department of Health & Human Services.

Gasper, J. T., & Reeves, A. (2011). Make it rain? Retrospection and the attentive electorate in the context of natural disasters. *American Journal of Political Science, 55*(2), 340–355. https://doi.org/10.1111/j.1540-5907.2010.00503.x

Gostin, L. O. (2002). Public health law in an age of terrorism: Rethinking individual rights and common goods. *Health Affairs, 21*(6), 79–93. https://doi.org/10.1377/hlthaff.21.6.79

Gostin, L. O., & Hanfling, D. (2009). National preparedness for a catastrophic emergency: Crisis standards of care. *Journal of the American Medical Association, 302*(21), 2365–2366. https://doi .org/10.1001/jama.2009.1780

Gostin, L. O., Sapsin, J. W., Teret, S. P., Burris, S., Mair, J. S., Hodge, J. G., Jr., & Vernick, J. S. (2002). The model state emergency health powers act: Planning for and response to bioterrorism and naturally occurring infectious diseases. *Journal of the American Medical Association, 288*(5), 622– 628. https://doi.org/10.1001/jama.288.5.622

Halverstadt, L. (2020, April 14). *Police are still citing the homeless, despite CDC and council guidance* [Organization]. Voice of San Diego. https://www.voiceofsandiego.org/topics/public-safety/pol ice-are-still-citing-the-homeless-despite-cdc-and-council-guidance

Hensel, W., & Wolf, L. (2011). Playing God: The legality of plans denying scarce resources to people with disabilities in public health emergencies. *Florida Law Review, 63*(3), 719. https://scholarship .law.ufl.edu/flr/vol63/iss3/5/

Hick, J. L., Hanfling, D., Wynia, M. K., & Pavia, A. T. (2020). Duty to plan: Health care, crisis standards of care, and novel coronavirus SARS-CoV-2. *National Academy of Medicine Perspectives.* https:// doi.org/10.31478/202003b

Hodge, J. G., Jr. (2006). Legal triage during public health emergencies and disasters. *Administrative Law Review, 58*(3), 627–644. https://www.jstor.org/stable/40711923

Hodge, J. G. (2017, January 27). *Public health emergency legal and ethical preparedness.* The Oxford Handbook of U.S. Health Law. https://doi.org/10.1093/oxfordhb/9780199366521.013.47

Hodge, J. G. (2018). Public health emergency legal preparedness and response. In *Public Health Law in a Nutshell* (3rd ed.). West Academic Publishing.

Hodge, J. G. (2020, September 30). *COVID-19 emergency legal preparedness primer.* The Network for Public Health Law. https://www.networkforphl.org/wp-content/uploads/2020/09/Western -Region-Primer-COVID-19-9-30-2020.pdf

Hodge, J. G., & Anderson, E. D. (2009). *Principles and practice of legal triage during public health emergencies* (SSRN Scholarly Paper ID 1335342). Social Science Research Network. https://papers.ssrn.com/ abstract=1335342

Hodge, J. G., Barraza, L., Weidenaar, K., Corbett, A., Measer, G., & Agrawal, A. (2015). Efficacy in emergency legal preparedness underlying the 2014 Ebola outbreak. *Texas A&M Law Review, 2,* 353–383. https://doi.org/10.37419/LR.V2.I3.1

Hodge, J. G., Mount, J. K., & Reed, J. F. (2005). Scope of practice for public health professionals and volunteers. *Journal of Law, Medicine and Ethics, 33*(4 Suppl.), 53–54. https://asu.pure.elsevier.com/ en/publications/scope-of-practice-for-public-health-professionals-and-volunteers

Hodge, J. G., Wetter, S. A., & White, E. N. (2019). Legal crises in public health. *The Journal of Law, Medicine & Ethics, 47*(4), 778–782. https://doi.org/10.1177/1073110519897792

Hoffman, S. (2009). *Preparing for disaster: Protecting the most vulnerable in emergencies. UC Davis Law Review, 42,* 1491. https://papers.ssrn.com/abstract=1268277

Homeland Security Act of 2002, Pub. L. No. 107–296, 116 Stat. 2135 (2002). https://www.dhs.gov/ho meland-security-act-2002

In re Certified Questions from U.S. Dist. Court, No. 161492___ (Michigan Supreme Court Oct. 2, 2020). https://courts.michigan.gov/Courts/MichiganSupremeCourt/Clerks/Recent%20Opinio ns/20-21%20Term%20Opinions/In%20re%20Certified%20Questions-OP.pdf

Institute of Medicine (US) Committee on Guidance for Establishing Standards of Care for Use in Disaster Situations. (2009). *Guidance for establishing crisis standards of care for use in disaster situations: A letter report* (B. M. Altevogt, C. Stroud, S. L. Hanson, D. Hanfling, & L. O. Gostin, Eds.). National Academies Press (US). http://www.ncbi.nlm.nih.gov/books/NBK219958

Jennings, B., & Arras, J. (2008). *Ethical guidance for public health emergency preparedness and response: Highlighting ethics and values in a vital public health service.* Centers for Disease Control and Prevention. https://www.cdc.gov/os/integrity/phethics/docs/white_paper_final_for_website _2012_4_6_12_final_for_web_508_compliant.pdf

The Joint Commission. (2016). *Emergency management standards supporting collaboration planning.* https://www.jointcommission.org/-/media/deprecated-unorganized/imported-assets/ tjc/system-folders/assetmanager/em_stds_collaboration_2016pdf.pdf?db=web&hash= 61306121B8D8EB2C53A4DAC313654B48

Kanu, F. A. (2020). Declines in SARS-CoV-2 transmission, hospitalizations, and mortality after implementation of mitigation measures—Delaware, March–June 2020. *MMWR. Morbidity and Mortality Weekly Report, 69*, 1691–1694. https://doi.org/10.15585/mmwr.mm6945e1

Kass, N. E. (2001). An ethics framework for public health. *American Journal of Public Health, 91*(11), 1776–1782. https://doi.org/10.2105/ajph.91.11.1776

Lister, S. (2011). *Public health and medical emergency management: Issues in the 112th Congress* (CRS Report for Congress). Congressional Research Service.

Model State Emergency Health Powers Act, §§ 104(m), 605(b). (2001). https://www.aapsonline.org/legis/msehpa.pdf

National Academies of Sciences, Engineering, and Medicine. (2020). *Rapid expert consultation on crisis standards of care for the COVID-19 pandemic.* The National Academies Press. https://doi.org/10.17226/25765

National Council of State Boards of Nursing, Inc. (n.d.). *Nurse Licensure Compact* [Organization]. NCSBN. https://www.ncsbn.org/nurse-licensure-compact.htm

National Emergencies Act. 50 U.S.C.A. §§ 1601, 1621, 1622, 1631, 1641, 1651 (West 2020).

Network for Public Health Law. (2015). *Table—Emergency declaration authorities across all states and D.C.* The Network for Public Health Law. https://www.networkforphl.org/wp-content/uploads/2020/01/Emergency-Declaration-Authorities.pdf

Network for Public Health Law. (2017). *Table—Legal liability protections for emergency medical/public health responses.* The Network for Public Health Law. https://www.networkforphl.org/wp-content/uploads/2020/01/Legal-Liability-Protections-for-Emergency-Medical-and-Public-Health-Responses.pdf

Obama, B. (2011, March 30). *Presidential policy directive/PPD-8: National preparedness.* Department of Homeland Security. https://www.dhs.gov/presidential-policy-directive-8-national-preparedness

Office of Civil Rights. (2020). *Civil Rights, HIPAA, and the Coronavirus Disease 2019 (COVID-19).* Department of Health and Human Services. https://www.hhs.gov/sites/default/files/ocr-bulletin-3-28-20.pdf

Pandemic and All-Hazards Preparedness Act, Pub. L. No. 109–417, 120 Stat. 2135 (2006).

Pennsylvania Department of State. (2020a). *Issuance of temporary licenses to health care practitioners not licensed in Pennsylvania to be expedited during coronavirus emergency.* https://www.dos.pa.gov/Documents/2020-03-18-Temporary-Licenses-Out-of-State-Practitioners.pdf

Pennsylvania Department of State. (2020b). *Temporary waiver of license reactivation requirements for additional health care practitioners during coronavirus emergency.* https://www.dos.pa.gov/Documents/2020-04-07-Summary-of-Additional-Health-Care-Practitioner-Waivers.pdf

Post-Katrina Emergency Reform Act of 2006, Pub. L. No. 109–295 § 513, 6 U.S.C. § 321b (2006).

Project BioShield Act of 2004, Pub. L. No. 108–276, 118 Stat. 835 (2004).

Public Health Security and Bioterrorism Preparedness Response Act, Pub. L. No. 107–188, 116 Stat. 594 (2002). https://www.govinfo.gov/content/pkg/PLAW-107publ188/pdf/PLAW-107publ188.pdf

Public Health Service Act. 42 U.S.C.A. § 201 et seq. (2020).

Schmit, C., & Reddick, A. (2016, January 1). *Pharmacist vaccination laws.* The Policy Surveillance Program. https://lawatlas.org/datasets/pharmacist-vaccination

Snoqualmie Tribal Code 10.1, §§ 4.0, 6.0 (2008). http://www.snoqualmietribe.us/sites/default/files/emergency_mgmt_act.10.1.codified.pdf

Stafford Disaster Relief and Emergency Assistance Act. 42 U.S.C.A. § 5121 et seq.

Sunshine, G. (2017). The case for streamlining emergency declaration authorities and adapting legal requirements to ever-changing public health threats. *Emory Law Journal, 67*(3), 397–414. https://www.ncbi.nlm.nih.gov/pmc/articles/PMC5956522

Sunshine, G., Barrera, N., Corcoran, A. J., & Penn, M. (2019). Emergency declarations for public health issues: Expanding our definition of emergency. *The Journal of Law, Medicine & Ethics : A Journal of the American Society of Law, Medicine & Ethics, 47*(2 Suppl.), 95–99. https://doi.org/10.1177/1073110519857328

Thomas, J. C., Sage, M., Dillenberg, J., & Guillory, V. J. (2002). A code of ethics for public health. *American Journal of Public Health, 92*(7), 1057–1059. https://doi.org/10.2105/ajph.92.7.1057

U.S. Army Corps of Engineers. (2006). *Performance evaluation of the New Orleans and Southeast Louisiana Hurricane protection system draft final report of the Interagency Performance Evaluation Task Force.* https://lccn.loc.gov/2006618548

U.S. Department of Health and Human Services. (2020a, March 17). *Declaration under the public readiness and emergency preparedness act for medical countermeasures against COVID-19* [Government]. Federal Register. https://www.federalregister.gov/documents/2020/03/17/2020-05484/declaration-under-the-public-readiness-and-emergency-preparedness-act-for-medical-countermeasures

U.S. Department of Health and Human Services. (2020b). *Fourth amendment to the declaration under the public readiness and emergency preparedness act for medical countermeasures against COVID-19 and republication of the declaration.* Department of Health and Human Services. https://www.federalregister.gov/documents/2020/12/09/2020-26977/fourth-amendment-to-the-declaration-under-the-public-readiness-and-emergency-preparedness-act-for

U.S. Department of Health and Human Services. (2020c, December 9). *Notice of declaration under the public readiness and emergency preparedness act for countermeasures against Marburgvirus and/or Marburg disease.* Federal Register. https://www.federalregister.gov/documents/2020/12/09/2020-26972/notice-of-declaration-under-the-public-readiness-and-emergency-preparedness-act-for-countermeasures

Wyoming Stat. Ann. § 19-13-115.

## Additional Resources

- **CDC's Public Health Emergency Law Online Training**
  https://www.cdc.gov/phlp/publications/topic/trainings/ph-emergencylaw.html
- **Public Health Law Academy Training: Public Health Threats & the U.S. Constitution**
  https://www.changelabsolutions.org/product/public-health-threats-us-constitution
- **The Network for Public Health Law's Legal Emergency Preparedness Resources**
  https://www.networkforphl.org/resources/legal-emergency-preparedness-resources
- **The Network for Public Health Law's Emergency Declaration Authorities Table**
  https://www.networkforphl.org/resources/emergency-declaration-authorities
- **CDC's Public Health Emergency Preparedness Clearinghouse**
  https://www.cdc.gov/phlp/publications/topic/emergency.html

# 12

# Global Health Law

Benjamin Mason Meier, Ana S. Ayala,* and Roojin Habibi

## Learning Objectives

By the end of this chapter, the reader will be able to:

- Discuss the importance of global health law in addressing global public health threats.
- Describe the World Health Organization's expansive authority to develop and implement international law to promote global public health, codifying global health law to address infectious disease (as seen in the International Health Regulations) and noncommunicable disease (as seen in the Framework Convention on Tobacco Control).
- Analyze how global health law can strengthen global health governance to foster international coordination and build public health capacity among state and nonstate actors.
- Conceptualize the promise of global health law as a foundation to realize global health with justice.

## Key Terminology

**Global Health:** Addressing public health in a globalizing world, global health looks beyond the efforts of individual nations to encompass the larger set of determinants that affect the health of the entire world. Global health recognizes that all countries are interconnected in facing public health threats, requiring collective global action to promote health and achieve equity in health for all people worldwide.

**Global Health Law:** Global health law describes legal frameworks that structure global public health. These frameworks encompass the legal institutions, processes, and instruments—both hard and soft law—that support global health and shape how a vast landscape of state and non-state actors engage in disease prevention and health promotion. This legal engagement is anchored in the fundamental premise that, in a globalizing world, threats to public health increasingly transcend national frontiers and require cross-border coordination.

**International Health Law:** The traditional approach to the application and use of international law to address public health challenges is driven solely by relationships among national governments (states). Historically, international health law structured multilateral cooperation (across multiple states) under international law to respond to public

---

*The views expressed are the author's own and do not reflect the views of the United States Government or the U.S. Department of Health and Human Services.

health threats. As compared to global health law, international health law does not include nonstate actors and does not necessarily focus on the promotion of justice in public health.

**International Health Regulations (IHR):** The IHR are an international legal agreement that aims to prevent, detect, control and provide a public health response to the international spread of disease. Overseen by the World Health Organization (WHO) and last revised in 2005, this legal instrument enshrines a broad range of state obligations, including the requirement that states build core public health capacities, that they maintain public health responses that are commensurate with the risk to human health, and that they acknowledge and act cooperatively in accordance with WHO guidance.

**International Human Rights Law:** International human rights law comprises a branch of international law focused on legal standards to address basic needs and establish necessary entitlements to uphold a universal moral vision for the advancement of dignity and justice. As a basis for global justice, international human rights obligations frame governmental responsibilities and facilitate legal accountability to realize the highest attainable standard of health for all.

**International Law:** International law is developed between national governments (states), often embodied in writing in a single treaty or related instruments, and is legally binding on governments party to the instrument. When governments seek to cooperate with other countries to confront a common health threat, international law often becomes central to crafting a coordinated approach.

**Public Health Emergency of International Concern (PHEIC):** Defined by Article 1 of the IHR, a PHEIC is as an extraordinary event which (1) poses a public health risk to other states, as seen through the international spread of disease; and (2) potentially requires a coordinated international response. Under the IHR, the legal authority to declare a PHEIC rests with the WHO Director-General, and is intended to alert states to the imperative for international cooperation and information exchange in a global public health response.

**Soft Law:** Soft law comprises a set of instruments that are not legally binding but express or lead to commitments with legal implications, as seen in codes of conduct, voluntary resolutions, and global declarations. As compared with legally binding hard law, soft law can be used, among other things, to reinforce legally binding commitments, serve as the basis for the future development of legally binding instruments, and interpret norms set out by legally binding treaties.

**State:** Under international law, a state is an organized political community, a nation or territory under one government, and capable of accepting binding obligations under international law. States are distinguished from nonstate actors—nongovernmental organizations, private businesses, and individual advocates that have power to effect change but are generally not bound by international law. A state that is bound by an international law is referred to as a "state party" to that law.

## Public Health Law Competencies

This chapter addresses the following competencies from the Public Health Law Competency Model (PHLCM; Ransom, 2016).

**1.1** Define basic constitutional concepts and legal principles framing the practice of public health across relevant jurisdictions.

**1.2** Identify and apply public health laws (e.g., statutes, regulations, ordinances, and court rulings) pertinent to practitioner's jurisdiction, agency, program, and profession.

**2.3** Recognize the legal authority and limits of critical system partners and others who influence health outcomes.

**Spark Questions**

1. How has globalization facilitated the global spread of disease? Think about ways that infectious diseases and noncommunicable diseases are determined by globalized forces. How have these global forces highlighted the importance of looking beyond domestic law to develop a global public health law response?
2. Where public health threats cross national boundaries and spread internationally, how can state and nonstate actors develop global health laws to address public health threats collectively and realize health equity worldwide?
3. How can the World Health Organization lead global health governance through global health law, ensuring a future of global health with justice?

## INTRODUCTION

**Global health law** describes legal frameworks that structure global public health. Globalization has exacerbated the spread of disease, affecting both fast-moving infectious diseases and—through transnational corporations and global markets—the influence of commercial determinants of health on noncommunicable diseases (NCDs). With globalization connecting societies in shared vulnerability, these forces have highlighted the limitations of domestic law in addressing global determinants of health (Aginam, 2005). Yet, if globalization has presented challenges to domestic disease prevention and health promotion efforts, global health law, as highlighted in Box 12.1, offers the promise of bridging national boundaries to alleviate public health inequities through the development of global norms and standards.

Arising out of **international health law**, which has structured multilateral cooperation under **international law** to respond to public health threats for over a century, global health law now seeks to structure the contemporary governance landscape for **global health**. To address the health harms of a globalizing world, global health law has sought to "evolve beyond its traditional confines of formal sources and subjects of international law" to realize "global health with justice" (Gostin & Taylor, 2008). This focus on global health has necessitated measures beyond individual nations and international laws, requiring both **state** and nonstate actors to come together to respond to globalized health challenges (Moon, 2018). Global health law seeks to frame this new global governance landscape to respond to the health challenges of the 21st century.

## BOX 12.1  AN IMPERATIVE FOR GLOBAL HEALTH LAW

"Health risks in the 21st century are beyond the control of any government in any country. In an era of globalization, promoting public health and equity requires cooperation and coordination both within and among states. Law can be a powerful tool for advancing global health, yet it remains substantially underutilised and poorly understood" (*Lancet* Commission report on Global Health and the Law, https://www.thelancet.com/commissions/legal-determinants-of-health).

Global health law has thus become a basis to describe the legal frameworks that seek to address the health challenges arising from an increasingly globalized world, reflecting a new set of public health threats, nonstate actors, and normative instruments that structure global health.

- New health threats—including emerging infectious diseases, NCDs, injuries, mental health, harmful commercial products, and other globalized health threats
- New health actors—including civil society, transnational corporations, private philanthropists, and other nonstate actors
- New health instruments—including international treaties, **soft law** instruments (codes of conduct, strategies, and resolutions), and other normative instruments of global health policy (Gostin, 2014).

Placing public health obligations on the global community of state and nonstate actors, these legal frameworks seek to realize justice in global health through sustainable global institutions that embrace values of equity, monitor progress, structure multisectoral engagement, and facilitate accountability to advance global public health (Magnusson et al., 2017).

This chapter introduces the field of global health law as a foundation to prevent disease and promote health in a globalizing world. Recognizing inequalities in public health throughout the world, the *Background* section considers the extent to which legal capacities and authorities differ across nations, undermining efforts to achieve equity in global health. To alleviate these global inequities, the *Analysis* sections (and accompanying *Hypothetical Case Studies*) look to global health governance as central to global health law, with the World Health Organization (WHO) exercising its legal authorities to prevent the international spread of infectious diseases and the underlying global determinants of NCDs. The *Discussion* section examines the rising importance of global health law to realize global health with justice, considering the influence of human rights law as a foundation for dignity in global health and the rise of new legal initiatives to alleviate global inequity. This chapter's *Conclusion* holds that engaging with public health law in a globalizing world will require global health law, establishing a basis for the global practice of public health law.

## BACKGROUND: AN IMPERATIVE FOR GLOBAL HEALTH LAW

Across countries, the legal frameworks anchoring disease prevention and health promotion are critically important in achieving global public health—including the prevention and control of vaccine-preventable diseases, access to safe water and sanitation, tobacco control, improved preparedness and response to epidemic threats, and control of neglected tropical diseases. Robust public health laws are essential to improving health outcomes and reducing health inequities throughout the world. Equity in global health envisions a world in which differences in health—within and across countries—are redressed through public health law in order to achieve optimal health for all population groups where they live, work, and play.

Law structures health outcomes by shaping the underlying determinants of the public's health, and these legal determinants of health equity provide a path to advance global health with justice. Yet, legal capacities and institutional authorities differ greatly across countries, weakening efforts to ensure equity in health across nations (Gostin et al., 2019).

The intersecting landscape of law, enforcement of law, and legal systems governing public health varies considerably from country to country. Public health law is unequal throughout the world, as seen in divergent national responses to the COVID-19 pandemic, with impactful differences across national laws to protect vulnerable populations. While there are laws that safeguard health as a human right, there are also laws that may result in punitive outcomes, stigma, or discriminatory harm, undercutting public health efforts. These inequalities in legal determinants of health have raised an imperative to address public health law at the global level.

Global health law has arisen as a framework to structure global health governance, encompassing, as detailed in Box 12.2, both international health law and "soft law" forms of global health policy. As the leading normative institution in global health governance, the WHO has the legal mandate under its constitution to propose conventions, regulations, and recommendations on any public health matter. Drawing on this global regulatory authority, states have engaged in lawmaking through the WHO to structure both infectious disease control and NCD prevention.

---

### BOX 12.2  GLOBAL HEALTH LAW: THE EXPANDING LEGAL LANDSCAPE TO PROMOTE GLOBAL HEALTH

- Global health law presents a legal framework to structure efforts by the global community to advance global health.
- Where global health has come to frame efforts to address common public health challenges across countries, law has become crucial to addressing the global health threats that have arisen in a rapidly globalizing world.
- This focus on global health, addressing global determinants of public health, demands an expanded scope and influence of public health law to meet the public health needs of a globalizing world, redressing health inequities within and across countries through global health law.
- Looking across countries, global health law has applied new sources of soft law to facilitate cooperation across state and nonstate actors, frame new institutions of global governance, and realize global health with justice.
- Shifting from international health law (applicable to states) to global health law (applied to both state and nonstate actors), a multilevel proliferation of international, national, nongovernmental, and corporate actors have come together to address a multisectoral array of determinants of health.
- Global health law frames this expanding landscape for global health, coordinating the global community of state and nonstate actors through institutions of global health governance.

---

### HYPOTHETICAL CASE STUDY #1: THE INTERNATIONAL HEALTH REGULATIONS: NATIONAL MEASURES TO RESPOND TO A PUBLIC HEALTH EMERGENCY

Roxana is a public health advisor to the Minister of Health and manages the IHR National Focal Point (NFP) in her country under the IHR. Her national government has recently received media reports of an unexplained outbreak of flu-like symptoms in a neighbouring island state, with the WHO already seeking prompt verification of these reports. Concerned about the repercussions of a weak national public health response, Roxana has been asked whether her country is permitted under the Article 43 of the IHR (See Box 12.3) to ban the arrival of noncitizen travellers from the implicated state.

1. Should the government implement immediate travel restrictions on the basis of currently available information?
2. Does your recommendation change if/when the WHO director-general declares the event a PHEIC?

## Analysis: The International Health Regulations (2005): An International Legal Agreement for Global Health Security

As reflected in Case Study #1, international travel connects people and places around the world more than ever before, where diseases anywhere can become a threat to people everywhere. The IHR recognize this interdependence, and strive to "prevent, protect against, control and provide a public health response to the international spread of disease" while avoiding "unnecessary interference with international traffic and trade." For more than a century, the IHR and their precursor legal agreements have sought to strike the appropriate balance between economic considerations (i.e., international trade and traffic) and a robust public health response to global health security threats (Habibi et al., 2020).

A core aim of the IHR is to encourage states to report potentially serious disease outbreaks to the WHO in a timely manner, without fear of the economic repercussions of international trade and travel restrictions. To this end, the IHR require that states notify the WHO (by way of their IHR National Focal Points) of any event that may constitute a PHEIC, referring to "an extraordinary event" that (a) poses a public health risk to other states, as seen through the international spread of disease; and (b) potentially requires a coordinated international response (WHO, 2005). (While the WHO may also receive reports of these events from nonofficial sources, as seen in the media reports in Case Study #1, the WHO must first verify such reports with the implicated state in accordance with the IHR.) The formal declaration of a PHEIC ultimately rests with the WHO Director-General, who must consider information provided by the implicated state, the views of an emergency committee of international experts, and the available scientific evidence. PHEIC declarations serve to alert member states about the gravity of the event and provide WHO recommendations to guide national responses. A PHEIC declaration can also serve to justify international action. Since the entry into force of the IHR (2005), six PHEICs have been declared by the WHO Director-General.

Article 43 of the IHR, excerpted in Box 12.3, guides states in their decisions to implement additional health measures (e.g., trade and travel restrictions) in response to public health risks. This IHR provision allows states to implement additional health measures only if they achieve the same or greater levels of health protection than recommendations issued by the WHO and only if states do the following:

1. Ensure that the additional health measure being considered is "no more restrictive of international traffic and not more invasive or intrusive to persons than reasonably available alternatives that would achieve the appropriate level of health protection;"
2. Determine additional health measures on the basis of scientific principles, available scientific evidence of risk to human health (or information from the WHO or other relevant intergovernmental organizations where such information is lacking), and guidance or advice from the WHO that may be available; and
3. Consider measures that are consistent with other provisions of the IHR, relevant national law, and *international law.*

The IHR do not further describe the sources and standards of evidence that states should consider when deciding to implement additional health measures, but they do note that such evidence must be generated by the "methods of science." However, when a PHEIC is declared, the WHO Director-General will issue temporary recommendations, informed by the views of the Emergency Committee, and while nonbinding, these recommendations provide guidance to states on health measures that have consensus support by technical and public health experts.

In Case Study #1, the government could avoid travel bans in the immediate term, considering that information gathered from media reports has not yet been officially verified with the implicated state. Reasonably available alternatives to travel restrictions in the immediate term could include consultations with the WHO, engaging in bilateral communications with the implicated state to gather more information, and increased surveillance efforts. Should the WHO

## BOX 12.3    ARTICLE 43 (ADDITIONAL HEALTH MEASURES)–INTERNATIONAL HEALTH REGULATIONS

1. These Regulations shall not preclude States Parties from implementing health measures, in accordance with their relevant national law and obligations under international law, in response to specific public health risks or public health emergencies of international concern, which:

   a. achieve the same or greater level of health protection than WHO recommendations; or

   b. are otherwise prohibited under Article 25, Article 26, paragraphs one and two of Article 28, Article 30, paragraph 1(c) of Article 31 and Article 33,

   provided such measures are other consistent with these Regulations.

   Such measures shall not be more restrictive of international traffic and not more invasive or intrusive to persons than reasonably available alternatives that would achieve the appropriate level of health protection.

2. In determining whether to implement the health measures referred to in paragraph one of this Article or additional health measures under paragraph two of Article 23, paragraph one of Article 27, paragraph 2 of Article 28 and paragraph 2(c) of Article 31, States Parties shall base their determinations upon:

   a. scientific principles;

   b. available scientific evidence of a risk to human health, or where such evidence is insufficient, the available information including from WHO and other relevant intergovernmental organizations and international bodies; and

   c. any available specific guidance or advice from WHO.

3. A State Party implementing additional health measures referred to in paragraph one of this Article which significantly interfere with international traffic shall provide to WHO the public health rationale and relevant scientific information for it. WHO shall share this information with other States Parties and shall share information regarding the health measures implemented. For the purpose of this Article, significant interference generally means refusal of entry or departure of international travellers, baggage, cargo, containers, conveyances, goods, and the like, or their delay, for more than 24 hours.

4. After assessing information provided pursuant to paragraph three and five of this Article and other relevant information, WHO may request that the State Party concerned reconsider the application of the measures.

5. A State Party implementing additional health measures referred to in paragraphs one and two of this Article that significantly interfere with international traffic shall inform WHO, within 48 hours of implementation, of such measures and their health rationale unless these are covered by a temporary or standing recommendation.

6. A State Party implementing a health measure pursuant to paragraph one or two of this Article shall within three months review such a measure taking into account the advice of WHO and the criteria in paragraph 2 of this Article.

7. Without prejudice to its rights under Article 56, any State Party impacted by a measure taken pursuant to paragraph one or two of this Article may request the State Party implementing such a measure to consult with it. The purpose of such consultations is to clarify the scientific information and public health rationale underlying the measure and to find a mutually acceptable solution.

8. The provisions of this Article may apply to implementation of measures concerning travellers taking part in mass congregations.

Director-General confirm media reports with the state implicated and determine that these reported events constitute a PHEIC on the basis of information received from the state and advice from the Emergency Committee, the government could, under IHR Article 43, base any additional health measures on (a) the temporary recommendations issued by the WHO Director-General; or (b) an assessment of the specific public health risks posed to the country, taking into account scientific principles, available scientific evidence, and other information from the WHO and relevant intergovernmental organizations. Travel bans that are not based on sound scientific evidence could result in unnecessary economic, social, and global health ramifications (e.g., stigmatization of the affected country, diverting resources from other public health measures critical to mitigating the PHEIC and disincentivizing the prompt reporting of outbreaks to the WHO in the future). The government could better prepare using less restrictive measures, for example, by developing protocols for the entry screening of travellers, establishing a robust contact-tracing program, scaling up widespread testing and diagnostics (if possible), mounting a risk communications campaign, and assessing the need and available supply of personal protective equipment. Should the government decide to implement travel restrictions on travellers from affected areas, it will be necessary for the government, in accordance with Article 43, to report these measures, and the public health rationale behind their decision, to the WHO within 48 hours of implementation and subsequently review the utility of travel restrictions to their national public health response within 3 months.

---

### HYPOTHETICAL CASE STUDY #2: THE FRAMEWORK CONVENTION ON TOBACCO CONTROL: IMPLEMENTING GLOBAL HEALTH LAW THROUGH DOMESTIC PUBLIC HEALTH LAW REFORMS

The national government is seeking to address the significant rise in flavored tobacco use among teens, particularly in low-income communities. Tobacco control researchers have found that corporations have purposefully sought to attract children and young adults to smoking through the marketing of tobacco flavors that appeal to children (including cotton candy, chocolate, cherry, grape, sour apple, and cinnamon roll), colorful packaging that appeals to young demographics, and individual packages at lower prices. In response, the Minister of Health is seeking to strengthen tobacco control laws and regulations. Anthony is a policy analyst for the Health Ministry, and the Minister of Health has asked him to analyze potential changes to policy, regulations, and guidance to translate the Framework Convention on Tobacco Control (FCTC) into domestic law and to consider the lessons that can be learned from other states' implementation of Articles 11 (see Box 12.4) and 16 (see Box 12.5) of the FCTC.

1. What is the state's legal obligation under the FCTC to support regulation of the sale of flavored tobacco products, particularly to prevent initiation by children and young adults?
2. What basic attributes should potential laws and regulations include to regulate the content, packaging, and labeling of flavored tobacco products, particularly with respect to children and young adults?

---

## Analysis: The Framework Convention on Tobacco Control (2003): Addressing NCDs Through International Law

NCDs pose unique challenges for global health, as Case Study #2 illustrates. Despite the vast global increase in NCD prevalence, NCDs lack the sense of urgency attendant to infection diseases, with NCDs being slow to develop, diffuse in their causes, and arguably founded on individual choice (Gostin & Wiley, 2016). Yet, in a globalizing world, NCDs are largely driven by the global market for commercial determinants of health, including tobacco, sugar-sweetened

## BOX 12.4 FCTC ARTICLE 11–PACKAGING AND LABELLING OF TOBACCO PRODUCTS

1. Each Party shall, within a period of three years after entry into force of this Convention for that Party, adopt and implement, in accordance with its national law, effective measures to ensure that:

   a. tobacco product packaging and labelling do not promote a tobacco product by any means that are false, misleading, deceptive or likely to create an erroneous impression about its characteristics, health effects, hazards or emissions, including any term, descriptor, trademark, figurative or any other sign that directly or indirectly creates the false impression that a particular tobacco product is less harmful than other tobacco products. These may include terms such as "low tar," "light," "ultra-light," or "mild"; and [...]

4. For the purposes of this Article, the term "outside packaging and labelling" in relation to tobacco products applies to any packaging and labelling used in the retail sale of the product.

## BOX 12.5 FCTC ARTICLE 16–SALES TO AND BY MINORS

1. Each Party shall adopt and implement effective legislative, executive, administrative or other measures at the appropriate government level to prohibit the sales of tobacco products to persons under the age set by domestic law, national law or eighteen. These measures may include:

   a. Requiring that all sellers of tobacco products place a clear and prominent indicator inside their point of sale about the prohibition of tobacco sales to minors and, in case of doubt, request that each tobacco purchaser provide appropriate evidence of having reached full legal age;

   b. Banning the sale of tobacco products in any manner by which they are directly accessible, such as store shelves;

   c. Prohibiting the manufacture and sale of sweets, snacks, toys or any other objects in the form of tobacco products which appeal to minors; and

   d. Ensuring that tobacco vending machines under its jurisdiction are not accessible to minors and do not promote the sale of tobacco products to minors.

2. Each Party shall prohibit or promote the prohibition of the distribution of free tobacco products to the public and especially minors.

3. Each Party shall endeavor to prohibit the sale of cigarettes individually or in small packets which increase the affordability of such products to minors.

beverages, high-calorie foods, and alcohol (Kickbusch et al., 2016). Globalization furthers the expansive trade of these commercial determinants, and as a result of these underlying determinants of health, transnational corporations and global markets have driven a meteoric increase in the prevalence of NCDs worldwide (Freudenberg, 2012). In parallel with the spread of infectious diseases, vulnerable and socially disadvantaged populations are often the most affected by NCDs, experiencing far greater prevalence than advantaged groups (WHO, 2014). These global determinants and social gradients raise key commonalities between infectious diseases and NCDs in a globalizing world, with the global implications of NCDs necessitating a global health law response.

Addressing the commercial determinants that underlie tobacco-related NCDs, the 2003 WHO FCTC has established a global legal framework to combat the globalization of the tobacco epidemic. The FCTC sets international standards to guide governments in reducing tobacco consumption, providing the foundation for the legal obligation that the government in Case Study #2 can implement at the local level to support regulation of the sale of flavored tobacco products.

Much like the IHR, the FCTC embraces a multisectoral approach to public health and calls on governments to adopt core measures for reducing tobacco demand: regulating the price of products, placing limitations on advertising, promoting education and communication, and raising the age of consumption (WHO, 2003). Importantly, the FCTC also fosters international cooperation to aid national implementation, highlighting the critical importance of linking global norms to national reforms. These national reforms require the implementation of domestic laws (both national and subnational) to ensure that the measures outlined in the FCTC are translated into public health impacts.

States like the government in Case Study #2 may take a range of measures to prevent the sale of tobacco products to minors under FCTC Article 16, including the use of legislation and regulatory enforcement mechanisms. The Minister of Health may use legislation to prohibit the flavoring of tobacco products, particularly those that would appeal to a younger demographic as well as to prohibit access to tobacco products in general. Governments can require retailers to use clear signage to indicate the age limit for purchasing tobacco products, to prohibit the sale of individual packages at lower prices, and to require purchasers to have government-issued documents proving their legal age. Extended by FCTC Article 11, governments can prohibit tobacco-product labeling and advertisements that are "false, misleading, deceptive or likely to create an erroneous impression about [the tobacco product's] characteristics, health effects, hazards or emissions." Governments can penalize companies for failing to limit access to tobacco products to minors or for knowingly misleading the public on the health effects of tobacco products.

## DISCUSSION: GLOBAL HEALTH WITH JUSTICE

As a legal foundation to advance public health in a globalizing world, global governance has become crucial in developing legal norms and implementing those norms through global institutions and national reforms. Operating through global health law, well-governed institutions can set global public health standards—coordinating disparate actors, forming partnerships with key stakeholders, and developing consensus on shared goals for global health. These new instruments of global health law provide global institutions with the legal norms to negotiate a shared vision of good governance for global health, collaborate with other organizations across sectors, and align domestic law with global health law (Gostin, 2014). Facilitating accountability for these global health goals, global health law can structure an institutional basis for developing benchmarks, monitoring progress, and enhancing compliance.

Global health law can thereby provide a normative framework for achieving global health with justice. In an increasingly globalized world—facing new global health threats and creating an imperative for global health institutions to meet an expanding set of global equity challenges to underlying determinants of health—global health law can codify normative frameworks to realize the human rights that underlie global health (Magnusson et al., 2017). Looking to human rights law as central to global health governance, stakeholders have engaged a diverse array of state and nonstate actors through the rise of new policy institutions beyond the WHO—governance institutions developed through their normative foundations in justice (Ruger, 2018). Global health law can codify these vital norms for justice across institutions, providing a legal basis for human rights in global health (Meier & Gostin, 2018).

As a path to realize justice in global governance through the human right to health, advocates have proposed a Framework Convention on Global Health (FCGH). This proposed treaty has been developed "as a mechanism to channel more constructive and cooperative action to address ... the health of the world's population" (Gostin, 2008, p. 383). Through a rights-based approach to global health law, the FCGH seeks to facilitate mutual responsibilities between donor and recipient nations, coordinate the efforts of governmental and nongovernmental actors, and catalyze financial support to strengthen global health governance. This FCGH effort seeks to create a human rights foundation for global governance of public health, developing a legal framework to implement the human right to health under global health law (Gable & Meier, 2013). The FCGH Alliance has brought together civil society organizations, marginalized communities, scholars, and practitioners to advocate for an FCGH as a legal basis to overcome an expanding array of governance challenges (Gostin et al., 2016). Focusing on shortcomings of weak accountability, inadequate funding, and decentralized governance, the FCGH Alliance supports an FCGH as a model for reinforcing the realization of human rights, particularly the right to health, under WHO leadership.

## CONCLUSION

Global health law is necessary to engage the public health threats, nonstate actors, and normative instruments that structure global health. Differences in legal capacity for public health across countries are driving inequities in global health. Global health law seeks to redress these inequities through global health governance. Leading global health governance, the WHO has developed international legal responses to address the global spread of infectious disease (as seen through the IHR) and commercial determinants of NCDs (as seen through the FCTC). In drawing from human rights law, global health law can structure new forms of global governance necessary to realize global health with justice.

## CHAPTER REVIEW

### Review Questions

1. Why does globalization raise an imperative for global health law?
2. The WHO director-general declares a PHEIC based upon a vote of member states. True/False
3. What is one example of a way a state can meet FCTC obligations to prohibit the sale of tobacco products to minors?
4. As a path to realize justice in global health, advocates have proposed a _____ based upon norms of _____.

### Essay Questions

1. Why is soft law necessary to regulate global public health?
2. Why do states come together to address infectious disease threats through international law? How does the IHR bind states together?
3. How are global health law responses distinct for infectious versus noncommunicable disease threats? How are they similar?
4. Why are human rights central to realizing global health with justice? How can global health law codify human rights obligations to realize equity and justice in global health?

## Internet Activities

1. How have states learned from other states in developing public health law?
   - See *Lancet*-O'Neill Commission on Global Health and the Law: https://www.thelancet
     .com/commissions/legal-determinants-of-health
2. How have states sought to meet their minimum core obligations under the IHR?
   - See Joint External Evaluation (JEE) mission reports: https://www.who.int/ihr/
     procedures/mission-reports/en
3. How have states applied the IHR decision instrument criteria in deciding whether to notify the WHO of a public health emergency in accordance with Article 6 of the IHR (2005)
   and Annex 2?
   - See IHR (2005); https://www.who.int/ihr/publications/9789241580496/en
4. How have states implemented the FCTC under domestic law?
   - See Campaign for Tobacco-Free Kids' Tobacco Control Laws and Litigation Database:
     https://www.tobaccocontrollaws.org
5. How would an FCGH realize global health with justice?
   - See Framework Convention Alliance: https://fcghalliance.org

## REFERENCES

Aginam, O. (2005). *Global health governance: International law and public health in a divided world.* University of Toronto Press.

Freudenberg, N. (2012). The manufacture of lifestyle: The role of corporations in unhealthy living. *Journal of Public Health Policy, 33*(2), 244–256. https://doi.org/10.1057/jphp.2011.60

Gable, L., & Meier, B. M. (2013). Global health rights: Employing human rights to develop and implement the framework convention on global health. *Health and Human Rights: An International Journal, 15,* 17–31. https://www.hhrjournal.org/2013/10/global-health-rights-employing-human-rights-to-develop-and-implement-the-framework-convention-on-global-health

Gostin, L. O. (2008). Meeting basic survival needs of the world's least healthy people: Toward a Framework Convention on Global Health. *Georgetown Law Journal, 96,* 331–392. https://scholarship.law.georgetown.edu/fac_lectures/11

Gostin, L. O. (2014). *Global health law.* Harvard University Press.

Gostin, L. O., Habibi, R., & Meier, B. M. (2020). Has global health law risen to meet the COVID-19 challenge? Revisiting the international health regulations to prepare for future threats. *The Journal of Law, Medicine and Ethics, 48,* 376–381. https://doi.org/10.1177/1073110520935354

Gostin, L. O., Monahan, J. T., Kaldor, J., DeBartolo, M., Friedman, E., Gottschalk, K., Kim, S. C., Alwan, A., Binagwaho, A., Burci, G. L., Cabal, L., DeLand, K., Evans, T. G., Goosby, E., Hossain, S., Koh, H., Ooms, G., Periago, M. R., Uprimny, R., & Yamin, A. E. (2019). The legal determinants of health: Harnessing the power of law for global health and sustainable development. *The Lancet, 393*(10183), 1857–1910. https://doi.org/10.1016/S0140-6736(19)30233-8

Gostin, L. O., & Taylor, A. L. (2008). Global health law: A definition and grand challenges. *Public Health Ethics, 1*(1), 53–63. https://doi.org/10.1093/phe/phn005

Gostin, L. O., & Wiley, L. (2016). *Public health law: Power, duty, and restraint.* University of California Press.

Habibi, R., Hoffman, S. J., Burci, G. L., de Campos, T. C., Chirwa, D., Cinà, M., Dagron, S., Eccleston-Turner, M., Forman, L., Gostin, L. O., Meier, B. M., Negri, S., Ooms, G., Sekalala, S., Taylor, A., & Yamin, A. E. (2020). The Stellenbosch Consensus on Legal National Responses to Public Health Risks. *International Organizations Law Review,* doi:10.1163/15723747-2020023.

Kickbusch, I., Allen, L., & Franz, C. (2016). The commercial determinants of health. *The Lancet, 4,* e895–e896. https://doi.org/10.1016/S2214-109X(16)30217-0

Magnusson, R. (2017). *Advancing the right to health: The vital role of law.* World Health Organization. https://apps.who.int/iris/bitstream/handle/10665/252815/9789241511384-eng.pdf?sequence=1.

Meier, B. M., & Gostin, L. O. (2018). *Human rights in global health: Rights-based governance for a globalizing world*. Oxford University Press.

Moon, S. (2018). Global health law and governance: Concepts, tools, actors and power. In G. L. Burci & B. Toebes (Eds.), *Research handbook on global health law* (pp. 24–54). Edgar.

Ransom, M. M. (Ed.). (2016). *Public health law competency model: Version 1.0*. https://www.cdc.gov/phlp/docs/phlcm-v1.pdf

Ruger, J. P. (2018). *Global health justice and governance*. Oxford University Press.

World Health Organization. (2003). Framework Convention on Tobacco Control. https://www.who.int/fctc/en

World Health Organization. (2005). *WHO guidance for the use of annex 2 of the International Health Regulations*. https://www.who.int/ihr/revised_annex2_guidance.pdf?ua=1

World Health Organization. (2014). *Global status report on noncommunicable diseases 2014*. https://apps.who.int/iris/bitstream/handle/10665/148114/9789241564854_eng.pdf?sequence=1

## Additional Resources

- **GLOBALink**
  https://www.globalink.org
- **Global Health Security Agenda**
  https://ghsagenda.org
- **Global Tobacco Control: Learning from the Experts 2007**
  https://www.globaltobaccocontrol.org/online_training
- **World Health Organization, Tobacco Free Initiative**
  https://www.who.int/tobacco/en

# 13

# The Evolution of Environmental Public Health and the Law

Montrece McNeill Ransom, Angela K. McGowan, Dana Reed Wise,
Nathan Roush, Jessika Douglas, and Priscilla Keith

## Learning Objectives

By the end of this chapter, the reader will be able to:

- Describe the evolution of environmental public health law.
- Define environmental public health law, as distinct from environmental law.
- Discuss the legal framework for addressing selected, contemporary environmental public health issues including healthy housing, climate change and mosquito-borne diseases, and the built environment.

## Key Terminology

**Built environment:** Those environments that are man-made or modified, including homes, schools, workplaces, highways, urban sprawl, and various mobile and stationary sources of air pollution.

**Climate change:** Climate change is the long-term alteration of temperature and typical weather patterns in a place (National Geographic, 2020). The World Health Organization (WHO) argues that climate change threatens good health including clean air, safe drinking water, food supply, and safe shelter.

**Command and control regulation:** The direct regulation in an industry or activity that states what is permitted and what is illegal (McManus, 2009).

**Environmental law:** "Regulations, statutes, local, national and international legislation, and treaties designed to protect the environment from damage and to explain the legal consequences of such damage towards governments or private entities or individuals" (Environmental Science.org, 2020).

**Environmental public health law:** Environmental laws that affect health by limiting exposures to disease-causing agents, targeting unhealthy features of the environment, influencing the creation and maintenance of community spaces for physical activity, and regulating the use and disposal of harmful industrial materials like lead (Temple University: Center for Public Health Law Research, 2017).

**Health Impact Assessment (HIA):** A systematic process that uses research, data, analysis, and stakeholder feedback to determine the possible health effects and their distribution of a policy, project, or plan and to recommend ways to maximize health.

**Healthy housing/home:** Housing that is designed, constructed, maintained, and rehabilitated in a manner that is conducive to good occupant health (Centers for Disease Control and Prevention [CDC], 2019a).

**Nuisance:** Condition, activity, or situation (e.g., a loud noise or foul odor) that interferes with the use or enjoyment
of property; especially a nontransitory condition or persistent activity that either injures the physical condition
of adjacent land or interferes with its use or with the enjoyment of easements on the land or of public highways
(Garner, 2009).

**Promulgate:** To publish; to announce officially; to make a law, whether statutory or administrative, public as important or
obligatory. See *Wooden v. Western New York & P. R. Co.* (Super. Ct.), 18 N. Y. Supp. 769. (The Law Dictionary
& Black's Law Dictionary Free [2nd ed.], n.d.).

**Vector-borne diseases:** Human illnesses caused by parasites, viruses, and bacteria that are transmitted by mosquitoes,
sandflies, triatomine bugs, blackflies, ticks, tsetse flies, mites, snails, and lice (https://www.who.int/news-room/fact
-sheets/detail/vector-borne-diseases).

**Zoning codes:** Local laws that designate areas for certain land uses, normally used for land planning; can designate areas
for residential and industrial uses, and can designate green space.

## Public Health Law Competencies

This chapter addresses the following competencies from the Public Health Law Competency Model (PHLCM; Ransom, 2016).

**1.1** Define basic constitutional concepts and legal principles framing the practice of public
health across jurisdictions.

**1.2** Identify and apply public health laws (e.g., statutes, regulations, ordinances, and court
rulings) pertinent to practitioner's jurisdiction, agency, program, and profession.

**2.1** Identify law-based tools and enforcement procedures available to address day-to-day
(nonemergency) public health issues.

---

### Spark Questions

1. Compare and contrast environmental public health law with environmental law.
2. What is one example of a law or policy designed to protect environmental public health?

---

## INTRODUCTION

There is an increasing recognition that where we live can have an important impact on health
and that zip codes may be as important as genetic codes in determining a population's health
(Robert Wood Johnson Foundation Commission, 2014). Environmental conditions can cause
asthma, create environments and social settings that challenge the ability of people to be
healthy (e.g., toxic situations, lead, violence, access to healthy foods), bring about natural disasters (e.g., hurricanes, floods, and fires), and cause deaths, illnesses, and billions of dollars of
damages each year. The WHO estimates that over 12 million deaths are caused each year due
to environmental risks to health, and that 23% of all deaths globally could be prevented with
healthier environments. Law and policy play a critical role in achieving these goals.

## DEFINING ENVIRONMENTAL PUBLIC HEALTH LAW

While some of the modern research in public health law addresses the role of law in specific
domains of environmental public health practice (e.g. lead poisoning, **climate change**, chemical exposures), there is very little literature exploring, in an integrated, comprehensive fashion,

the role of law in environmental public health efforts. One reason for this gap may be the narrow way **environmental law** has been traditionally characterized. Environmental law has been defined as the "collective body of rules and regulations, orders and statutes, constraints and allowances that are all concerned with the maintenance and protection of the natural environment of a country."

The WHO defines the environment as it relates to health as "all the physical, chemical, and biological factors external to a person, and all the related behaviors" (2006). *Healthy People*, an initiative that describes the national health goals of the United States, further explains environmental health to include "preventing or controlling disease, injury, and disability related to the interactions between people and their environment" (HealthyPeople.gov, 2020). **Environmental public health law**, which should be considered a subset or extension of public health law, can be defined as those laws and policies that seek to protect the environment and its inhabitants from activities and conditions that may negatively impact or endanger the environment or health of the population. These laws are also used to promote healthier behavior and deter activity that creates health risks. In this context, "environment" includes (a) the natural environment, (i.e., air, water, soil, and the physical, biological, and social features and surroundings); (b) the man-made or **built environment;** and, (c) the social environment (i.e., lifestyle factors like diet, exercise, and socioeconomic status).

Like all public health laws, environmental public health laws are derived from: federal and state constitutions; statutes and other legislative enactments; agency rules and regulations; judicial rulings and case law; and policies of public bodies. (See Box 13.2 later in this chapter for a discussion of selected cases relevant to the three eras described in Part II). Accordingly, the body of laws that make up environmental public health include environmental law as well as transportation law, administrative law, land use law, housing law, energy law, business law, and **nuisance** law. In choosing this terminology, the authors considered the historical foundations of environmental public health efforts and the evolving, interconnected nature of the field. This terminology also embraces the shift in the environmental public health community from a primary focus on adverse exposure to pollutants and toxins, to a more sharpened concentration on the relationship between the environments where we live, work, and play, and the impact of those environments on our health outcomes. Effectively addressing modern environmental public health concerns requires that federal, Tribal, state, and local public health practitioners and their partners understand this broader definition and its component laws and policies including legislation, regulations, and court opinions, as well as how these laws can be used to achieve public health goals.

This chapter provides an overview of the evolution of environmental public health law and aims to define and characterize the field. Using hypothetical case studies, this chapter discusses the legal framework for addressing selected, contemporary environmental public health concerns including **healthy housing**, climate change, **vector-borne diseases**, and the built environment.

## THE EVOLUTION OF ENVIRONMENTAL PUBLIC HEALTH LAW

### Sanitation Era: 1800s to Early 1900s

*The condition of perfect public health requires such laws and regulations as will secure to man associated in society the same sanitary enjoyments that he would have as an isolated individual and will protect him from injury from and influences toward his locality, his dwelling house, his occupation… or from any other causes.*

SIR EDWIN CHADWICK
Report of the Sanitary Condition of the Labouring
Population of Great Britain, 1842

The foundation for the field of public health can be traced to the 19th century "sanitation movement." The public health concerns of this era included infectious diseases due to unsafe waste disposal; contaminated water, food, and air; crowded living environments; and the proximity of housing to industry. Other issues in the Sanitation Era included disease associated with poor nutrition, poor maternal and infant health, and injuries associated with unsafe workplaces. As late as 1850, the urban life expectancy in the United States was approximately 25 years and environmentally related diseases were a major cause of mortality. Between 1800 and 1850, epidemics from smallpox, yellow fever, cholera, typhoid, and typhus were rampant, and the leading causes of death during this period were influenza, pneumonia, diphtheria, tuberculosis, and gastrointestinal infections (Institute of Medicine, 1988).

In 1842, Edwin Chadwick, an English lawyer and secretary to the Poor Law Commission, compiled the renowned Report of the Sanitary Condition of the Labouring Population of Great Britain. This report brought into focus the dangerous, unhealthy living conditions of the poor, drew significant attention to environmental conditions as determinants of health, and served as a foundation for similar, subsequent reports. Perhaps the most recognized example of such a subsequent report in the United States is the Shattuck Report. Formally entitled Report of the Sanitary Commission of Massachusetts, this report was published in 1850 and was the first to systematically use vital records data and other demographic data to describe the health of the population. The recommendations became the foundation of the sanitation movement in the United States, which laid the framework for the dramatic increase in life expectancy that occurred in the next 150 years. As an example, in the United States, life expectancy at birth over the 110 years from 1900 to 2010 went from 47.3 to 78.7 years (CDC/National Center for Health Statistics [NCHS], 2013). The Shattuck Report recommended the establishment of a state health department and local health boards and resulted in the first attempt to write a comprehensive public health code.

Following the Civil War, many states and localities adopted these recommendations ultimately resulting in the public health system that exists today (The Climate Change and Public Health Law Site, n.d.). By 1900, 40 of the 45 states had established health departments. The first county health departments were established in 1908 (Hinman, 1990). These health departments were responsible for almost all environmental health legislation until the mid to late 1900s, and this legislation was based on the principles of public health. From the 1930s through the 1950s, state and local health departments made substantial progress in disease prevention activities, including sewage disposal, water treatment, food safety, organized solid waste disposal, and public education about hygienic practices (e.g., food handling and handwashing). Federal environmental public health legislation was seriously limited during this era.

## The *Silent Spring* Era: Late 1950s to 1990s

> *The most alarming of all man's assaults upon the environment is the contamination of air, earth, rivers, and sea with dangerous and even lethal materials.*
>
> RACHEL CARSON
> Silent Spring (1962)

The strong tradition of state and local environmental public health and sanitary services was maintained until the 1960s, when environmental concerns about air pollution, exposure to toxic chemicals, and the degradation of natural resources began garnering more attention. The 1962 publication of Rachel Carson's *Silent Spring*, an examination of chlorinated hydrocarbon pesticides and the environmental damage caused by their use, highlighted a broad range of actual and potential hazards in the natural environment and catalyzed public interest and activism. This era is often called the peak of the "environmental movement." These times were marked by rapidly escalating concerns about industrial waste and emissions, toxic chemicals, air and drinking water pollutants, and motor vehicle pollutants. Although the control of infectious and waterborne diseases remained an essential component of environmental public health practice, prevention and national policy efforts began to shift toward the identification and control of adverse effects from toxic pollutants in the environment and to the preservation of natural resources; legal efforts began to shift from a common law approach to a much more comprehensive, **command and control regulatory** scheme.

What most would identify as contemporary environmental law came into fruition during the **Silent Spring Era**. Until this time, the role of the federal government was to offer research, funding, and guidelines for state and local efforts. The public outcry brought about by Silent Spring, and a growing recognition of the interstate nature of pollutants, shifted this thinking. Congress quickly responded by convening committees and holding hearings, which culminated in the creation of the Environmental Protection Agency (EPA) by presidential executive order in 1970 (U.S. EPA, 2018). The EPA's mandate was to focus on legal and engineering strategies related to air and water pollution, as well as species and land protection. During this era, the U.S. government passed more than 100 environmental laws—including acts addressing solid waste disposal, air and water pollution, the protection of endangered species, and the conservation of land. (See Table 13.1 for a list of selected laws.)

As a former EPA administrator put it, there is no more significant success story in the realm of public policy in our recent history than U.S. environmental regulation (https://archive.epa.gov/epa/aboutepa/epa-twenty-years-young.html). The laws enacted during this era have made dramatic progress in reducing certain kinds of pollution, particularly emissions from large industrial point sources. "Aggregate emissions of the six principal air pollutants monitored since 1970 (also called criteria pollutants): nitrogen dioxide ($NO_2$), ozone ($O_3$), sulfur dioxide ($SO_2$), particulate matter (PM), carbon monoxide (CO) and lead (Pb), have decreased by 25 percent" (U.S. EPA, 2005). Waterways once again support healthy aquatic ecosystems suitable for recreation. Two-thirds of the nation's surveyed waters are currently safe for fishing and swimming, compared to half that number in the early 1970s (U.S. EPA, ND). Waste disposal, especially the disposal of hazardous wastes, is closely regulated, and the inactive and abandoned waste dumps that were ubiquitous during this era are being cleaned up.

Yet, in many ways, the regulatory scheme and legal framework developed during the Silent Spring Era have led to the detachment of public health principles from many aspects of environmental regulation, decision-making, and education. Arguably, the collection of environmental laws birthed in the Silent Spring Era have been constrained, at least to some degree, by traditional legal structures, and as such, traditional environmental law has been limited in its ability to fully adopt an approach that appreciates the interconnections between the health of our planet, biodiversity, and humans. This is true on a global scale. Scholars note that the 2019 SARS-CoV-2 virus (COVID-19) pandemic has its origins in this detachment and can be attributed, at least in part, to the limited ability of the international community to effectively use law and policy to protect our forests and wildlife and to govern land use, which have led to the disappearance of the traditional buffer zones that used to separate humans from animals and their pathogens (Duvic-Paoli, 2020).

The legal enactments of the Silent Spring Era have also contributed to a significant change in the structure and function of many public health programs in the United States, resulting in more of a patchwork approach and the compartmentalization of the disciplines of environmental health, public health, and policy. This was a significant paradigm shift away from

## TABLE 13.1  SILENT SPRING ERA: Selected Federal Environmental and Environmental Public Health Laws (Listed in Alphabetical Order)

| YEAR | LAW | CITATION | DESCRIPTION |
|---|---|---|---|
| 1970; Amended 1990 | Clean Air Act | 42 U.S.C. 7401 et seq. | Required the EPA (created in 1970) to develop National Ambient Air Quality Standards to protect public health and public welfare and to regulate emissions of hazardous air pollutants from various sources. 1990 amendments focused on the ozone layer, reducing acid rain and toxic pollutants, and improving air quality and visibility. Cite: EPA https://www.epa.gov/clean-air-act-overview/progress-cleaning-air-and-improving-peoples-health |
| 1972 | Clean Water Act | 33 U.S.C. § 1251 et seq. | Establishes the basic structure for regulating discharges of pollutants into U.S. waters and regulating quality standards for surface waters. The basis of the Act was the 1948 Federal Water Pollution Control Act. |
| 1980 | Comprehensive Environmental Response, Compensation and Liability Act (CERCLA) | 42 U.S.C. § 103 | Commonly known as Superfund, CERCLA was enacted December 11, 1980. This law taxed the chemical and petroleum industries and provided federal authority to respond to releases or threatened releases of hazardous substances that could endanger public health or the environment. |
| 1986 | Emergency Planning and Community Right-to-Know Act (EPCRA) | 42 U.S.C. § 11001 et seq. | Assists communities to protect the public health, safety, and environment from chemical hazards; states must have a State Emergency Response Commission and local planning committees. There are 4 main sections:<br>■ Emergency planning (sections 301-303)<br>■ Emergency release notification (section 304)<br>■ Hazardous chemical storage reporting requirements (sections 311-312)<br>■ Toxic chemical release inventory (section 313) |
| 1973 | Endangered Species Act | 16 U.S.C. ch. 35 § 1531 et seq. | Protects threatened and endangered plants, animals, and their habitats. Managed by the U.S. Fish and Wildlife Service of the Department of the Interior. |
| 1969; (Enacted 1/1/70) | National Environmental Policy Act (NEPA) | 42 U.S.C. § 4321 et seq. | Reaction to a century of economic expansion, population growth, and urbanization, which had environmental costs. Law requires government to research and assess potential environmental impacts of major (important) federal actions including environmental assessments and environmental impact statements; established President's Council on Environmental Quality. CITE: *RB Jai Alai, LLC v. Secretary of the Florida Department of Transportation*, 112 F.Supp.3d 1301, 1307-1308 (M. D. Fla. 2015). |
| 1972 | Noise Control Act | 42 U.S.C. § 4901 et seq. | Created a national policy to prevent noise that is potentially harmful to health and welfare. The Act also serves to (1) coordinate federal research and activities; (2) authorize federal noise emission standards for products distributed in commerce; and (3) inform the public about noise emission and noise reduction for these products. |

*(continued)*

**TABLE 13.1  SILENT SPRING ERA: Selected Federal Environmental and Environmental Public Health Laws (Listed in Alphabetical Order; *continued*)**

| YEAR | LAW | CITATION | DESCRIPTION |
|---|---|---|---|
| 1970 | Occupational Safety and Health | 29 U.S.C. ch. 15 § 651 et seq | Sets and enforces safer workplace conditions in the U.S. Established the Occupational Safety and Health Administration (OSHA), which sets workplace health and safety standards, and the National Institute for Occupational Safety and Health, which researches and advises on work-related illnesses and injuries. |
| 1990 | Pollution Prevention Act | 42 U.S.C. § 13101 et seq. | Attempts to lower environmental pollution by changing or preventing amount of pollution created; encouraged recycling. |
| 1976 | Resource Conservation and Recovery Act | 42 U.S.C. ch. 82, § 6901 et seq. | Amended the 1965 Solid Waste Disposal Act to set goals for protecting human and environmental health from waste disposal, energy conservation and natural resources, and recycling and management of waste. Joint federal and state effort; principal federal law in the United States governing the disposal of solid waste and hazardous waste. |
| 1974 | Safe Drinking Water Act | 42 U.S.C. § 300f | Authorizes the EPA to establish standards for sources of water— above and underground—designated for human consumption (both health and nuisance standards). |
| 1976; Amended 2016 | Toxic Substances Control Act (Amended-2016) Frank R. Lautenberg Chemical Safety for the 21st Century Act | 15 U.S.C. § 2601 et seq. Pub. L. No: 114-182 | Provides for requiring reporting, testing, regulating, and screening chemicals and chemical mixtures for consumers. Required EPA to evaluate chemicals with clear deadlines and make risk-based chemical assessments providing chemical information to the public; provided funding for the EPA to enforce. |

public health principles and practice toward a command and control framework. Because most of the actual implementation of environmental services occur on the state and local levels, the major federal laws, in many ways, provided a blueprint for states to follow when organizing state and local environmental health efforts. As such, state health agencies were no longer the primary governmental entities addressing health concerns related to air quality, drinking water, food safety, and solid waste management. It is during this era that we see the emergence of state and local departments of environmental control and protection as distinct and separate agencies.

## Sustainability Era: Late 1990s to the Present

*[The sustainability movement] insists on a whole-systems approach, whereas the environmental movement has focused on the human impact upon non-human systems, and the new age movement has focused on spirituality and personal growth.*

GILMAN, R.
Sustainability: The State of the Movement (1990)

Today, as we move into the *Sustainability Era*, which began in the late 1990s, environmental health and protection responsibilities are part of the mission of a dozen major federal departments and agencies. Within the executive branch, there are those agencies responsible for developing environmental regulations (e.g., EPA), those charged with enforcing environmental laws

## BOX 13.1 ENVIRONMENTAL PUBLIC HEALTH LAW AND HEALTH EQUITY

What other major social movement emerged during the latter part of the Silent Spring Era?

*Environmental justice* (EJ) represents the convergence of two of the greatest social movements of the latter half of the 20th century: the environmental movement and the civil rights movement. Environmental justice is defined by EPA as the fair treatment and meaningful involvement of all people regardless of race, color, national origin, or income, with respect to the development, implementation, and enforcement of environmental laws, regulations, and policies. In 1994, with the signing of executive order 12898, federal executive branch agencies became responsible for making "achieving justice part of its mission by identifying and addressing, as appropriate, disproportionately high and adverse human health or environmental effects of its programs, policies, and activities on minority populations and low-income populations." This landmark order was the first major federal action on environmental justice in the United States. It brought legitimacy and attention to the EJ movement in the United States and acknowledged that low-income communities and communities of color bear a disproportionate burden of environmental pollution and its health effects.

*Source:* Executive Order 12898, 59 FR 7629.

and regulations (e.g., Agency for Toxic Substances and Disease Registry), those subjected primarily to the law's requirements (e.g., Department of Transportation), and those concerned primarily with the budgetary and economic impact of environmental laws and regulations (e.g., Office of Management and Budget). State efforts are just as complex and have varying, diverse approaches to addressing environmental public health issues. In fact, according to one source, more than 90% of state and local environmental health programs are assigned to agencies other than health departments (Association for State and Territorial Health Officials, 2014).

Many Silent Spring Era federal and state environmental laws are not aimed at many of the causes of 21st-century environmental problems. For example, nonpoint source pollution—runoff from roads, driveways, parking lots, and roofs associated with land development—is the cause of nearly half of the nation's water quality problems. "Urban sprawl has resulted in habitat destruction, air pollution from cars stuck in traffic, the disappearance of open space, and the decline in quality of community life" (Nolon, 2002). In 2018, more than 141 million Americans still live in counties where pollution levels exceed the national ambient air quality standards,

## BOX 13.2 KEY ENVIRONMENTAL PUBLIC HEALTH LAW CASES

Litigation, as discussed in Chapter 5, can be a powerful tool in public health and in advancing environmental public health goals. As illustrated by the following six cases, lawsuits can help inform our understanding of guidelines and standards, result in positive or negative environmental change, and create barriers to or set precedents for a more sustainable future.

### SANITATION ERA
*Missouri v. Illinois and the Sanitary District of Chicago*, **200 U.S. 496 (1906)**
The city of Chicago was dumping raw, untreated sewage into Lake Michigan, which was also the source of drinking water for Chicago residents. An outbreak of cholera resulted, and the city began dumping its sewage into the Mississippi River instead. The Mississippi

BOX 13.2 *(continued)*

River was the source of drinking water for the residents of St. Louis, and shortly after the dumping began, typhoid deaths in St. Louis increased by 77%. In its lawsuit against Illinois, the state of Missouri argued that this dumping was a public health nuisance because it created "an unreasonable interference with a right common to the general public." Since this was a dispute between states, this case was ultimately decided by the U.S. Supreme Court. Interestingly, the Supreme Court found for Illinois. It looked at the scientific evidence available at the time and concluded that any bacteria being released in Chicago would be dead by the time they reached St. Louis. Missouri could also not establish that their water quality had declined due specifically to Chicago's dumping. The Supreme Court noted that there were cities in Missouri upstream of St. Louis that also were dumping sewage in the Mississippi. The Court recommended that St. Louis filter its water if it was concerned about disease.

*Village of Euclid, Ohio v. Ambler Realty Co.*, 272 U.S. 365 (1926)
In upholding the right of the Village of Euclid to impose zoning restrictions on property owners, in 1926 the U.S. Supreme Court established the constitutionality of zoning laws to regulate *land use*. Ambler Realty owned land that was significantly reduced in value when the Village of Euclid adopted a comprehensive zoning code that limited what and how Ambler Realty could build on their property. Ambler Realty sued the city and this case was ultimately heard by the Supreme Court. In a landmark decision, the Court ruled in favor of the Village of Euclid and declared zoning codes are a valid extension of a local government's right to regulate land uses in the name of protecting public health, safety, and welfare. This case gave way for what is called "Euclidean zoning." Euclidean zoning segregates residential from commercial and other uses and is the most common form of land-use regulation in the United States today. While it has been used by local jurisdictions to prevent and control health hazards such as noise, glare, and pollution, in many communities, this zoning has also effectively made it impractical for many residents to walk or bicycle to school, work, grocery stores, social events, and healthcare facilities. Even where zoning does permit mixed-use, it often restricts the density required to support retail establishments. Euclidean zoning has resulted in communities where access requires a personal vehicle and where the mixed-use neighborhoods contemplated in the 21st-century Sustainability Era are violations of zoning ordinances or otherwise discouraged.

*SILENT SPRING ERA*
*Sierra Club v. Morton*, 405 U.S. 727 (1972)
This case centered around a planned Disney ski resort development in the Mineral King Valley in the Sequoia National Forest. The Sierra Club opposed the construction, arguing it would negatively impact wildlife and the surrounding forest area. This case made it all the way to the U.S. Supreme Court, where the standing (right to sue) of the Sierra Club was challenged. During the time it took for the Sierra Club to amend its complaint and demonstrate its right to sue, the National Environmental Policy Act was passed. In order to comply with this act, Disney had to write an environmental impact statement outlining what impact the ski resort would have on the local wildlife and forest area. After conducting this assessment, Disney recognized the significant impact the resort would have on the ecology and backed out.

*Chevron, U.S.A., Inc. v. Nat. Res. Def. Council, Inc.*, 467 U.S. 837 (1984)
The Clean Air Act (CAA) Amendments of 1977 required states that had not achieved national air quality standards to establish a permit program regulating new or modified major stationary sources of air pollution. At that time, a permit generally would not be

*(continued)*

BOX 13.2 *(continued)*

issued for such sources unless stringent conditions were met. The EPA passed a regulation in 1981 under the CAA allowing states to treat all pollution-emitting devices in the same industrial grouping as though they were encased in a single "bubble." Plants may, using the bubble provision, install or modify one piece of equipment without the need for a permit if the alteration did not increase the total emissions of the plant. The U.S. Court of Appeals for the D.C. Circuit set aside the regulations embodying the "bubble concept" as contrary to law, and recognized that the CAA did not explicitly define what Congress envisioned as a stationary source to which the permit program should apply and the issue was not squarely addressed in the legislative history; they concluded the plant-wide definition was inappropriate, while stating it was mandatory in programs designed to maintain existing air quality. The U.S. Supreme Court reversed the D.C. Circuit ruling, holding that the bubble regulation was a reasonable interpretation of the term "stationary source" in the CAA. Furthermore, it held that Congress did not have a specific intention for the term and the EPA's regulation was a reasonable policy choice, as it provided reasonable accommodations for the many competing interests (economic interest in permitting capital improvements to continue and environmental interest in improving air quality) affected by the CAA.

### SUSTAINABILITY ERA
#### Massachusetts v. EPA, 549 U.S. 497 (2007)
In 2007, the U.S. Supreme Court weighed in on the debate around whether the government has an obligation to regulate the release of carbon dioxide and other harmful gases. In this case, the Bush Administration argued that it would be acting beyond the scope of its authority for the federal government to regulate carbon emissions, including tailpipe emissions from cars and trucks, under the CAA. The Supreme Court disagreed, noting that it needed to be proven that greenhouse gasses do not contribute to climate change, or a reasonable explanation should be provided as to why the government would be incapable of restricting pollution. The high Court's findings definitively stated that action was necessary to combat climate change and underscored its urgency. This ruling set the precedent for others that followed and reiterated the importance of government regulation to better the environment and public health.

#### Deepwater Horizon Litigation, 2010 to the Present
In 2010, due to negligence on the part of oil and gas company British Petroleum (BP), the Deepwater Horizon drilling rig exploded on the Gulf of Mexico, killing 11 people and spilling the equivalent of nearly 5 million barrels of oil into the Atlantic Ocean. The BP oil spill presented an unprecedented disaster and had a profound impact on nearby people. More than 25% of locals suffered from mental illness in the wake of the event, and the accident had a global impact. BP pled guilty in November of 2012, reaching a settlement with the U.S. Dept. of Justice to pay $4.5 billion. However, the costs have been astronomical compared to that amount. To date, BP has paid more than $28 billion in cleanup costs and claims, and it is subject to $18 billion more in penalties. This case set a clear example and made it clear to oil companies that they have a responsibility to conduct their business in a way that considers and protects the environment and public health.

and while total emissions of six common air pollutants dropped by 68% over the last decades, carbon monoxide emissions have increased by 12% since 1980 (U.S. EPA, 2019).

These and other issues highlight the potential limits of the command and control regulatory scheme put in play in the Silent Spring Era and point to the need for a more holistic, cross-sectoral approach to U.S. environmental policy. The Sustainability Era responds to this need and is undergirded by a recognition that our health and environmental woes are interwoven. Sustainability has been defined as "… the need to ensure a better quality of life for all, now and into the future, in a just and equitable manner [while] living within the limits of supporting ecosystems (Kollmuss & Agyeman, 2002). The concept of living within "available biophysical (including land, sea, and air) limits, prioritizing well-being over growth, and running our society on recyclables and renewables" is increasingly important for engaged citizens (Caradonna, 2015). This has created an opportunity to develop a more holistic approach when implementing programs to improve and protect public health.

The Sustainability Era serves as a reminder that local governments often are the best entity to prioritize which issues to address in their own communities, and know how to use law to do so. Unless preemption applies, with the proper resources, as the following hypothetical case studies indicate, cities and counties are uniquely situated to respond to community health threats. Local governments can employ a myriad of legal tools to address the 21st-century environmental public health issues at the center of the Sustainability Era, including *healthy homes*, climate change, and the *built environment*.

## HYPOTHETICAL CASE STUDIES

---

### HYPOTHETICAL CASE STUDY #1: HEALTHY HOMES

Jasmin is an inspector, and she works in the environmental health division of her local health department. She responds to a complaint from Helen, a resident of a small apartment building and a recipient of a Housing Choice Voucher, about the smell of tobacco smoke from an adjacent unit. Helen is particularly concerned because her 5-year-old daughter suffers from asthma. This apartment complex is privately owned, and each of the 10 units is rented individually. Upon arrival at the complex, Jasmin smells tobacco smoke coming from one of the units and observes peeling paint on the walls in the common areas as well as sewage and trash in the hallways. She also notices a broken handrail along the stairway and dead insects and rodent droppings on the stairs. Upon inspection of Helen's apartment, in addition to dead insects and rodent droppings, Jasmin finds a large water stain on the ceiling tile and mold in the bathroom, not only around the shower tile, but also on the floor.

1. What are the elements of a healthy home?
2. What public health concerns are raised by this hypothetical case study?
3. What is the legal framework for achieving healthy homes in the United States?

---

### Healthy Homes: Selected Public Health Issues

The WHO considers healthy housing strategies among those critical to sustainable development. According to the National Center for Healthy Housing (2018), a healthy home is "housing that is designed, constructed, maintained, and rehabilitated in a manner that is conducive to good occupant health." As described in Box 13.3, housing stability, quality, safety, and affordability all have a significant impact on health outcomes. Public health practitioners have identified seven principles of a healthy home: (a) Keep it Clean; (b) Keep it Dry; (c) Keep it Pest-Free; (d) Keep it Safe; (e) Keep it Contaminant Free; (f) Keep it Ventilated; and (g) Keep it Maintained (Healthy Homes Coalition of West Michigan, 2018; National Center for Healthy Housing, 2020). As an inspector for the environmental health division, Jasmin, in Hypothetical Case Study #1, is responsible for ensuring that residential housing meets these standards.

## BOX 13.3 HOUSING STABILITY, QUALITY, AND SAFETY IMPACT HEALTH

Stability
- Over 550,000 are homeless each night in the United States or 0.17% of population (Department of Housing and Urban Development [HUD], 2018).
- 6,000 people are evicted from their homes daily (Robert Wood Johnson Foundation, 2019 Annual Message: Our Homes Are Key to Our Health).

Quality and Safety
- Lead—In the United States, ≥ 4 million households have children exposed to high levels of lead (CDC, 2018). Half a million children ages 1 to 5 have blood lead levels above 5 µg/dL.
- Asthma—7.9% of the U.S. population currently has asthma (CDC, 2019b). Triggers can include tobacco smoke, dust and pests, mold, and air pollution.
- Overcrowding can lead to physical injuries, infectious disease, and mental illness.

Housing Affordability
- 31% of households spent over 30% of their incomes for housing in 2017.
- 15% spent over 50% of their incomes on housing in 2017 (Joint Center for Housing Studies. The State of the Nation's Housing 2019 Harvard University).

Rental housing is more likely to be in substandard condition than owner-occupied housing. Depending on the type and location of rental units, tenants like Helen and her daughter can frequently be at risk of significant health problems. The public health issues identified in this Hypothetical Case Study #1 involve habitability, lead paint, vector (e.g., mosquito, rodent, pets and fleas), ground water, and other safety issues. Studies show that myriad health conditions, including asthma, elevated blood lead levels in children, pesticide poisonings, falls, and other injuries are associated with the housing conditions identified in Hypothetical Case Study #1. For example, despite laws banning its use, many houses built before 1978 still have lead-based paint. If the paint is stable and not deteriorating, lead may not be an issue. However, in Hypothetical Case Study #1, Jasmin sees peeling paint, which raises concerns for the health of Helen's daughter. Lead exposure is particularly harmful to children ages 6 years or younger, with developing nervous systems and rapid metabolism, which are particularly vulnerable to the adverse effects of lead. Because lead exposure can seriously harm a child's health—including damage to the brain and nervous system, slowed growth and development, learning and behavioral problems, and hearing and speech problems—prompt attention would be required.

## Healthy Housing: Selected Legal Frameworks

### FEDERAL APPROACHES

#### Residential Lead-Based Paint Hazard Reduction Act and the Lead Disclosure Rule

In 1992, Congress passed the Residential Lead-Based Paint Hazard Reduction Act, which authorized the HUD and EPA to **promulgate** the Lead Disclosure Rule, which requires the disclosure of any known information concerning lead-based paint hazards before the sale or lease of residential housing built before 1978 (42 U.S. Code § 4852d). Because of the requirements under this regulation, one of Jasmin's questions for Helen might be whether her landlord informed her of the potential lead hazards in the home. To comply, Helen's landlord would have had to have provided Helen with an EPA-approved information pamphlet, informed her of any known lead-based paint hazard on the property, added a signed lead disclosure statement to the lease agreement, and kept a record of this disclosure for at least 3 years.

## HUD Regulations and Policies

National standards for informing residents about lead-based paint hazards just discussed apply to all housing. While similar far-reaching laws do not exist for other housing-related health hazards, there are several HUD regulations that are applicable to Hypothetical Case Study #1. It is mentioned in Hypothetical Case Study #1 that Helen is the recipient of a Housing Choice Voucher, and this means her landlord must comply with the HUD Housing Quality Standards (HQS; 24 CFR § 982.401 HQS, April 1, 2010). "The Housing Choice Voucher program, formerly known as the Tenant-Based Section 8 Voucher is the federal government's major program for assisting very low-income families, the elderly, and the disabled, allowing them to afford decent, safe, and sanitary housing in the private market" (Baltimore County Government, 2020). Participants, like Helen, are free to choose any housing that meets the requirements of the program and are not limited to units located in subsidized housing projects. These standards define housing quality as it relates to things like food preparation and refuse disposal, thermal environment, interior air quality, electricity, water supply, and lead-based paint. According to HUD Housing Quality Standards, Helen's home should have been inspected before she moved in, once a year after she has moved in, and—as is the case here—any time there is a complaint about health or safety conditions at the property. While statewide landlord–tenant law and the lease requirements are applied to determine the steps and timing for repairs, landlords should be vigilant about making necessary repairs for these properties because they may be reviewed by the local public housing authority and HUD.

### STATE AND LOCAL APPROACHES

For all other housing, state or local health, housing, and building codes may be the only occupant protections in place. The authority to inspect owner- and renter-occupied single or multifamily homes or apartments is often provided by state law or local ordinance. Generally, these laws authorize the public health officer or the local public health department to enforce the local housing and sanitation code. For example, the King County Board of Health Code authorizes the director of the health department to enforce violations of any public health rule or regulation (King County Board of Health Code). Such codes are usually comprehensive and provide varying departments and agencies with broad authority to control public nuisances or health hazards in a community.

Some communities have used this authority to create Proactive Rental Inspection (PRI) programs. Unlike rental code enforcement, which is complaint-based, PRI programs ensure inspections of covered properties are mandatory and periodic. PRIs have proven to be more effective in protecting tenants' health and safety, and tenants (who might not feel safe lodging complaints against landlords) no longer need to worry about initiating inspections or any subsequent repairs (ChangeLab Solutions, 2020). In addition, a few localities have incorporated HUD standards into their housing or building codes (HUD, 2009). For example, the San Francisco Department of Public Health (n.d.) has implemented an Apartment Inspection Program that conducts routine inspections of multiunit housing, conducts home inspections for asthma patients and lead-poisoned children, and evaluates complaints of other public health nuisances.

In most local jurisdictions, the hazards Jasmin identified would be violations of a local ordinance, or housing code. Following the inspection, a notice would be sent to the property owner so that they may be provided an opportunity to correct the problem. For example, in Bloomington, Minnesota, deadlines to remediate or correct local code violations are usually 10 days. If the violations are not corrected, further action may be taken and the property owner may be billed or fined (City of Bloomington, Minnesota, 2020). In some jurisdictions, 30 days are allowed to correct housing code violations that are nonemergencies. Local governments use varied approaches to address these situations. For example, the Philadelphia Lead Court—a partnership between the health department, the Office of the City Solicitor, and the Court of Common Pleas—has been able to work together to help to provide a process to deal with violations, provide incentives for addressing hazards, and expeditiously manage, enforce, and resolve these cases (Temple University: Center for Public Health Law Research, 2013). Depending on the jurisdiction, if the health hazards are so severe that the home is deemed uninhabitable, Helen and the other tenants may be given the opportunity to move.

---

**HYPOTHETICAL CASE STUDY #2: CLIMATE CHANGE AND VECTOR-BORNE DISEASES**

It is mosquito season in a major southern city. Alyx is a homeowner who travels for long periods of time and is often away from home. While on a long trip for work, Alyx's neighbor complains to the mosquito and vector control division of the local health department about an abandoned boat that Alyx has in her backyard. The neighbor says there is standing water, and she believes that this boat is a source of mosquito breeding. Upon inspection, the city inspector finds that there is indeed standing water and issues a notice to Alyx that she must remove the standing water from her property within 5 days. Alyx fails to do so and is issued a citation and a fine.

1. Why are standing water and vector-borne diseases a public health concern?
2. What is the connection between climate change and vector-borne diseases?
3. What is the legal framework for mosquito control on the local level?

---

## Climate Change and Vector-Borne Diseases

*Climate change* impacts public health in a variety of ways, and environmental public health practitioners play a vital role in helping communities address its health effects. As the climate continues to change, communities will be susceptible to a number of health threats, including heat-related conditions, allergens, food and waterborne diseases, air pollution, and even mental health and stress-related disorders; additionally, there will be increased exposure to mosquito- and other vector-borne diseases (VBDs). VBDs, including those listed in Box 13.4, are diseases that are transmitted to humans through the bites of insects that carry disease-causing pathogens.

---

### BOX 13.4 VECTOR-BORNE DISEASES

Arboviral—viruses spread by mosquitoes and ticks:
- Chikungunya
- West Nile
- Yellow fever
- Zika
- Malaria

Bacterial Diseases—bacteria spread by ticks and fleas:
- Lyme disease
- Plague
- Tularemia

Dengue viruses—spread by mosquitoes

Rickettsial Zoonoses—bacteria spread primarily by ticks, lice, and fleas
- Q fever
- Rocky Mountain spotted fever
- Typhus fevers

*Source*: Centers for Disease Control and Prevention. (2019a). *Division* of *Vector-Borne Diseases: About the Division of Vector-Borne Diseases*. https://www.cdc.gov/ncezid/dvbd/about.html

Globally, the WHO reports more than 1 billion cases of VBDs annually, and over 1 million of those infections result in death. Mosquitos, along with ticks and flies, are common vectors, and due to their widespread occurrence and their sensitivities to their environments, VBDs are some of the best-studied diseases associated with climate change. Climate change creates new risks, particularly in the United States, for human exposure to VBDs. For example, studies have found that warming temperatures coupled with more humid days have elongated mosquito seasons in 76% of major cities in the United States since the 1980s, and the CDC reports that mosquito-borne illnesses have increased almost tenfold nationally from 2004 to 2016 (Rosenberg et al., 2018).

Climate change also creates new uncertainties about the spread of these and other VBDs, by altering the conditions that affect the development and dynamics of the disease vectors and the pathogens they carry. For example, *Aedes aegypti,* the species that transmits Zika, dengue, yellow fever, and chikungunya, has moved northward in the United States by roughly 150 miles per year. By 2050, researchers predict almost half the world's population will be exposed to at least one of two major disease-carrying mosquitoes (Zhu, 2019). Scientists are also concerned about the growing threat of resistance, which undercuts the effectiveness of insecticides. This creates a critical need for local mosquito control and abatement programs.

## Legal Framework for Mosquito Control and Abatement

In Hypothetical Case Study #2, the concern is that the standing or stagnant water on Alyx's property can present safety and health hazards if left untreated. As her neighbor's concern indicates, such standing water can serve as a breeding ground for mosquitoes and other insects, particularly in the summer. Mosquito control is a consummate goal of public health, and as result of our system of federalism, a wide variety of state and local government agencies can have authority for mosquito control including those listed in Box 13.5. For example, according to research conducted by Pepin and Penn, in Georgia, the health department has primary authority to control the mosquito population in certain situations, such as at large gatherings or in response to the management of solid waste. But, the department of natural resources has the primary authority over things like the management of mosquitoes at scrap tire businesses (Pepin & Penn, 2017). The department of agriculture also has the authority to issue licenses for pesticide applicators. In other states, either mosquito control districts or a single state agency may be tasked broadly with mosquito control. In states like Alabama and Indiana, counties and cities take the lead in mosquito control activities (Pepin & Penn, 2017).

In recent years, in preparation for VBDs such as West Nile virus and Dengue fever, many state and local governments have taken steps to enhance their mosquito abatement programs, often through mosquito control districts. Today, there are more than 700 mosquito-abatement districts in the United States, each with a different set of authorities. But there are at least four common characteristics across jurisdictions:

1. The legal authority to exist and operate as a public entity
2. General or specific definition of the function of the agency
3. Enforcement authority
4. Funding authority

### BOX 13.5 GOVERNMENT AGENCIES THAT MIGHT BE RESPONSIBLE FOR MOSQUITO CONTROL

- Mosquito Control Agency/District/Commission
- Health Department
- Environmental/Natural Resources
- Agriculture (Pesticides)

## BOX 13.6  OVERVIEW OF PUBLIC HEALTH NUISANCE

**New Hampshire (NH)**

A local health officer's authority to abate public nuisances is an important tool in protecting public health. In general, a nuisance is defined as a "condition, activity, or situation (such as a loud noise or foul odor) that interferes with the use or enjoyment of property; esp., a nontransitory condition or persistent activity that either injures the physical condition of adjacent land or interferes with its use or with the enjoyment of easements on the land or of public highways" Garner (2009).

When this interference substantially and unreasonably affects the use and enjoyment of a single or small group of properties, it is considered a "private nuisance" (*Dunlap v. Daigle*, 1982). When an activity unreasonably interferes "with a right common to the general public," it is considered a "public nuisance" (*Robie v. Lillis*, 1972). As such, a public nuisance is a "behavior that unreasonably interferes with the health, safety, peace, comfort or convenience of the general community" (*Robie v. Lillis*, 1972).

A public nuisance could include public health threats such as pest infestations, unsanitary living conditions, smoke from outdoor wood boilers, or properties with an unreasonable accumulation of garbage. At times, conduct may be both a private and a public nuisance if it causes both a particular harm to a specific property and a more generalized harm to the greater community (*Urie v. Franconia Paper Co.*, 1966).

However, the local health officer's focus is to play an important role in addressing the health threat presented by public nuisances (Association of State and Territorial Health Officials, 2018; NH Public Health Nuisance Task Force & Network for Public Health Law Eastern Region, 2014).

Usually, local governments have the authority to abate *nuisances* that can impact the health of their citizens. This is true, for example, in New Hampshire, where state statute authorizes the local health officer to abate a nuisance, defined as a "condition, activity, or situation (such as a loud noise or foul odor) that interferes with the use or enjoyment of property ..." As shown in Box 13.6, the statute goes on to specifically mention "public health threats such as pest infestations, unsanitary living conditions ..." In this case, Alyx's local health department might decide to enforce a nuisance law or other rules that require that properties not include hazards like pools of water that are public health threats since they can be breeding grounds for mosquitoes.

While approaches may vary, in Hypothetical Case Study #2, it is likely that the monitoring and abatement of mosquitoes would be the responsibility of a local mosquito control program. In Indianapolis, Indiana, for example, the Mosquito Control Program is a unit of the Marion County Public Health Department. The most visible and popular elements of the program include larviciding (controlling mosquito larvae and pupae in standing water) and adulticiding (controlling adult mosquitoes via truck-mounted ultra-low volume sprayers). The program also routinely tests for West Nile virus to ensure expedited control measures are taken when the presence of mosquito-borne illnesses is detected in the community, and performs resistance testing to confirm resistance is not occurring in the mosquito population. Staff is also responsible for retrieving waste tires throughout the city.

## Local Environmental Public Health Practitioners, Climate Change, and COVID-19

An increase in mosquito and other vector-borne diseases is just one example of how climate change impacts health. Arguably, the global spread of infectious diseases, including COVID-19, is closely linked to the climate crisis. Both climate change and COVID-19 are of environmental origin, and both impact those of lower socioeconomic status and other vulnerable populations the hardest, thereby highlighting (and potentially increasing) not only health disparities, but racial and economic inequality generally. Both also provide salient examples of how essential local environmental health practitioners are to the response to emerging public health threats. In the wake of the spread of COVID-19, the National Environmental Health Association (NEHA) distributed rapid needs assessments to assess environmental health activities and needs (NEHA, 2020). While it found that all environmental public health sectors—federal, state, and local—reported being actively involved in the COVID-19 response, the highest reported sector was local (NEHA, 2020). This is an example of police powers in action and underscores the importance of building the legal capacity of the local environmental public health workforce so that they are better prepared to address emerging health threats across the spectrum.

---

### HYPOTHETICAL CASE STUDY #3: BUILT ENVIRONMENT

Jennifer is an environmental public health professional who likes to bike and/or walk to work. She has just started a new job, and much to her dismay, there are no bike lanes available for her to ride her bike and sidewalks are nonexistent. Thus, she must drive to work. She is pleased to learn that there is a gym onsite because there are no recreational facilities within five miles of her home. Jennifer has committed to healthier eating, but with her busy work schedule, she often lacks the time to drive to the nearest grocery store. Most nights her dinner comes from one of the many fast-food restaurants near her home. Although she tries to choose one of the few healthy options on the menu, it is not an easy task. Crime in her neighborhood and a cul-de-sac of vacant homes also make Jennifer apprehensive about taking the after-dinner walk her doctor has suggested she needs to lose weight and lower her blood pressure. Jennifer knows that living closer to her job would be ideal, but affordable housing is not available and new housing is years away from being developed.

1.  What are some of the health concerns related to Jennifer's built environment?
2.  What are zoning codes and how are they used to shape the built environment?
3.  How can zoning and land-use decisions impact health disparities?

---

## The Built Environment's Impact on Health

The built environment includes those environments that are man-made or modified, including homes, schools, workplaces, highways, urban sprawl, and various mobile and stationary sources of air pollution. The relationship between community design and health was well-established in the 18th and 19th century Sanitation Era, when Frederick Law Olmstead designed Central Park to be the "lungs of the city" and critical for physical activity and recreation (Central Park Conservancy, 2020). Still, despite these examples and substantial evidence of how the built environment influences health, for many decades the health and built environment relationship went largely unappreciated.

Recently there has been increasing collaboration between planners and civic officials, and renewed consideration and awareness about how community design intricacies and urban-planning processes can lead to environments that either reduce or exacerbate health inequities. Decisions about where grocery stores, recreational facilities, homes, schools, and churches are built have a significant impact on an individual's choices, behavior, access, and ultimately, their health. One response to this is the "New Urbanism movement." New Urbanism is a planning and development approach based on principles grounded in public health, but with a focus on sustainability. The New Urbanism movement encompasses the idea of improving the built environment so that an individual's default choices and behaviors are healthier, and in ways that increase their connectivity and access. New Urbanism principles include: walkability; connectivity; mixed-use development of housing, shops, restaurants, and workplaces; mixed-housing types within closer proximities; and quality architecture and urban design focused on aesthetics, comfort, and creating a sense of place. New Urbanism also places an emphasis on smart or green transportation, such as pedestrian routes and high-quality trains, sustainability such as increased local production, and increasing the overall quality of life in communities (New Urbanism, n.d.).

## Zoning Codes and Land-Use Planning

**Zoning codes** and ordinances determine where various categories of land use may occur, thereby systematically influencing the location of resulting environmental and health impacts. Zoning is not a new tool in the public health toolbox. In 1926, the U.S. Supreme Court in *Village of Euclid v. Ambler Realty Co.* recognized zoning ordinances as a proper exercise of the state's police power to protect community health and safety, citing the previous case of *Jacobson v. Massachusetts* where governmental actions to protect the public's health were validated. Many state and county codes and ordinances provide that one purpose of zoning is to promote health and general welfare in determining how land is used and developed.

As illustrated in Hypothetical Case Study #3, zoning codes and associated decision-making processes can determine how close people are able to live to business areas, the proximity of daily services to residential districts, and where different types of uses (e.g., industry, retail, housing) may be located. Studies show that local zoning codes can affect human exposure to pollution and access to potential hazards such as alcohol and fast-food. Land-use decisions can influence the use of transit by promoting public transit options and transit-oriented development, requiring bicycle parking and pedestrian and bike lanes, and limiting automobile parking.

## Zoning, the Built Environment, and Health Disparities

Zoning codes and ordinances can also be determinants of environmental injustice and impact the distribution of harms and amenities throughout the city and among populations by race, class, age, or disability status. These elements form and shape the patterns of daily interaction and can significantly influence health and contribute to health inequities. Research on the connections between health and the built environment has shown that the burden of illness is greater on minority and vulnerable populations and on those of low socioeconomic status. The high prevalence of noxious land uses and ready availability of tobacco products and inexpensive, unhealthy foods in communities where low-income families and people of color are more likely to live, work, and play provide salient examples of how the built environment can impact health and exacerbate health disparities. To effectively address the influences of the *built environment* on health disparities in healthcare service delivery and planning requires public health practitioners to have a good understanding of the barriers to equitable access to high quality of care and specific needs of health-disadvantaged populations, particularly as they relate to policy and decision-making processes involved in local zoning efforts.

One tool communities, stakeholders, and practitioners may use to evaluate the potential positive and negative effects of proposed policies such as local zoning efforts is the **Health Impact Assessment (HIA)**. Also discussed in Chapter 18, an HIA is a pragmatic tool that can help communities and decision-makers collaborate to identify the potential health effects of policy decisions in multiple sectors; how those impacts might disproportionately affect different racial, income, geographic, and other groups; and how that distribution can influence health outcomes. HIAs then use those findings to develop recommendations that can help maximize health benefits and minimize preventable risks, such as chronic disease and injuries (Pew Charitable Trusts, 2019).

HIAs involve six steps and should involve communities, individuals that may be affected, policymakers, and other stakeholders throughout the process. These steps are the following:

1. Screening. The HIA team and stakeholders determine whether an HIA is needed, can be accomplished in a timely manner, and would add value to the decision-making process.

2. Scoping. The HIA team and stakeholders identify the potential health risks and benefits, and develop a plan for completing the assessment, including specifying their respective roles and responsibilities.
3. Assessment. The HIA team evaluates the proposed project, program, policy, or plan and identifies its most likely health effects using a range of data sources, analytic methods, and stakeholder input to answer the research questions developed during scoping.
4. Recommendations. The HIA team and stakeholders develop practical solutions that can be implemented within the political, economic, or technical limitations of the project or policy to minimize identified health risks and maximize potential health benefits.
5. Reporting: The HIA team distributes information including the HIA's purpose, process, findings, and recommendations to a wide range of stakeholders.
6. Monitoring and evaluation. The HIA team and stakeholders evaluate the HIA according to accepted standards of practice. They also propose a plan for monitoring and measuring the HIA's impact on decision-making and the effects of the implemented decision on health (Pew Charitable Trusts, 2019).

HIAs are distinguishable from other health assessment methodologies that may be used during or after an HIA. Some of the most common health assessments tools are the following:

1. *Community Health Needs Assessment (CHNA).* A CHNA is a systematic examination of the health status indicators for a given population that is used to identify key problems and assets in a community. The ultimate goal of a community health assessment is to develop strategies to address the community's health needs and identified issues. Data obtained on health status and community health needs and assets during a community health assessment can be used in an HIA to describe the existing health status of the affected population.
2. *Cost-benefit analysis.* Cost-benefit analysis is a type of economic evaluation that measures both costs and benefits (i.e., negative and positive consequences) associated with an intervention in dollar terms. Because an HIA typically does not examine the costs associated with its recommended strategies to promote health and mitigate adverse health impacts, a cost-benefit analysis could be conducted to help decide which HIA recommendations are the most feasible.
3. *Environmental Impact Assessment (EIA).* In the United States, the National Environmental Policy Act (NEPA) requires federal agencies to integrate environmental values into their decision-making processes by considering the environmental impacts of their proposed actions and reasonable alternatives to those actions. To meet the NEPA requirements, federal agencies first prepare an environmental assessment (EA) to determine whether a more thorough environmental impact statement (EIS) is needed. Although the NEPA does not refer to the HIA as a separate requirement, the HIA can be an appropriate way to meet statutory requirements for health effects analysis when conducted within the context of an interdisciplinary EIA.
4. *Human Health Risk Assessment.* A human health risk assessment is a quantitative, analytic process to estimate the nature and risk of adverse human health effects associated with exposure to specific chemical contaminants or other hazards in the environment, now or in the future. Human health risk assessments are not comprehensive and tend to focus on biophysical risks from exposure to hazardous substances. Results from a human health risk assessment can be used within an HIA to predict human health effects of specific exposures.
5. *Public Health Assessment.* A public health assessment is formally defined as "The evaluation of data and information on the release of hazardous substances into the environment in order to assess any past, current, or future impact on public health,

develop health advisories or other recommendations, and identify studies or actions needed to evaluate and mitigate or prevent human health effects" (Source: 42 C.F.R. §90.8 [1990]). See the Agency for Toxic Substances and Disease Registry (ATSDR) *Public Health Assessment Guidance Manual* for more information. ATSDR developed the public health assessment process for evaluating the public health implications of exposures to environmental contamination. Findings from a public health assessment can be used within an HIA to predict human health effects of specific exposures (CDC, 2016).

The "TransForm Baltimore" project of Baltimore, Maryland lends insight to three domains for how the *built environment* influences health and health disparities: (a) content within the zoning code and processes that may promote or inhibit health, (b) the role health considerations play in zoning decisions, and (c) how the land-use planning and zoning rewrite process encourages or suppresses inclusion of health. TransForm Baltimore brought together professionals from the Baltimore Department of Health, the Baltimore Department of Planning, and Johns Hopkins Bloomberg School of Public Health to conduct an HIA and to ensure health considerations were included in the rewrite of the Baltimore zoning code (Johnson Thornton et al., 2013). In its report, this group included recommendations for how zoning codes could best promote health.

Many of these recommendations from the TransForm Baltimore report would benefit communities like Jennifer's, described in Hypothetical Case Study #3. In the TransForm Baltimore report, in addition to advocating for the inclusion of public health experts in zoning advisory committees, the group recommended the following:

1. The purpose statement of the zoning code could more clearly articulate the role of public health in zoning, such as providing the opportunity for all communities to be healthy now and in the future.
2. Walkability and access to daily services could be promoted by allowing more mixed-use areas (a combination of retail and residential uses) and design standards, such as windows on the first floor of businesses and landscaping, which make areas more attractive to pedestrians.
3. Food access could be enhanced by reducing the required lot size for food stores, allowing farmers' markets, community gardens, and urban agriculture throughout the city.
4. Crime could be addressed by limiting the concentration of off-premises alcohol outlets and requiring a conditional use permit for any new mixed-income areas.
5. Residential segregation could be decreased by allowing a greater mix of housing types throughout residential districts and reducing the minimum lot size for detached homes. Specific guidance is needed about how zoning boards and planning commissions determine whether a proposed project promotes health and welfare.
6. Outreach in any zoning or land-use planning process should include a variety of perspectives by framing zoning for lay citizens and describing how reworking zoning provisions might positively affect the health of their neighborhoods.

Zoning and its attendant legal and policy-making processes can be essential tools for public health practitioners seeking to improve public health and addressing community health disparities. Land-use planning efforts and rewrites such as those described in the TransForm Baltimore effort have the potential to greatly influence future urban design and the *built environment*, and in turn the public's health. Assessments like those previously described, which can assess the impact of policy decisions on health, the environment, and communities, for example, can be beneficial in determining how to prioritize spending limited resources. The more public health researchers and practitioners can build their capacity to understand the language and practices of urban planning, particularly zoning law, the better they can contribute to such efforts on the local level.

## CONCLUSION

Law and policy can be important tools to protect and improve our environmental and health conditions. As this discussion of history of environmental public health law described, there have been significant changes in the environmental and policy issues that need to be addressed in this field. Humans have often caused a great deal of change and damage to our physical environment in the name of progress, and it resulted in many environmental and health consequences. With the *Silent Spring Era*, law and policy were increasingly used to regulate and monitor environmental actions and to protect the natural environment and human health. Progress has been made in improving environmental conditions and reducing hazards. Over the last three decades, thinking has turned to addressing long-term issues such as sustainability, preventing climate change, and new and creative multisectoral partnerships that have at times created innovations and improved conditions. Challenges remain in continuing to address the built environment and continuing to focus on environmental justice issues. As we look toward the future—as environmental public health law must face new and different issues, diseases, and conditions—one thing remains clear: laws and policies can have an important impact on environmental health.

## CHAPTER REVIEW

### Review Questions

1. Define environmental public health.
2. List the three major eras in the evolution of environmental public health law.
3. Why might a PRI program be more effective in protecting tenants' health and safety than a periodic inspection program?
4. Which one of these diseases is *not* a VBD?

   a. Rocky Mountain Spotted Fever
   b. Plague
   c. Anthrax
   d. Dengue
   e. Zika

5. Which of these government agencies might be responsible for mosquito control?

   a. Mosquito Control Agency/District/Commission
   b. Health Department
   c. Environmental/Natural Resources
   d. Agriculture
   e. All of the above

6. What 1926 case recognized zoning ordinances as a proper exercise of the state's police power to protect community health and safety?

### Essay Questions

1. You are brought in as an environmental policy fellow with your local mayor's office. The city is trying to determine what laws or policies might be implemented to help mitigate the impacts of climate change in the community. Specifically, you have been asked to ensure the approach considers environmental justice principles, as many of the neighborhoods impacted are older and have large minority populations. What public health issues

would you consider as you decide what laws or policies might need to be addressed? How is that issue related to climate change? What is one local law you might suggest to address this issue?

2.  Of the laws passed during the *Silent Spring Era*, which would you argue has made the greatest impact on promoting environmental health (or alternately, with our current environmental issues, what law do you think needs to be expanded or modified)?

3.  Consider the three main eras in the evolution of environmental public health. For each era, describe the three major public health issues, and identify one law that has been or is currently being used to address them.

## Internet Activities

1.  Using your local health department's website, identify one of the major environmental risks in your own community (e.g., heat, lead in the water, drought, and hurricane). Research and describe how that issue impacts health outcomes and offer one state or local law that has been used to address this issue.

2.  Conduct an internet search for the environmental code enforcement unit for your local community. What issues does that unit handle? What are the steps you must take to file a housing hazard–related complaint?

3.  Nonprofit hospitals are required to do a CHNA every 3 years and post their report on their website or make it available to the public. Identify a nonprofit hospital in your local community and find its website. See if you can find the hospital's CHNA. What are three issues identified in the CHNA? What are the strategies outlined to address those issues? Based on the information provided, what is the role of the community or community engagement programs?

## REFERENCES

24 CFR § 982.401 Housing Quality Standards (HQS), April 1, 2010.

42 C.F.R. § 90.8 (1990).

42 U.S. Code § 4852d.

Association of State and Territorial Health Officials. (2014). *Profile of state environmental health: Summary and analysis of workforce changes from 2010-2012.* https://www.astho.org/Profile-of-State-Environmental-Health-Workforce

Association of State and Territorial Health Officials. (2018). *ASTHO report: Analysis of express legal authorities for mosquito control in the United States, Washington, D.C., and Puerto Rico.* https://www.astho.org/ASTHOReports/Analysis-of-Express-Legal-Authorities-for-Mosquito-Control-in-the-US-DC-and-PR/10-12-18

Baltimore County Government. (2020, January 9). *Housing choice voucher program.* https://www.baltimorecountymd.gov/Agencies/housing/dsssec8.html

Caradonna, J. L. (2015). *10 successes of the sustainability movement to date.* https://www.resilience.org/stories/2015-09-11/10-successes-of-the-sustainability-movement-to-date

Carson, R. (1962). *Silent spring.* Houghton Mifflin Company.

Centers for Disease Control and Prevention. (2016, October 21). *Healthy places: Health Impact Assessment: Different types of health assessments.* https://www.cdc.gov/healthyplaces/types_health_assessments.htm

Centers for Disease Control and Prevention. (2018). State blood lead testing laws requiring 5 ug/dL & CDC reference rule. https://www.cdc.gov/phlp/docs/laws-bll.pdf

Centers for Disease Control and Prevention. (2019a). Division of Vector-Borne Diseases: About the Division of Vector-Borne Diseases. https://www.cdc.gov/ncezid/dvbd/about.html

Centers for Disease Control and Prevention. (2019b). Most recent national asthma data. https://www.cdc.gov/asthma/most_recent_national_asthma_data.htm

Centers for Disease Control and Prevention/National Center for Health Statistics. (2013). *Health, United States, 2012: With special feature on emergency care.* https://www.cdc.gov/nchs/data/hus/hus12.pdf

Central Park Conservancy. (2020). *How public health influenced the creation, purpose, and design of Central Park.* https://www.centralparknyc.org/articles/how-public-health-influenced-the-creation -purpose-and-design-of-central-park

ChangeLab Solutions. (2020). *Healthy housing through proactive rental inspection: A summary and guide for implementing PRI programs.* https://www.changelabsolutions.org/product/healthy -housing-through-proactive-rental-inspection

City of Bloomington, Minnesota. (2020). *Residential property code compliance.* https://www .bloomingtonmn.gov/eh/residential-property-code-compliance

The Climate Change and Public Health Law Site. (n.d.). *Historic public health reports: The Shattuck Report.* https://biotech.law.lsu.edu/cphl/history/books/sr

*Dunlap v. Daigle,* 122 N.H. 295, 298 (1982).

Duvic-Paoli, L. (2020, March). *Covid-19 symposium: The COVID-19 pandemics and limits of International Environmental Law.* https://opiniojuris.org/2020/03/30/covid-19-symposium-the -covid-19-pandemic-and-the-limits-of-international-environmental-law

Environmental Science.org. (2020). *Environmental law: Government and public policy towards the environment.* https://www.environmentalscience.org/environmental-law

Garner, B. A. (2009). *Black's law dictionary* (9th ed.). West Publishing Company.

Gilman, R. (1990). *Sustainability: The state of the movement.* https://www.context.org/iclib/ic25/ gilman/#:~:text=However%2C%20there%20are%20important%20ways,on%20spirituality%20 and%20personal%20growth

Harvard University Joint Center for Housing Studies. (2019). *The state of the nation's housing 2019.* https://www.jchs.harvard.edu/sites/default/files/Harvard_JCHS_State_of_the_Nations _Housing_2019.pdf

Healthy Homes Coalition of West Michigan. (2018). *For families: What is a healthy home?* http:// www.healthyhomescoalition.org/what-is-a-healthy-home

HealthyPeople.gov. (2020). *2020 topics & objectives: Environmental health.* https://www.healthypeople .gov/2020/topics-objectives/topic/environmental-health#one

Hinman, A. R. (1990). 1889 to 1989: A century of health and disease. *Public Health Reports, 105*(4), 374–380. https://www.ncbi.nlm.nih.gov/pmc/articles/PMC1580071

Institute of Medicine (US) Committee for the Study of the Future of Public Health. (1988). *The future of public health: A history of the public health system.* National Academies Press (US). https://www .ncbi.nlm.nih.gov/books/NBK218224

Johnson-Thornton, R. L., Greiner, A., Fichtenberg, C. M., Feingold, B. J., Ellen, J. M., & Jennings, J. M. (2013). Achieving a healthy zoning policy in Baltimore: Results of a health impact assessment of the TransForm Baltimore zoning code rewrite. *Public Health Reports, 128*(Suppl. 3), 87–103. https://doi.org/10.1177/00333549131286s313

Kollmuss, A., & Agyeman, J. (2002). Mind the gap: Why do people act environmentally and what are the barriers to pro-environmental behavior? *Environmental Education Research, 8*(3), 239–260. https://doi.org/10.1080/13504620220145401

The Law Dictionary & Black's Law Dictionary Free (2nd ed.). (n.d.). *What is promulgate?* https:// thelawdictionary.org/promulgate

The Law Dictionary, 'What is Environmental Law?' https://thelawdictionary.org/environmental -law/

McManus, O. (2009). *Environmental regulation* (Section 4852d). Elsevier.

National Center for Healthy Housing. (2018, May). *Healthy homes maintenance checklist.* https:// nchh.org/resource-library/healthy-homes-maintenance-checklist_english.pdf

National Center for Healthy Housing. (2020). *The principles of a healthy home.* https://nchh.org/ information-and-evidence/learn-about-healthy-housing/healthy-homes-principles

National Environmental Health Association. (2020, April). NEHA issues key findings in *Covid-19 rapid needs assessment.* https://www.neha.org/node/61327

National Fair Housing Alliance. (2017). *The case for fair housing: 2017 fair housing trends report.* https:// nationalfairhousing.org/wp-content/uploads/2017/07/TRENDS-REPORT-2017-FINAL.pdf

National Geographic. (2020). *Resource library: Encyclopedic entry: Climate change.* https://www .nationalgeographic.org/encyclopedia/climate-change

New Hampshire Public Health Nuisance Task Force & the Network for Public Health Law Eastern
Region. (2014, October). *Public health nuisance guidance document.* https://www.dhhs.nh
.gov/dph/holu/documents/hom-nuisance-guidance.pdf

New Urbanism.org. (n.d.). *New Urbanism: Principles of urbanism.* http://www.newurbanism.org/
newurbanism/principles.html

Nolon, J. (2002, January 1). *Introduction: Considering the trend toward local environmental law.* https://
digitalcommons.pace.edu/cgi/viewcontent.cgi?article=1176&context=lawfaculty

Pepin, D., & Penn, M. (2017). Legal authority for mosquito control and pesticide use in the
United States. *Public Health Reports, 132*(3), 389–391. https://journals.sagepub.com/eprint/
X3zE3Jnj9D8uNxCyXXKF/full

Pew Charitable Trusts. (2019, February 28). *Do health impact assessments promote healthier decision-
making?* https://www.pewtrusts.org/en/research-and-analysis/issue-briefs/2019/02/do-health
-impact-assessments-promote-healthier-decision-making

Robert Wood Johnson Foundation. (2019). *2019 annual message: Our homes are key to our health.* https://
www.rwjf.org/en/library/annual-reports/2019-annual-message.html

Robert Wood Johnson Foundation Commission. (2014, November 4). *Improving health by
investing in communities.* https://medium.com/@RWJFCommission/to-improve-our-health-lets
-transform-the-places-we-live-7f85d97c51b9

*Robie v. Lillis,* 112 N.H. 492, 495 (1972).

Rosenberg, R., Lindsey, N. P., Fischer, M., Gregory, C. J., Hinckley, A. F., Mead, P. S., Paz-Bailey, G.,
Waterman, S. H., Drexler, N. A., Kersh, G. J., Hooks, H., Partridge, S. K., Visser, S. N., Beard, C.
B., & Petersen, L. R. (2018). Vital signs: Trends in reported vectorborne disease cases—United
States and Territories, 2004-2016. *Morbidity and Mortality Weekly Report, 67*(17), 496–501. https://
doi.org/10.15585/mmwr.mm6717e1

San Francisco Department of Public Health. (n.d.). *Environmental health.* https://www.sfdph.org/
dph/EH/Housing/healthy.asp

Temple University: Center for Public Health Law Research. (2013, May 16). *Philadelphia lead court
effectively reduces lead hazards.* http://publichealthlawresearch.org/news/2013/12/philadelphia
-lead-court-effectively-reduces-lead-hazards

Temple University: Center for Public Health Law Research. (2017). *Environmental health.* http://
publichealthlawresearch.org/topic/environmental-health

Urban Institute. (2018, October 18). *Research report: Strategic housing code enforcement and public
health.* https://www.urban.org/research/publication/strategic-housing-code-enforcement-and
-public-health

*Urie v. Franconia Paper Co.,* 107 N.H. 131, 133(1966).

U.S. Department of Housing and Urban Development. (2009). *Healthy homes strategic plan – 2009.*
https://www.hud.gov/sites/documents/DOC_13701.PDF

U.S. Environmental Protection Agency. (2005, January). *Recommendations to the Clean Air Act Advisory
Committee.* https://www.epa.gov/sites/production/files/2015-05/documents/aqm_report1
-17-05.pdf

U.S. Environmental Protection Agency. (2018, November 19). *EPA history: The origins of EPA.* https://
www.epa.gov/history/origins-epa

U.S. Environmental Protection Agency. (2019, July 8). *Air quality: National summary.* https://www
.epa.gov/air-trends/air-quality-national-summary

World Health Organization. (2006). *Preventing disease through healthy environments.* WHO Press.

Zhu, J. J. (2019). *Man vs. mosquito: The local agencies at the front lines of climate change.* https://
www.pri.org/stories/2019-09-20/man-vs-mosquito-local-agencies-front-lines-climate
-change#:~:text=By%202050%2C%20researchers%20predict%2C%20almost%20half%20the%20
world%E2%80%99s,of%20insecticides.%20Mosquitoes%20are%20not%20a%20new%20enemy

## Additional Resources

- **Center for Parent Information and Resources**
  https://www.parentcenterhub.org/ohi-lead
- **National Center for Healthy Housing**
  https://nchh.org
- **Mosquito Control Capabilities in the United States**
  https://www.naccho.org/uploads/downloadable-resources/Mosquito-control-in-the-U.S.
  -Report.pdf
- **Health Impact Project: Health Impact Assessments**
  https://www.pewtrusts.org/en/projects/health-impact-project/health-impact-assessment
- **NCSL: Environment and Natural Resources**
  https://www.ncsl.org/research/environment-and-natural-resources.aspx
  Environmental Health State Bill Tracking Database: https://www.ncsl.org/research/
  environment-and-natural-resources/environmental-health-legislation-database.aspx
- **CDC – National Center for Environmental Health**
  https://www.cdc.gov/nceh
- **CDC – Public Health Law Program: Environmental Health Law**
  https://www.cdc.gov/phlp/publications/topic/environmental.html
- **Environmental Protection Agency (Environmental Topics)**
  https://www.epa.gov/environmental-topics
- **Healthy People Initiative (national health goals and objectives)**
  - **Environmental Health**
    https://health.gov/healthypeople/objectives-and-data/browse-objectives/
    environmental-health
  - **Social Determinants of Health**
    https://health.gov/healthypeople/objectives-and-data/social-determinants-health

# 14

# Public Health Law and American Indians and Alaska Natives

Aila Hoss and Michelle Castagne (Sault Ste. Marie Tribe of Chippewa Indians)

## Learning Objectives

By the end of this chapter, the reader will be able to:

- Discuss the historical context underlying the legal principles of Tribal public health law.
- Describe Tribal sovereignty and Tribal inherent authority to promote public health.
- Analyze the legal principles governing the legal relationships between Tribes, states, and the federal government in the context of public health practice.
- Verify the source of legal authority for an action taken regarding American Indian (AI)/Alaska Native (AN) public health.

## Key Terminology

**Federal Indian Law:** The body of law governing the rights, relationships, and responsibilities of Tribes, states, and the federal government (Fletcher, 2016, § 3).

**Indian/Tribal/Urban Health System (I/T/U):** The three-tiered healthcare delivery system that includes Indian Health Service facilities, Tribal health programs, and urban Indian health centers (National Indian Health Board, 2014, p. 1).

**Inherent Authority:** The innate authority of Tribes as sovereigns to govern their people and lands (*United States v. Wheeler*, 1978).

**Tribal Consultation:** The requirement for federal agencies to consult with Tribes when taking actions that impact Tribes or American Indian and Alaska Native people (Clinton, 1994, pp. 936, 937).

**Tribal Law:** The laws of each individual Tribe (Newton, 2012, § 4).

**Tribal Set-Aside:** A term used by federal agencies for funds allocated to AI/AN programs to differentiate from funding for programs available to all populations (U.S. Commission on Civil Rights, 2018, p. 26). "For example, a program may be funded at $100 million; from the $100 million the amount of $5 million or 5 percent might be specifically

---

This chapter refers to the Indigenous populations of the United States as American Indian and Alaska Natives. In other contexts, the terms Native, Tribal, Indian, and Indigenous are also used. The term "Indian," for example, is the term used under federal law. Under federal law, Native Hawaiians are not considered "Indians" and are thus subject to other federal laws and policies not discussed in this chapter. While the legal framework regarding Native Hawaiians is distinct, the United States also colonized the Hawaiian Islands, which remain occupied today. The authors thank Delight Satter, MPH (Confederated Tribes of Grand Ronde) and Dawn Pepin, JD, MPH for their thoughtful comments to this chapter.

targeted, or set aside, for AI/ANs" (U.S. Commission on Civil Rights, 2018, p. 26; U.S. Environmental Protection Agency [EPA], n.d.-a, n.d.-b; Office for Victims and Crime, 2020).

**Tribal Sovereignty:** The inherent right of Tribes to make their own laws and be ruled by them (*Williams v. Lee,* 1959).

**Trust Responsibility:** The fiduciary and moral obligation of the federal government, based on treaties, agreements, case law, and statutes, to protect Tribal treaty rights, lands, and assets (U.S. Department of the Interior, Indian Affairs, n.d.).

## Public Health Law Competencies

This chapter addresses the following competencies from the Public Health Law Competency Model (PHLCM; Ransom, 2016).

**1.1** Define basic constitutional concepts and legal principles framing the practice of public health across relevant jurisdictions.

**2.3** Recognize the legal authority and limits of critical system partners and others who influence health outcomes.

---

### Spark Questions

1. How does political jurisdiction relate to public health activities?
2. How have Tribes used culture as a public health tool? Can law be used as a tool to promote and protect culture?
3. How can law and policy be structural determinants of health for particular communities?
4. As a public health practitioner, what is your role in promoting American Indian and Alaska Native health?
5. As a public health practitioner, how can you support Tribal inherent authority to promote public health?

---

## INTRODUCTION

Tribes have existed as distinct sovereign nations on the land that is now called the United States since time immemorial (Pevar, 2012, p. 3). Tribal governments exercise the authorities and responsibilities of a nation-state (Pevar, 2012, p. 81), including protecting the health and welfare of their citizens (Hoss, 2019, pp. 119, 120). European colonization and the subsequent founding of the United States led to the development of a unique framework under federal law that governs the legal relationships between Tribes, the federal government, and states (Fletcher, 2016, p. 3). This chapter describes the historical context and legal foundations for the modern-day practice of Tribal public health. It also discusses the diversity of health systems that support American Indian and Alaska Native health, including Tribal governments, Urban Indian Health Centers, and Federal Indian Health Programming. Finally, this chapter ends with discussing legal strategies for intergovernmental relations in Tribal public health.

## Foundations of Tribal–U.S. Relations

Estimates suggest that prior to European contact, tens of millions of Indigenous people living in what is now the United States were members of hundreds of distinct Tribal nations (Pevar, 2012, p. 1). Colonization resulted in the death—from infectious disease, violence, systematic genocide—of millions of Indigenous people (Dunbar-Ortiz, 2014, pp. 39–42). By the

## BOX 14.1  HEALTH INEQUALITIES AND AI/AN POPULATIONS

American Indians and Alaska Natives experience a variety of health inequalities, including higher rates of heart disease, motor vehicle injuries, and certain cancers (Indian Health Services, 2019). As stated in a recent report from the U.S. Commission on Human Rights:

"The efforts of the federal government have been insufficient to meet the promises of providing for the health and wellbeing of tribal citizens, as a vast health disparity exists today between Native Americans and other population groups. The life expectancy for Native peoples is 5.5 years less than the national average" (U.S. Commission on Civil Rights, 2018, p. 65).

### Health Resiliencies

Despite these health inequalities, Tribal cultural practices can be used to promote public health. Tribal promotion of traditional tobacco use has been a tool to reduce commercial tobacco use (National Native Network, n.d.). For additional examples, visit the webpage of the Centers for Disease Control and Prevention (CDC) "Tribal Practices for Wellness in Indian Country" (https://www.cdc.gov/healthytribes/tribalpractices.htm).

## BOX 14.2  THE MARSHALL TRILOGY

The first three Supreme Court cases related to Tribal interests are referred to as the "Marshall Trilogy." The opinions, written by Chief Justice Marshall, describe the scope of Tribal rights according to the federal government. These cases both recognize Tribal sovereignty and limit the scope of Tribal rights. They remain controversial but also the foundation of modern federal Indian law.

*Johnson v. M'Intosh* (21 U.S. 543, 1823): In this controversy between landowners, the plaintiffs purchased the land from a Tribe and the defendant via a land grant from the federal government. The court found that the doctrine of discovery allowed for the conquest of the Indigenous lands in what is now the United States.

*Cherokee Nation v. Georgia* (30 U.S. 1, 1831): Following the state of Georgia's efforts to regulate within Cherokee Nation's lands, the Supreme Court heard a case from the Cherokee Nation challenging the state's asserted jurisdiction. The Court did not hear the case on the merits but found that Tribes were not foreign nations but domestic dependent nations. The relationship between the Tribes and the United States was described as that of a guardian and a ward.

*Worcester v. Georgia* (31 U.S. 515, 1832): Following continued attempts by the state of Georgia to regulate on Tribal lands, the Supreme Court found that the state did not have jurisdiction. Tribes are sovereign nations.

time the U.S. Articles of Confederation were ratified in 1781, the Indigenous population had been greatly reduced (Dunbar-Ortiz, 2014, pp. 39–42) and assimilation policies that sought to displace American Indians from their communities continued to be a tool used to undermine Tribal governments and people (Pevar, 2012, pp. 8–10).

Despite this history, the resiliency of Tribes and Native people has resulted in thriving Tribal governments and vibrant communities. Today, there are 574 Tribes recognized by the United States (Indian Entities Recognized, 2020). Not mutually exclusive from federal recognition, there are over 80 state-recognized Tribes with government-government relationships with states (National Conference of State Legislatures, 2020). There are also numerous

## BOX 14.3  CULTURAL SOVEREIGNTY

Every Tribe has its own unique history, cultures, and practices. Political sovereignty ensures that Tribes can protect their cultures.

"The concept of cultural sovereignty encompasses the spiritual, emotional, mental, and physical aspects of our lives. Because of this, only Native people can decide what the ultimate contours of Native sovereignty will be."

*Wallace Coffey, Former Chairman, Comanche Nation*
*Rebecca Tsosie, Professor of Law, University of Arizona*

Tribes that do not have any federal or state recognition.[1] There are over five million people who identify as American Indian or Alaska Native (Norris et al., 2012), although this number is underreported (Tribal Epidemiology Centers, 2013, p. 131). It is important to note that the United States has not recognized the sovereign rights of all Indigenous communities within its borders, such as Native Hawaiians (Getches et al., 2011, pp. 946–948).

Tribal, state, and federal government relationships are governed by a body of law called **federal Indian law** (Fletcher, 2016, p. 3). At the core of this body of law is the principle of **Tribal sovereignty**, which is not based on federal law but instead recognized by it (Pevar, 2012, p. 81). Sovereignty refers to the authority of Tribes to exercise jurisdiction over their land and govern their people (*Williams v. Lee*, 1959, p. 271). As distinct nations, each Tribal government and its law are unique and reflective of their histories and cultures (Newton, 2012, § 4). Tribal sovereignty is also a means to protect each Tribe's cultures, practices, and teachings (Coffey & Tsosie, 2001, p. 196).

---

### HYPOTHETICAL CASE STUDY #1: TRUST RESPONSIBILITY AND FEDERAL AGENCIES

After severe hurricanes hit several jurisdictions across the southern United States, including two states and a federally recognized Tribe, the rains and heavy winds have resulted in flooding and road and building damage. Thousands of people have been displaced from their homes and hundreds are needing emergency response. As authorized by law, each jurisdiction issues an emergency declaration and begins response activities. One state emergency management official authorizes emergency crews to enter Tribal lands without notifying the Tribe. The Federal Emergency Management Agency (FEMA), whose mission is to reduce life and property loss in disasters across the United States, sends several teams to provide ground support following the hurricanes to the two states. It fails to send support to the Tribe, with one official stating that it is the responsibility of the agencies like Indian Health Service (IHS) and the Bureau of Indian Affairs to provide support to Tribes.

- To what extent do states have jurisdiction on Tribal lands?
- Does the state have authority to send emergency crews to Tribal lands?
- Is FEMA correct in relying solely on certain federal agencies to provide services and programming to Tribes?
- Does it violate the trust responsibility when a federal agency fails to provide services and programming to Tribes?

---

[1] The federal recognition process has been used as a political tool and includes an arduous administrative process today. Because of this, some Tribes have had their federal recognition terminated or have been unable or unwilling to secure federal recognition (Pevar, 2012, pp. 271–274).

Jurisdictional issues between Tribes and state and federal governments are remarkably complex. Hypothetical Case Study #1 raises the question of the extent to which states have jurisdiction on Tribal lands. The general rules include that Tribes maintain jurisdiction over their people, especially on Tribal lands (Pevar, 2012, pp. 128, 149), that states generally do not have jurisdiction on Tribal lands (Pevar, 2012, pp. 128, 149); and the federal government maintains concurrent jurisdiction on Tribal lands (Pevar, 2012, pp. 128, 149) with Tribal jurisdiction only diminished by explicit acts of Congress (Pevar, 2012, pp. 128–148).

In general, criminal jurisdiction is based on various case law and statutes and depends on the crime, the identity of the parties, and the location of the crime (Newton, 2012, § 9). Civil jurisdiction is based largely on a two-prong test established by the Supreme Court in 1981. This *Montana test* recognizes Tribal inherent authority to maintain jurisdiction over nonmembers on reservation lands when individuals or entities engage in commercial dealing, contracts, leases, or other consensual relationships, or if the conduct threatens the political integrity, the economic security, or the health or welfare of the Tribe (Newton, 2012, § 9). As such, in Hypothetical Case Study #1, it is likely that the state does not have the authority to send emergency crews to Tribal lands without some previously contemplated agreement entered into by the Tribe. The state generally would not have automatic jurisdiction on Tribal lands unless there is a prior agreement or an explicit act of Congress. Tribes and states can and do create mutual aid agreements for emergency response purposes.

Based on history, treaties, agreements, case law, and legislation, the federal government maintains a **trust responsibility** towards Tribes (*United States v. Mitchell*, 1980; *Menominee v. United States*, 1968; *Passamaquoddy v. Morton*, 1975). The *trust responsibility* is both a fiduciary duty and a moral duty to protect Tribal treaty rights, lands, and resources (U.S. Department of the Interior, Indian Affairs, n.d.). Part of the responsibility includes federal agency consultation with Tribes prior to action that impacts Tribes or American Indian and Alaska Native communities (Clinton, 1994, pp. 936, 937). This consultation requirement is mandated by executive order (Executive Order No. 13084, 1998; Executive Order No. 13175, 2000; Memorandum for the Heads of Executive Departments and Agencies, 2009). While there are particular federal agencies with an exclusive mission to support tribes, the trust responsibility permeates all federal agencies and all of the federal government. In Case Study #1, the trust responsibility may be implicated because FEMA has a responsibility to protect the lands and resources of the Tribe in parity with its responsibility to the states impacted by the hurricanes.

The Supreme Court has also found that the U.S. Congress holds a plenary power to legislate on all issues in regard to Tribes or American Indian and Alaska Natives (*Ex Parte Crow Dog*, 1883; *United States v. Kagama*, 1886). While plenary power allows for a federal preemption of Tribal authority or abrogation of Tribal treaty rights (*Ex Parte Crow Dog*, 1883; *United States v. Kagama*, 1886), the use of this power to undermine Tribal sovereignty or to absolve federal responsibilities outlined in treaties is strongly disfavored. Any limiting of Tribal sovereignty under federal statute requires specific authorization by Congress (*Ex Parte Crow Dog*, 1883; *United States v. Kagama*, 1886).

The Indian health system is influenced by the history of colonization by the federal government. Indian affairs were originally managed by the Department of War and so, in order to minimize infectious disease transmission between Indians and the military, physicians and missionaries treated Indians for smallpox in the early 19th century (Newton, 2012, § 22.04[1]). This was formalized in 1832, when Congress passed a law allowing the military to administer smallpox vaccines to Indians (Indian Vaccination Act, 1832).

Tribal–U.S. treaties also required the federal government to provide health services to Tribes in exchange for their ceded territories (Newton, 2012, § 22.04[1]). These treaties were largely not complied with, as there were only four hospitals and 77 physicians servicing Indians by 1880 (Newton, 2012, § 22.04[1]) and infectious disease continued to spread on reservations and Indian boarding schools (Meriam, 1928; Native Voices, n.d.), culminating in the passage of the Snyder Act in 1921 (25 U.S.C. § 13). This act appropriated healthcare funds to serve Tribes (25 U.S.C. § 13). Following additional reorganizations and restructuring of the agencies responsible for providing Indian healthcare, these services were eventually housed under the U.S. Department of Health and Human Services (HHS) under the agency called "Indian Health Service" (IHS) (42 U.S.C. § 2001 et seq.; Newton, 2012, § 22.04[1]).

## SYSTEMS SUPPORTING AMERICAN INDIAN AND ALASKA NATIVE HEALTH

A variety of governments and organizations support the health of American Indians and Alaska Natives, including Tribal governments, inter-Tribal organizations, nonprofit corporations, state and local governments, and federal agencies, among others (Tribal Public Health Institute Feasibility Project, 2013, p. 5). Law provides authority for or impacts the practice of public health for each of these contributors. Additionally, many Tribal cultures approach health holistically, acknowledging that cultural, spiritual, environmental, and community heath are inextricably linked (National Tribal Public and Environmental Health Think Tank, n.d.). Thus, many programs supporting American Indian and Alaska Native health can incorporate cultural practices or environmental protection activities. This chapter offers details related to Tribal, federal, and urban Indian health systems. However, many other entities can support or serve as a barrier to American Indian and Alaska Native public health.

### Tribal Public Health Systems

The foundation of Tribal public health systems is Tribal governments (Hoss, 2019, pp. 119, 120). Tribal sovereignty includes an inherent authority to promote the health and welfare of their people (Hoss, 2019, pp. 119, 120). Some Tribal constitutions outline the responsibility of the Tribe to support community health (Hoss, 2019, pp. 126, 127), like that of the Standing Rock Sioux Tribe, which states that the Tribal Council "shall … promote and protect the health, education and general welfare of the members of the Tribe" (Standing Rock Sioux Tribe Const. art. IV, § 1[c]).

---

### HYPOTHETICAL CASE STUDY #2: TRIBAL PUBLIC HEALTH SERVICES

A Tribe would like to open a syringe service program at their government center. One of their attorneys, a junior associate at a local firm, begins researching the issue and finds that the Tribe does not have a public health department. Additionally, there is no authorizing language in the health code for syringe service programs, which instead outlines the responsibility of the human services department to conduct health programming to reduce incidence of infectious disease.

- Does the Tribe need to have a specifically designated public health department in order to operate a syringe service program?
- Must all Tribal public health activities be managed by health-related agencies?
- How might a Tribe use law and their sovereign authority to create harm reduction or other public health programming, such as emergency preparedness?

---

Hypothetical Case Study #2 raises the question of whether the Tribe needs to have a specifically designated public health department in order to operate a syringe service program. The answer depends on Tribal governmental structure and **Tribal law**. Under federal law, Tribal agencies that are responsible for conducting public health activities by official government mandate are considered public health authorities (45 C.F.R. § 164.501). However, as sovereign nations, all Tribes have inherent authority to engage in public health activities governed by *Tribal law* and in accordance with the Tribal government structure (Hoss, 2019, pp. 119, 120). Thus, a Tribe that centralizes public health activities in one or two departments or one that decentralizes them across multiple government entities, may maintain public health jurisdiction (Hoss, 2019, pp. 119, 120). While explicit Tribal authorization may not be necessary, specific authorization in Tribal codes can still be useful to operationalize and fund public health programming (Hoss, 2019, p. 127). In Hypothetical Case Study #2, if a syringe service program does not conflict with existing Tribal laws, the Tribe does not need to have a designated public health department to operate such a program.

Although the structures of Tribal governments vary (Fletcher, 2016, p. 235), many Tribes have chosen to create designated health agencies responsible for providing health services and programming (Knudson et al., 2012). As outlined by Tribal code, the Navajo Nation's Department of Health, for example, is responsible for ensuring "quality comprehensive and culturally relevant healthcare and public health services are provided on the Navajo Nation" (Navajo Department of Health Act, 2014, §602). The code also outlines specific powers of the Department of Health including regulating and enforcing health codes and epidemiological surveillance (Navajo Department of Health Act, 2014, §602). As another example, the Little Traverse Bay Bands of Odawa Indians Code of Law establishes a Tribal health department (Waganakising Odawa Tribal Code of Law tit. XV, ch. 12, 15.1201) that allows the department to conduct a variety of activities including the following:

1. Promote, design, and implement health programs for each facet of our Tribal community.
2. Strive to improve and enhance the understanding of health-related issues within our community and in the greater community.
3. Assist with annual community events that incorporate health and well-being.
4. Provide services and programs that increase health and well-being.
5. Administer health-based programs, grants, and projects that assist our Tribal Citizens with an awareness of the unique needs of our Tribal Citizens.
6. Establish more interactive resources for [T]ribal citizens that utilize the most current and feasible technologies.
7. Administer all Indian Health Services' health-related programs and funding received by the Tribe, as appropriate.
8. Administer all funds and grants to the Tribe related to health matters, as appropriate.
9. Establish appropriate programs such as health clinic, dental clinic, contract health, healthy start, community outreach, diabetes self-management, substance abuse, mental health, and any other applicable health-related opportunities (Waganakising Odawa Tribal Code of Law tit. XV, ch. 12, 15.1204).

It is also important to note that Tribal public health activities, like other jurisdictions, are not always relegated to health-related agencies. For example, Tribal environmental management agencies protect not only the environment, but also human health. The Swinomish Tribal Code provides the Tribe's Department of Environmental Protection to study, assess, and develop procedures to protect the environment (Swinomish Indian Tribal Community, n.d., Chapter 1). For example, it regulates pollution to ensure that there is clean air to breathe by limiting open burning (Swinomish Indian Tribal Community, n.d., Chapter 2).

Hypothetical Case Study #2 illustrates an area where Tribes are actively using their sovereign authority to pass laws to create harm reduction programs for people who use drugs. For example, the Eastern Band of Cherokee Indians has a law establishing a syringe service program to reduce the incidence of HIV and viral hepatitis (Eastern Band of Cherokee Indians, Tribes and Tribal Nations, 2021, Sec. 130A-113.27). These programs also engage in other activities to support participants including distributing naloxone, an opioid overdose reversal drug, and providing substance use disorder treatment referrals (Eastern Band of Cherokee Indians, Public

Health and Human Services, n.d.). Other Tribes also engage in similar harm reduction programming. The Blackfeet Nation operates a syringe service program (Blackfeet Tribal Health Department, 2017; North American Syringe Exchange Network, n.d.) and the Assiniboine and Sioux Tribes of the Fort Peck Reservation have also offered syringe services (Montana Healthcare Foundation, n.d.).

Tribal governments also use their authority to engage in emergency preparedness activities (Hoss & Sunshine, 2017). Snoqualmie Indian Tribe's Emergency Management Department Act creates the agency responsible for emergency preparedness and response activities. Responsibilities for the department include developing emergency management plans, conducting emergency response exercises, and recruiting response volunteers (Hoss & Sunshine, 2017). The COVID-19 pandemic provides numerous examples of Tribal exercise of their emergency preparedness authorities. Many Tribes declared emergencies to respond to the crisis, including the Colorado River Indian Tribes, San Carlos Apache Tribes, Karuk Tribe, and the Lac Courte Oreilles Band of Lake Superior Chippewa Indians (Karuk Tribe, n.d.; Lac Courte Oreilles Band of Lake Superior Chippewa Indians, n.d.; Utacia Krol & Silversmith, 2020). Stay-at-home orders were also implemented by many Tribes (Baker, 2020; Nicholson, 2020).

## Federal Indian Healthcare Systems

The Indian health system, much like the U.S. health system, is a complex web of treatment and prevention services available to AI/ANs. Though Tribes have employed various health and wellness services since time immemorial, the current Indian health system is a merger of traditional Tribal wellness practices and Westernized medicine rooted in the trust responsibility. While over 20 federal agencies provide services to AI/ANs (U.S. Commission on Civil Rights, 2018, p. 6), coordinated healthcare services are largely housed under the HHS IHS (42 U.S.C. § 2001 et seq.; Newton, 2012, § 22.04[1]). Public health services are integrated with the clinical services provided by IHS, but advocates say the system has long been overburdened and underfunded (Tribal Budget Formulation Workgroup, 2019, p. 14). Increasingly, support for mental health and public health services within the Indian health system have been supplemented with new funding from the Substance Abuse and Mental Health Services Administration (SAMHSA) and the CDC.

## I/T/U System

The IHS is one of six core federal healthcare systems[2] (Corrigan et al., 2003, p. 28). In the mid-1970s, Congress ushered in an era of self-determination for Tribal nations with the passage of the Indian Self-Determination and Education Assistance Act (ISDEAA) of 1975 (25 U.S.C. § 5301) and the Indian Health Care Improvement Act (IHCIA) of 1976 (Public Law 94–437). ISDEAA is the basis for Tribes assuming management of many IHS services and directs the Secretary of HHS to enter into compacts and contracts at the request of any Tribe (25 U.S.C. § 5321). The IHS now has the authority to provide healthcare and public health services in a variety of ways: directly through agency-operated programs; indirectly through Tribally-contracted and operated health programs; and indirectly through services purchased from private providers. Approximately 60% of the IHS budget is now managed directly by Tribes under ISDEAA (Indian Health Service, 2016). The IHS also

---

[2] The six major government healthcare programs: Medicare, Medicaid, the State Children's Health Insurance Program (SCHIP), the Department of Defense TRICARE and TRICARE for Life programs (DOD TRICARE), the Veterans Health Administration (VHA) program, and the Indian Health Service (IHS).

## BOX 14.4  ALASKA TRIBAL HEALTH COMPACT

Alaska Natives have a unique relationship with the U.S. government, different from even the Tribal nations in the lower 48 states. Given that the 229 federally recognized Tribes live across over 500,000 square miles of mostly roadless land in Alaska, an innovative health system was created to serve the Native and non-Native peoples living in remote areas. The Alaska Tribal Health Compact (ATHC) was formed in 1994, creating infrastructure for Tribes and Tribal health organizations to assume nearly all functions previously provided by IHS (Alaska Native Health Board, n.d.). It is the only multiparty compact in the I/T/U system (Alaska Native Health Board, n.d.).

provides funding for urban Indian organizations (UIOs) that serve AI/ANs living outside Tribal lands through 41 urban nonprofit organizations (Indian Health Care Improvement Act, Title V). The varied system of delivery is collectively referred to as "the I/T/U" (IHS, Tribal, and Urban) system (National Indian Health Board, 2014, p. 1). Because each Tribal nation is a sovereign government, there are nuances even within the I/T/U system of how healthcare and public health services are delivered. For example, the Tribes in Alaska have a uniquely compacted system to provide for the health of AI/ANs in the state. See Box 14.4. Further, not all AI/ANs solely utilize health services in the Indian health system—many also have employer-sponsored insurance, federal coverage like Medicaid, or receive services elsewhere.

The IHCIA was permanently reauthorized in the Patient Protection and Affordable Care Act (ACA). IHCIA greatly increased funding for disease prevention, data analysis, and workforce development programming to serve American Indian and Alaska Natives (Patient Protection and Affordable Care Act Summary of Indian Health Provisions, n.d.).

### Organization

The *I/T/U system* collectively employs approximately 15,370 persons (IHS, 2020). These employees provide services such as inpatient, ambulatory, emergency, dental, public health nursing, and preventive care. Specialty cases are referred to providers outside the system through a program called "Purchased/Referred Care" (IHS, n.d.-c).

The IHS is organized into Administrative Facilities, Training Facilities, Research Facilities, and Treatment Facilities. Administrative Facilities include a national headquarters and 12 regional facilities called "Area Offices" (Figure 14.1). The Area Offices administer services through a system of 170 IHS and Tribally managed Service Units (IHS, 2020).

### Funding Mechanisms

Over 20 federal agencies receive appropriations to provide services to AI/ANs, including the IHS. The federal budget process begins with federal agencies developing budget requests that are then sent to the president. Federal budgets related to AI/ANs are often developed with Tribal input or through formal **Tribal consultations**. The president submits a budget request to Congress which ultimately determines the federal budget through the appropriations process. Two-thirds of the federal budget consists of mandatory spending, which is required funding that supports programs like Medicare and Medicaid, and one-third consists of discretionary spending (Levit et al., 2015, p. 1). Discretionary funding, determined by Congress each year, supports other programs and services, including the HHS appropriations. The IHS is funded mostly through discretionary funding, but also receives mandatory funding through reimbursements from Medicare, Medicaid, and uniquely, a grant program entitled the "Special Diabetes Program for Indians" (IHS, 2018, p. 10). See Box 14.5.

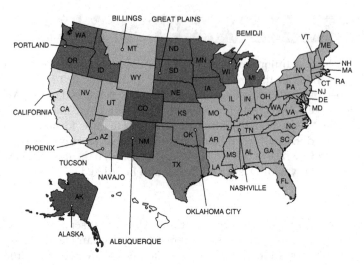

**FIGURE 14.1** Indian Health Service Regions.

*Source:* Indian Health Service. (n.d.). *The Federal Health Program for American Indians and Alaskan Natives.*
https://www.ihs.gov/foodhandler/staff

---

### BOX 14.5 SPECIAL DIABETES PROGRAM FOR INDIANS (SDPI)

SDPI is a grant program that provides $150 million in funding to about 300 I/T/U programs for diabetes prevention and treatment services. The program was established by Congress in the 1997 Congressional Budget Act in response to rising prevalence rates of diabetes in the AI/AN adult population (IHS, n.d.-a). SDPI also funds national training, technical support, clinical tools, and data collection and analysis. SDPI has contributed to standardizing diabetes care management and treatment in the I/T/U system (Department of Health and Human Services, Office of the Assistant Secretary for Planning and Evaluation [DHHS, ASPE], 2019, p. 4).

There have been no further increases in the prevalence[3] (DHHS, ASPE, 2019, p. 2) of diabetes since 2011 in AI/AN adults; there was an over 50% decrease of diabetes-related end-stage renal disease in AI/AN adults between 1996 and 2013 (Bullock et al., 2017, p. 27). No other program has improved access to diabetes treatment and prevention resources as much as SDPI over the last two decades (DHHS, ASPE, 2019, p. 5).

---

Other federal agencies with discretionary funding may identify **Tribal set-aside** funding to ensure the health needs of AI/ANs are being met. For example, the EPA provides the "Drinking Water Infrastructure GrantsTribal Set-Aside Program" (EPA, n.d.-b) and "Clean Water Indian Set-Aside Program," (EPA, n.d.-a) and the Office for Victims of Crime provides the "Office of Victims and Crime Tribal Set-Aside" (Office for Victims and Crime, 2020).

ISDEAA requires the secretary of HHS to consult with Indian Tribes in developing the budget for the IHS (25 U.S.C. § 5325). Based on feedback received from Tribes, Tribal-serving organizations, and UIOs, the secretary formulates an annual IHS budget to be submitted first to the president and then to Congress (25 U.S.C. § 5325). Within the IHS, the Budget Formulation Workgroup, comprised of Tribal leaders, consults annually with Tribes to prepare budget recommendations for the agency (IHS, 2006, Sec. 12).

---

[3] "*Prevalence* is a measure of the total number of individuals with a given condition at a point in time, while *incidence* is a measure of the number of individuals that are newly diagnosed with a condition over a period of time."

## Urban Indian Health Programs

While Tribal public health systems provide infrastructure and services for AI/ANs living in Tribal communities, over 70% of AI/ANs live in urban areas (Norris et al., 2012, p. 12, 13; U.S. Census Bureau, 2012, Table PCT2). Urban Indian Health Programs (UIHP) hold a unique and vital role in the fabric of public health services for American Indians and Alaska Natives living in urban areas. Some UIHPs create an infrastructure to do so by working with nearby Tribal governments, local public health agencies, private industries, and others to provide public health services such as disease prevention and education, wellness promotion activities, and connection to other federal or state benefits like Women, Infants, and Children (WIC) or Medicaid resources (Indian Health Service, n.d.-b, Ch. 19 §3-19.1 [A-J]).

## Intergovernmental Coordination and Public Health

Public health crises are not contained by political borders, whether Tribal, state, or international. Thus, intergovernmental coordination is an essential component to effective public health practice. A variety of tools exist to promote intergovernmental coordination, including mutual aid agreements, and can be used to share resources and information and outline responsibilities across governments. For example, Tribes and local governments across the Olympic Peninsula in Washington agreed to provide cross-governmental support in the event of an emergency. The mutual aid agreement, entitled the "Olympic Regional Tribal-Public Health Collaboration and Mutual Aid Agreement," specifies that assistance can include support in instances of isolation or quarantine activities and personnel sharing.

Inter-Tribal health boards provide another example of intergovernmental coordination. There are at least 12 Inter-Tribal health boards, most operating as a nonprofit organization with distinct and responsive missions. For example, the Southern Plains Health Board serves 44 Tribes across Kansas, Oklahoma, and Texas. Its mission is to improve health outcomes through advocacy and education. Many Tribal Epidemiology Centers (TECs; see Box 14.6) are housed within these health boards. TECs are located in each IHS region and provide public health surveillance and evaluation, among other activities, to the Tribes in their area. In order to address challenges in data collection, the 2010 reauthorization of IHCIA designated TECs as Health Insurance Portability and Accountability Act (HIPAA) public health authorities. This allows access to identifiable health information for public health purposes just like state, local, and Tribal agencies. This reauthorization also requires HHS and CDC to provide technical assistance to TECs in their public health surveillance activities.

Federal and state governments also establish groups to support intergovernmental cooperation. Federal advisory committees are groups that can be established by statute, the president, or agencies to provide advice and recommendations on matters of interest to the federal government (Federal Advisory Committee Act, § 3). Several agencies, including the DHHS and the CDC, have Tribal Advisory Committees (TACs). TACs advise agencies on strategies and policies impacting AI/AN health. Representatives generally include Tribal elected officials from each IHS region (CDC, n.d.).

Many states have commissions to better understand and support AI/AN interests. Indiana law, for example, establishes the Native American Indian Affairs Commission (Ind. Code 4-23-32-3). The commission is charged with providing recommendations to government agencies on a variety of issues, including "[h]ealth issues affecting Native American Indian communities, including data collection, equal access to public assistance programs, and informing health officials of cultural traditions relevant to health care" (Ind. Code 4-23-32-7). Recent commission activities have included studying health access issues for AI/ANs in Indiana, a state without federal Indian health facilities (Indiana Native American Indian Affairs Commission, 2018).

## BOX 14.6 FUNCTIONS OF TRIBAL EPIDEMIOLOGY CENTERS

In consultation with Tribes, TECs offer functions that include:

1. collect[ing] data relating to, and monitor[ing] progress made toward, meeting each of the health status objectives of the Service, the Indian [T]ribes, [T]ribal organizations, and urban Indian organizations in the Service area;
2. evaluat[ing] existing delivery systems, data systems, and other systems that impact the improvement of Indian health;
3. assist[ing] Indian [T]ribes, [T]ribal organizations, and urban Indian organizations in identifying highest priority health status objectives and the services needed to achieve those objectives, based on epidemiological data;
4. mak[ing] recommendations for the targeting of services needed by the populations served;
5. mak[ing] recommendations to improve healthcare delivery systems for Indians and urban Indians;
6. provid[ing] requested technical assistance to Indian [T]ribes, [T]ribal organizations, and urban Indian organizations in the development of local health service priorities and incidence and prevalence rates of disease and other illness in the community; and
7. provid[ing] disease surveillance and assist[ing] Indian [T]ribes, [T]ribal organizations, and urban Indian communities to promote public health.

(25 U.S.C. § 1621m[b], 2010).

## CONCLUSION

Tribal health systems are complex and include a variety of entities including Tribal, federal, and nonprofits. As this chapter has described, Tribes are sovereign nations that maintain a nation-to-nation relationship with the United States. There are 574 federally recognized Tribes, and more than 80 state-recognized Tribes with government-to-government relationship with states. Tribes have the duty and inherent authority to promote the public health and welfare of their communities, and there are many examples of Tribes exercising their sovereignty in this way. Federal Indian law is the body of law that governs the jurisdictional relationships between Tribes, states, and the federal government. In the context of public health, federal Indian law can be implicated in funding and implementation of programs. In order to work more effectively with Tribal governments, public health practitioners should be aware of the legal tools that exist to better serve AI/AN communities and promote intergovernmental coordination across Tribes, states, and the federal government while respecting Tribal sovereignty.

## CHAPTER REVIEW

### Review Questions

1. What is Tribal sovereignty? What impact does it have on Tribal public health?
2. What does I/T/U? refer to? Distinguish between them.
3. What funding mechanisms exist to support Indian healthcare and public health services delivery?
4. What mechanisms exist to support intergovernmental coordination on Tribal public health issues?
5. How has the Patient Protection and Affordable Care Act impacted the AI/AN public health?

## Essay or Discussion Questions

1.  What is the relationship between political and cultural sovereignty? How does this impact Tribal public health?
2.  How can culture be used as a tool to support Tribal public health? What role does law play in supporting and protecting culture?
3.  What is the relationship between public health and healthcare systems?

## Internet Activities

1.  **Exploring Tribal Codes**: The National Indian Law Library's Tribal Law Gateway (https://www.narf.org/nill/triballaw/index.html) houses over 100 Tribal codes. Can you find Tribal code provisions related to public health?
2.  **Federal Legislation**: The National Indian Health Board (NIHB) and the National Council of Urban Indian Health (NCUIH) are nonprofit organizations that research, convene, and advocate for Indian health issues on behalf of Tribes and AI/ANs living in urban settings. The NIHB and NCUIH conduct extensive legislative tracking on federal legislation impacting AI/ANs. Review some of the NIHB's legislative alerts at: https://www.nihb.org/legislative/legislative.php or NCUIH legislative alerts at: https://www.ncuih.org/legislativetracker. What are some of the pressing issues?

## REFERENCES

45 C.F.R. § 164.501.

25 U.S.C. § 13.

25 U.S.C. § 5301.

25 U.S.C. § 5321.

25 U.S.C. § 5325.

42 U.S.C. § 2001 et seq.

Alaska Native Health Board. (n.d.). Alaska Tribal Health Compact. http://www.anhb.org/tribal-resources/alaska-tribal-health-compact

Baker, B. (2020). *Northern Cheyenne Tribe extends stay-at-home order.* The Billings Gazette. https://billingsgazette.com/news/local/northern-cheyenne-tribe-extends-stay-at-home-order/article_f8745932-4d6e-5ead-83a7-40ea3cb465c2.html

Blackfeet Tribal Health Department. (2017). Blackfeet Reservation community health assessment 2017. https://www.cheerequity.org/uploads/3/7/9/4/37948891/0_full_cha_final_4.12.17.pdf

Bullock, A., Burrows, N. R., Narva, A. S., Sheff, K., Lekiachvili, A., Cain, H., & Espey, D. (2017, January 13). Vital signs: Decrease in incidence of diabetes-related end-stage renal disease among American Indians/Alaska Natives – United States, 1996-2013. *Morbidity and Mortality Weekly Report, 66*(1). https://www.cdc.gov/mmwr/volumes/66/wr/pdfs/mm6601e1.pdf

Centers for Disease Control and Prevention. (n.d.). Tribal Advisory Committee. https://www.cdc.gov/tribal/consultation-support/tac/index.html.

Clinton, W. J. (1994, April 29). *Memorandum on government to government relations with native American tribal governments.* https://www.justice.gov/archive/otj/Presidential_Statements/presdoc1.htm

Coffey, W., & Tsosie, R. A. (2001). Rethinking the Tribal sovereignty doctrine: Cultural sovereignty and the collective future of Indian Nations. *Stanford Law and Policy Review, 12*, 191–221.

Corrigan, J. M., Eden, J., & Smith, B. M. (Eds.). (2003). *Leadership by example: Coordinating government roles in improving health care quality.* The National Academies Press

Department of Health and Human Services, Office of the Assistant Secretary for Planning and Evaluation. (2019, May 10). The Special Diabetes Program for Indians: Estimates of Medicare savings. https://aspe.hhs.gov/system/files/pdf/261741/SDPI_Paper_Final.pdf

Dunbar-Ortiz, R. (2014). *An indigenous peoples' history of the United States*. Beacon Press.

Eastern Band of Cherokee Indians, Public Health and Human Services. (n.d.). Syringe services program: Safe disposal and counseling. https://cherokee-phhs.com/syringe-services/index.html

Eastern Band of Cherokee Indians, Tribes and Tribal Nations. (2021). Code of ordinances. https://library.municode.com/tribes_and_tribal_nations/eastern_band_of_cherokee_indians/codes/code_of_ordinances?nodeId=THCHCO_CH130APUHEHUSE_ARTIIICLNEEXOTHEPRTAPR_S130A-113.27NEHYSYEXOTHEPRPRAULIIM

Ex Parte Crow Dog, 109 U.S. 556, 572 (1883).

Exec. Order No. 13084 (May 14, 1998); Exec. Order No. 13175 (Nov. 6, 2000); The White House (Nov. 5, 2009). Memorandum for the Heads of Executive Departments and Agencies.

Federal Advisory Committee Act. 5 U.S.C.A. App. 2.

Fletcher, M. L. M. (2016). *Federal Indian law*. West Academic.

Getches, D. H., Wilkinson, C. F., Williams, R. A., & Fletcher, M. L. M. (2011). *Cases and materials on federal Indian law* (6th ed.). West Academic.

Hoss, A. (2019). A framework for Tribal public health law. *Nevada Law Journal, 20*(1), 113–144.

Hoss, A., & Sunshine, G. (2017, March 2). *Tribal emergency preparedness law*. https://www.cdc.gov/phlp/docs/brief-tribalemergency.pdf

Indian Entities Recognized and Eligible to Receive Services From the United States Bureau of Indian Affairs. (2020). Fed. Reg. 83, 4235.

Indian Health Care Improvement Act, PL 94-437.

Indian Health Service. (n.d.-a). About SDPI. https://www.ihs.gov/sdpi/about

Indian Health Service. (n.d.-b). Indian health manual. https://www.ihs.gov/IHM/pc/part-3/p3c19/#3-19.1) *and* https://www.ihs.gov/urban

Indian Health Service. (n.d.-c). Purchased/Referred Care (PRC). https://www.ihs.gov/prc

Indian Health Service. (2006, January 18). HS Circular No. 2006-01. (2006, January 18). https://www.ihs.gov/IHM/circulars/2006/tribal-consultation-policy

Indian Health Service. (2016, July). Tribal self-governance. https://www.ihs.gov/newsroom/factsheets/tribalselfgovernance

Indian Health Service. (2018). Indian Health Service: Spending levels of IHS and three other federal dealth care programs. https://www.gao.gov/assets/700/695871.pdf

Indian Health Service. (2019). Disparities. https://www.ihs.gov/newsroom/factsheets/disparities

Indian Health Service. (2020). Fact sheets: IHS profile. https://www.ihs.gov/newsroom/factsheets/ihsprofile

Indiana Code 4-23-32-3.

Indiana Code 4-23-32-7.

Indiana Native American Indian Affairs Commission. (2018). *2018 annual report*. https://www.in.gov/inaiac/files/2018-annual-report.pdf

Indian Vaccination Act (1832).

Karuk Tribe. (n.d.). Karuk Tribe coronavirus (COVID-19) emergency response team. https://www.karuk.us/index.php/information/coronavirus-covid-19-information

Knudson, A., Hernandez, A., Kronstadt, J., Allis, P., Meit, M., Popat, S., Klug, M. G., & Francis, C. (2012, June). *A profile of tribal health departments*. http://www.norc.org/PDFs/Walsh%20Center/Research%20Briefs/Research%20Brief_W18_KnudsonA_Profile_2012.pdf

Lac Courte Oreilles Band of Lake Superior Chippewa Indians. (n.d.). Covid-10 tribal information. https://www.lcotribe.com/covid-19-tribal-information

Levit, M. R., Austin, D. A., & Stupak, J. M. (2015). Mandatory spending since 1962. https://fas.org/sgp/crs/misc/RL33074.pdf

*Menominee v. United States*, 391 U.S. 404 (1968)

Meriam, L. (1928). The problem of Indian administration: Report of a survey made at the request of Honorable Hubert Work, Secretary of the Interior, and submitted to him, February 21, 1928. https://files.eric.ed.gov/fulltext/ED087573.pdf

Montana Healthcare Foundation. (n.d.). Needle Exchange Program. https://mthcf.org/grantee/fort-peck-tribal-health-department

National Conference of State Legislatures. (2020). Federal and state recognized tribes. http://www.ncsl.org/research/state-tribal-institute/list-of-federal-and-state-recognized-tribes.aspx

National Indian Health Board. (2014, July). Indian health care 101. https://www.nihb.org/docs/01132015/Indian%20Health%20Care%20101.pdf

National Native Network. (n.d.). Traditional tobacco. https://keepitsacred.itcmi.org/tobacco-and-tradition/traditional-tobacco-use

The National Tribal Public and Environmental Health Think Tank. (n.d.). https://apha.org/topics-and-issues/environmental-health/partners/think-tank

Native Voices. (n.d.). 1921: Congress funds American Indian health care. https://www.nlm.nih.gov/nativevoices/timeline/427.html.

Navajo Department of Health Act. (2014, November 6). http://www.navajo-nsn.gov/News%20Releases/OPVP/2014/nov/Navajo%20Department%20of%20Health%20Enacted.pdf

Newton, N. J. (Ed.). (2012). *Cohen's handbook of federal Indian law*. LexisNexis.

Nicholson, K. (2020). *Southern Ute Indian Tribe sticks with stay-at-home order until further notice*. https://www.denverpost.com/2020/04/23/southern-ute-indian-tribe-stay-at-home-order

Norris, T., Vines, P. L., Hoeffel, E. M. (2012). The American Indian and Alaska native population: 2010. *2010 Census Briefs*. https://www.census.gov/history/pdf/c2010br-10.pdf

North American Syringe Exchange Network. (n.d.). SSP locations. https://www.nasen.org/map

Office for Victims and Crime. (2020). Tribal Victim Services Set-Aside. https://www.ovc.gov/news/tribal-set-aside.html

*Passamaquoddy v. Morton*, 528 F.2d 370 (1st Cir. 1975)

Patient Protection and Affordable Care Act; Summary of Indian Health Provisions. (n.d.). https://www.nihb.org/docs/12082016/Affordable_Care_Act_Provisions_Summary.pdf

Pevar, S. L. (2012). *The rights of Indians and tribes*. Oxford University Press.

Public Law 94–437.

Ransom, M. M. (Ed.). (2016). *Public health law competency model: Version 1.0*. CDC. https://www.cdc.gov/phlp/docs/phlcm-v1.pdf

Standing Rock Sioux Tribe Constitution. http://indianaffairs.nd.gov/image/cache/standing_rock_constitution.pdf [https://perma.cc/KZT3-EDMW]

Swinomish Indian Tribal Community. (n.d.). Title 19 – Environmental protection. https://swinomish.org/government/tribal-code/title-19-environmental-protection.aspx

Tribal Budget Formulation Workgroup. (2019, April). *The national Tribal Budget Formulation Workgroup's recommendations on the Indian Health Service fiscal year 2021 budget*. https://www.nihb.org/docs/04242019/307871_NIHB%20IHS%20Budget%20Book_WEB.PDF

Tribal Epidemiology Centers. (2013). *Best bractices in American Indian & Alaska Native public health: A report from the Tribal Epidemiology Centers*. http://itcaonline.com/wp-content/uploads/2014/03/TEC_Best_Practices_Book_2013.pdf

Tribal Public Health Institute Feasibility Project. (2013, January). https://redstarintl.org/wp-content/uploads/2018/12/tphi_findings_report.pdf

*United States v. Kagama*, 118 U.S. 375, 384-85 (1886).

*United States v. Mitchell*, 445 U.S. 535 (1980).

*United States v. Wheeler*, 435 U.S. 313 (1978).

U.S. Census Bureau. (2012, December). American Indian and Alaska Native summary file: 2010 census of polution and housing (Table PCT2). https://www.census.gov/content/dam/Census/library/publications/2012/dec/c2010br-10.pdf

U.S. Commission on Civil Rights. (2018). Broken promises: Continuing federal funding shortfall for Native Americans. https://www.usccr.gov/pubs/2018/12-20-Broken-Promises.pdf

U.S. Department of the Interior, Indian Affairs. (n.d.). Frequently asked questions. http://www.bia.gov/FAQs/index.htm

U.S. Environmental Protection Agency. (n.d.-a). Clean Water Indian Set-Aside Program. https://www.epa.gov/small-and-rural-wastewater-systems/clean-water-indian-set-aside-program

U.S. Environmental Protection Agency. (n.d.-b). Drinking Water Infrastructure Grants - Tribal Set-Aside Program. https://www.epa.gov/tribaldrinkingwater/drinking-water-infrastructure-grants-tribal-set-aside-program

Utacia Krol, D., & Silversmith, S. (2020). Coronavirus in Arizona: Several tribes declare a state of emergency; many shut down gaming. *Arizona Republic*. https://www.azcentral.com/story/

news/local/arizona/2020/03/15/arizona-tribes-respond-covid-19-emergency-declarations
-and-testing/5055702002

Waganakising Odawa Tribal Code of Law. http://www.ltbbodawa-nsn.gov/TribalCode.pdf [https://
perma.cc/25C5-NU29]

*Williams v. Lee*, 358 U.S. 217 (1959).

## Additional Resources

- **Tribal Public Health Law Resources**
  https://www.cdc.gov/phlp/publications/topic/tribal.html
- **Tribal Nations and the United States: An Introduction**
  http://www.ncai.org/tribalnations/introduction/Tribal_Nations_and_the_United_States_An
  _Introduction-web-.pdf
- **A Profile of Tribal Health Departments. (2012, June 29)**
  http://www.norc.org/PDFs/Walsh%20Center/KnudsonA_Profile_Tribal_Health_Dept
  _FINAL_2012.pdf
- Blackhawk, M. (2019). Federal Indian law as paradigm within public law. *Harvard Law Review*.
  https://harvardlawreview.org/2019/05/federal-indian-law-as-paradigm-within-public-law
- Bryan, R. T., Schaefer, R. M., DeBruyn, L., & Stier, D. D. (2009). Public health legal preparedness
  in Indian country. *American Journal of Public Health, 99*, 607–614. https://doi.org/10.2105/
  AJPH.2008.146522
- Strommer, G. D., Roels, S. K., & Mayhew, C. P. (2019). Tribal sovereign authority and self-
  regulation of health care services: The legal framework and the Swinomish tribe's dental health
  program. *Journal of Health Care Law and Policy, 21*(2). https://digitalcommons.law.umaryland
  .edu/jhclp/vol21/iss2/2
- Sunshine, G., & Hoss, A. (2015). Emergency declarations and tribes: Mechanisms under tribal
  and federal law. *Michigan State International Law Review, 24*(1), 33–44. https://www.ncbi.nlm.nih
  .gov/pmc/articles/PMC4703113
- Warne, D., & Frizzell, L. B. (2014). American Indian health policy: Historical trends and
  contemporary issues. *American Journal of Public Health, 104*(S3), S263–S267. https://doi
  .org/10.2105/AJPH.2013.301682

# 15

# Public Health, LGBTQ Populations, and the Law

Heather A. Walter-McCabe and M. Killian Kinney

## Learning Objectives

By the end of this chapter, the reader will be able to:

- Define the role of public health law in promoting health thriving for LGBTQ communities.
- Apply knowledge of the LGBTQ community to public health law to promote health equity within healthcare systems.
- Appraise the inclusion/exclusion and equity of LGBTQ communities in the current public health laws.

## Key Terminology

**ASAB** (assigned sex at birth): The sex assigned to a child when born, which is based on primary sex characteristics and chromosomes.

**AFAB:** Assigned female at birth.

**AMAB:** Assigned male at birth.

**Cisgender:** A category for persons whose gender identity aligns with their sex assigned at birth.

**Cisnormativity:** Systemic prejudice that assumes most people are cisgender and works in favor of cisgender people.

**EMR/EHR** (electronic medical/health records): A digital or online version of patient health information (Centers for Disease Control and Prevention [CDC], 2019).

**Gender expression:** The physical (e.g., clothing, hairstyle), behavioral (e.g., mannerisms, vocal intonation), and relational (e.g., pronouns, chosen name) ways in which someone expresses their gender and engages with others to have their gender seen.

**Gender identity:** An individual's internal sense of self that may be a man or transgender man, woman or transgender woman, nonbinary (e.g., genderqueer, genderfluid, agender), or another gender; it is crucial to note the distinction of gender from sex, which is rooted in biological indicators (e.g., primary sex characteristics and chromosomes).

**Heteronormativity:** Systemic prejudice that assumes most people are heterosexual and works in favor of heterosexual/ straight people.

---

See UC Davis Health LGBTQ+ Glossary at https://health.ucdavis.edu/diversity-inclusion/LGBTQI/LGBTQ-Plus.html

**LGBTQ:** The acronym for the community of lesbian, gay, bisexual, transgender, queer, and additional sexual and gender minorities.

**Nonbinary:** A collection of genders that are not exclusively a man/masculine or woman/feminine, including genderqueer, gender fluid, and agender.

**Transgender:** A category for persons whose gender identity does not align with their sex assigned at birth; an umbrella term to describe all gender-diverse individuals, although not all gender-diverse individuals may use this language (e.g., some nonbinary individuals do not identify as transgender).

## Public Health Law Competencies

This chapter addresses the following competencies from the Public Health Law Competency Model (PHLCM; Ransom, 2016):

1.2  Identify and apply public health laws (e.g., statutes, regulations, ordinances, and court rulings) pertinent to the practitioner's jurisdiction, agency, program, and profession.

2.2  Identify law-based tools and enforcement procedures available to address day-to-day (nonemergency) public health issues.

■ Note that this chapter seeks to assist the reader in understanding how to examine the laws and organizational policies that might disparately impact the *LGBTQ* community. This chapter provides a lens through which one can examine laws for social determinants of health impacts.

---

### Spark Questions

1. How can public health practitioners in public law create a more inclusive and affirming space for LGBTQ individuals?
2. What current public health laws can you think of that impact the LGBTQ community, positively or negatively?

---

### BOX 15.1  HEALTH EQUITY/DISPARITIES STATISTIC, QUOTES, LEGAL PRINCIPLES

"Research suggests that LGBT individuals face health disparities linked to societal stigma, discrimination, and denial of their civil and human rights. Discrimination against LGBT persons has been associated with high rates of psychiatric disorders, substance abuse, and suicide. Experiences of violence and victimization are frequent for LGBT individuals, and have long-lasting effects on the individual and the community. Personal, family, and social acceptance of sexual orientation and **gender identity** affects the mental health and personal safety of LGBT individuals."

Office of Disease Prevention and Health Promotion. (n.d). *Lesbian, gay, bisexual, and transgender health.* https://www.healthypeople.gov/2020/topics-objectives/topic/lesbian-gay-bisexual-and-transgender-health

## INTRODUCTION

Public health law has a significant impact on the lives of **LGBTQ** individuals, where it can either promote health equity or create barriers to quality of life. The goal of this chapter is to provide initial insight into the role of public health practitioners in public health law to assess and propose policies for LGBTQ equity in policies impacting health inequity for this community.

An explicit goal of the Office of Disease Prevention and Health Promotion's (ODPHP) *Healthy People 2020* is to "improve the health, safety, and well-being of lesbian, gay, bisexual, and transgender (LGBT) individuals" (ODPHP, n.d., para. 1). The long-lasting impact of stigma and discrimination can contribute to diminished mental health (Deitz, 2015; Nadal et al., 2016; Su et al., 2016), maladaptive coping through substance use (Keuroghlian et al., 2015), and even suicide (Herman et al., 2014). *It is critical to note that the suicide attempt rate of the LGB community is at two to three times that of the general population, while the transgender community experiences suicide attempts at nearly nine times the general population* (Haas et al., 2010; James et al., 2016). This risk, as well as the disparate risk of being the victim of hate-based violence, both call for a strong public health practice and policy intervention (Blake & Hatzenbuehler, 2019; Johns et al., 2019)

In addition to general discrimination against sexual and gender minorities, **transgender** and nonbinary individuals face increased frequency of misgendering, which is positively correlated with psychological distress, including depression, stress, and felt stigma, all of which were already higher among those who felt more stigmatized based on their gender (McLemore, 2018). This population also experiences microaggressions around being asked to explain their gender, being called a former name, and frequent erasure in documentation (Brown & Burill, 2018). Trans-affirming healthcare providers play a significant role in mental health for transgender and nonbinary individuals (Pitts et al., 2009). In a study of sexual minorities (*N* = 914), living in a community of high structural stigma was found to decrease life expectancy by approximately 12 years compared to those living in low structural stigma environments (Hatzenbuehler et al., 2014). Increasingly, the role of the environment is being recognized as an important contributing factor and is an issue that is ripe for advocacy for improved conditions.

## ANTIDISCRIMINATION LAWS AS A TOOL OF PUBLIC HEALTH FOR LGBTQ POPULATIONS

Social determinants of health, defined by the World Health Organization, are "the conditions in which people are born, grow, live, work and age, including the health system" (WHO, 2008, p. 1) and have an impact on population health. The social and political structures that support or seek to change these conditions can be an important place for public health to intervene. Antidiscrimination laws have the potential to positively impact LGBTQ health outcomes. Stigma researchers have recognized that social stigma and discrimination have, as mentioned previously, a negative impact resulting in poor mental health (particularly anxiety and depression), increased substance use, disproportionate rates of sexually transmitted infections, and increased suicide rates (Blake & Hatzenbuehler, 2019; James et al., 2016; Kelleher, 2009; Meyer & Frost, 2012; Meyer & Northridge, 2007). Here, through the lens of hypothetical case studies, we discuss three specific areas of law that may have an impact on LGBTQ communities positively or negatively, depending on how they are written and enforced.

---

### HYPOTHETICAL CASE STUDY #1: HOUSING DISCRIMINATION

Olivia is a 25-year-old transgender woman who uses "they, them, theirs" pronouns. They have recently moved from their small hometown to the big city and are excited about the opportunities this new phase of life presents. Finding an apartment was difficult. When discussing this challenge with friends, Olivia learns that they are being quoted higher security deposits and different move-in costs than their **cisgender** friends. Despite this difficulty, Olivia is able to find a rental unit near their new job.

During a trip to the apartment complex mailbox, Olivia's landlord stops them and tells them that neighbors are complaining and that they should avoid dressing in women's clothing in the common areas of the property. Olivia heads back to their apartment, feeling anxious and depressed.

1. Are there federal housing laws that might protect Olivia from the discrimination described in Case Study #1?
2. How might state laws address the discrimination in housing faced by Olivia and others in the LGBTQ population?

## Housing Laws

Housing laws at the federal level (see the Title VIII of the Civil Rights Act of 1968, 42 U.S.C. §§ 3601-3619) do not have specific protections for sexual or gender minorities, like Olivia in Hypothetical Case Study #1. Housing insecurity can be a driver of poor health outcomes (Bierman & Dunn, 2006). At this time, the Department of Housing and Urban Development (HUD) has a history of providing some protection for the LGBTQ community through interpreting the protections against sex discrimination as protection against discrimination for failing to conform with gender stereotypes (U.S. Department of Housing and Urban Development, n.d.). In Hypothetical Case Study #1, the landlord's request that Olivia not wear women's clothing in the common areas might be considered a violation of the Fair Housing Act's prohibition against sex discrimination.

Depending on the state in which they reside, Olivia may also be able to file a claim under state antidiscrimination laws. State laws can provide protections by explicitly passing statutes naming sexual orientation and **gender identity** as protected classes in housing laws. Currently, as shown in Table 15.1, 26 states provide no protection in housing law to persons on the basis of sexual orientation or gender identity (Movement Advancement Project, n.d.). Without state laws providing such protections, the LGBTQ community is largely without recourse when they experience housing discrimination.

---

### HYPOTHETICAL CASE STUDY #2: EMPLOYMENT DISCRIMINATION

Robin has been working for a large corporation for more than a year. She is a stellar employee and has recently received top ratings on her performance review, leaving her feeling confident and secure in her professional future. Up until this point, she has kept her work area pretty sparse, but she decides it is time to personalize her cube. She keeps it minimal but brings in photos of her family. One day, her boss walks by her desk and sees a photo of Robin sharing a kiss with her girlfriend during a birthday celebration. Less than 2 weeks later, she is fired. As the family breadwinner, Robin is concerned about how she will cover basic family needs, including healthcare, as she starts the hunt for a new job.

1. Are there federal laws protecting employees from discrimination based on sexual orientation or gender identity in the United States?
2. How might state laws address employment discrimination such as that faced by Robin and others in the LGBTQ population?

**TABLE 15.1  State Housing Nondiscrimination Laws: Variations and Distinctions**

| | |
|---|---|
| Alabama, Arizona, Florida, Georgia, Idaho, Indiana, Kansas, Kentucky, Louisiana, Mississippi, Missouri, Montana, Nebraska, North Dakota, Ohio, Oklahoma, South Carolina, South Dakota, Texas, Virginia, West Virginia, Wyoming, U.S. Territories | There is no housing nondiscrimination law covering sexual orientation or gender identity. |
| Arkansas, North Carolina, Tennessee | States have a law preventing passage or enforcement of local nondiscrimination laws. |
| California, Colorado, Connecticut, Delaware, Hawaii, Illinois, Iowa, Maine, Maryland, Massachusetts, Minnesota, Nevada, New Hampshire, New Jersey, New Mexico, New York, Oregon, Rhode Island, Utah, Vermont, Washington | Housing nondiscrimination law covers sexual orientation and gender identity. |
| Michigan | State law does not explicitly enumerate sexual orientation or gender identity, but the Michigan Civil Rights Commission has stated it explicitly interprets the state's existing protections against sex discrimination to include protections for both sexual orientation and gender identity. |
| Missouri | There is no housing nondiscrimination law covering sexual orientation or gender identity; Supreme Court is considering two cases regarding whether the state's prohibition on sex discrimination includes discrimination based on sexual orientation or gender identity. |
| Pennsylvania | There is no housing nondiscrimination law covering sexual orientation or gender identity; state agency explicitly interprets existing sex protections to include both sexual orientation and gender identity. |
| Wisconsin | Housing nondiscrimination law covers only sexual orientation. |

*Source:* Adapted from Movement Advancement Project. (n.d.). *Nondiscrimination laws.* https://www.lgbtmap.org/equality-maps/non_discrimination_laws

## Employment Laws

Federal employment laws provide protections for specific categories of persons against employment discrimination. Current categories include race, religion, sex, national origin, disability, genetic information, and age. Though there is no protection explicitly for sexual orientation or gender identity and expression, as discussed in what follows, the courts have sometimes interpreted sex discrimination as including discrimination on the basis of sexual orientation or gender identity and expression failing to comply with gender stereotypes. In fact, 26 states are in jurisdictions that have interpreted federal laws in this way (Movement Advancement Project, n.d.). Under this principle, in Hypothetical Case Study #2, Robin may have a claim under federal law for gender discrimination, but this remains unclear. The U.S. Supreme Court heard three cases this session asking them to rule whether or not this interpretation is correct. As of the time of this writing, the Supreme Court is deliberating and should be rendering a verdict in the late spring of 2020.

Whether or not the federal government determines that federal law provides these protections, some states and even municipalities are providing protection to discrimination against LGBTQ workers. Twenty-six states have no statewide employment protection for either sexual orientation or gender identity (Movement Advancement Project, n.d.). Some states, even where municipalities might choose to provide additional protections, preempt local governments from doing so.

---

### HYPOTHETICAL CASE STUDY #3: PUBLIC ACCOMMODATION DISCRIMINATION

Sam is a transgender young man who is a high school student. He lives in a state where a "bathroom bill" is being considered. He has recently been called to the principal's office because he has been using the boy's bathroom. The principal warns Sam that he is not allowed to use the boy's bathroom and that he must use the bathroom corresponding with the sex assigned to him at birth. Sam was told that if he uses the boy's restroom again, he will be suspended from school indefinitely. Sam decides that his only choice is to avoid using the restroom and hold his urine throughout the school day.

1. Under federal law, must Sam use the bathroom associated with the sex he was assigned at birth?
2. Are there state laws protecting people like Sam from discrimination in public accommodations?
3. What are "bathroom bills," and how do they impact health?

---

## Public Accommodation Laws

Public accommodation laws provide protections for vulnerable groups in public spaces. Federal protections, as with the aforementioned, do not provide specific protection for sexual orientation or gender identity and expression. National attention was brought to this issue as the *Masterpiece Cakeshop* case made its way through the court system. In this case, the cake shop refused to make a cake for a same-sex couple for their private celebration following the wedding. This case implicated the right to public accommodation, though the court case was decided on a very narrow basis. In the end, it did not provide a decision applicable broadly on public accommodations with regard to LGBTQ populations (see what follows for additional details).

Another public accommodation topic that has been under consideration in state policy, as illustrated in Hypothetical Case Study #3, is "bathroom bills." In March 2016, North Carolina passed House Bill 2 (NC HB2; Public Facilities Privacy & Security Act, 2017), often referred to as a bathroom bill. NC HB2 required transgender and nonbinary people to use the bathroom that aligned with their sex assigned at birth (Kralik, 2017). NC HB2 passed after several trans-affirming bathroom bills that allowed transgender individuals to use the bathroom according to their gender identity (Drum, 2016). Although now repealed, since that time, 16 other states have proposed, but failed to pass, similar legislation (Kralik, 2017).

The report of the 2015 U.S. Transgender Health Survey (James et al., 2016) provides evidence that bathrooms are becoming increasingly dangerous spaces for transgender persons as this type of legislation remains under active discussion in state legislatures. Hypothetical Case Study #3 raises the issue of how these bills impact health. Transgender and nonbinary persons have reported issues around bathroom use, including being denied access, harassed (verbally and physically), and even sexually assaulted. Fifty-nine percent of transgender persons reported that they avoided public restrooms in the last year, and 32.0% limited fluid intake to limit necessary bathroom use. Furthermore, as highlighted in Hypothetical Case Study #3, eight percent of transgender persons reported urinary tract infection or related infections in the past year associated with avoidance of restroom use in public (James et al., 2016). Though it has been argued that bathroom bills limiting restroom use to assigned sex at birth would protect women and children from dangers posed by transgender persons in the bathrooms (Steinmetz, 2016), there have been no recorded cases of assault in a bathroom by a transgender person in the United States (Dastagir, 2016). As states continue to determine how they will approach this issue, it will be critical for public health persons to understand the implications of such bills.

## COURT CASES

### Medicaid Coverage of Transgender Health Services

Medicaid coverage of hormone therapy and gender-affirming surgeries have been in the courts across the nation. There has been activity at the state and federal levels. In May of 2016, the Department of Health and Human Services promulgated a rule interpreting Section 1557 of the Affordable Care Act (ACA), defining nondiscrimination in certain healthcare activities of the ACA to include gender identity as a protected group. Within a month of the rule, Franciscan Alliance, Inc. challenged the rule in the Northern District of Texas, submitting that the rule violated the Religious Freedom Restoration Act. In December of 2016, the court granted a temporary nationwide injunction against enforcing the rule. In January of 2017, the Trump administration issued an executive order entitled Minimizing the Economic Burden of the Patient Protection and Affordable Care Act Pending Repeal. This order was a step toward lowering the enforcement of components of the ACA. In July of 2017, Franciscan Alliance agreed to stop further court proceedings to allow the DHHS to reconsider its interpretation and guidance on Section 1557. In the spring of 2019, Franciscan Alliance renewed its motion for summary judgment, and the Department of Justice filed a brief in support of returning to the "longstanding tradition" of sex as its plain biological meaning and not inclusive of gender identity and expression. In May of 2019, the DHHS put forth a new proposed rule that explicitly excluded the inclusion of gender identity as a protected group. In October of 2019, the Northern District of Texas vacated the 2016 rule and remanded the interpretation back to the DHHS for further consideration in compliance with the law.

State Medicaid laws are also being challenged. For example, in Iowa, a line of cases has challenged state regulations, which would keep state Medicaid from funding gender-affirming surgeries. In *Pinneke v. Preisser* (1980), the court found the Iowa Department of Human Services' (IDHS) blanket ban on gender-affirming surgeries for "categorically needy" Medicaid enrollees was an "arbitrary denial based on diagnosis, type of illness, or condition." They also found that IDHS did not follow appropriate administrative procedures or seek input from medical providers in promulgating the rule. Following the case, IDHS promulgated a new rule using the required administrative procedures and seeking input from care providers (though none with expertise in transgender healthcare). Under the new rule, the state continued the practice of denying gender-affirming surgeries for the treatment of gender dysphoria. The *Smith v. Rasmussen* (2001) case challenged the rule under §1983, claiming unconstitutional discrimination. The court ruled that because the state followed administrative procedures and at least some medical professionals and evidence had been used, the rule was not arbitrary and could stand. Following *Smith*, Iowa added the category of gender identity to the Iowa Civil Rights Act (ICRA; 2009). The Iowa Supreme Court relied on the ICRA when ruling in the *Good v. Iowa Dept. of Human Services* (2019) that the IDHS rule banning gender-affirming surgeries could not stand. The court declined to rule on whether the ruling would be permissible under federal law since it was in violation of state law. Following the *Good* case, the Iowa legislature used the state budget bill to deny funding for gender-affirming surgeries for gender dysphoria in the state. This legislation is currently being challenged in court (*Covington, Vasquez, & One Iowa v. Reynolds*, 2020 WL 4514691, Iowa Ct. App.). Iowa is merely one example of state-level activity.

## Public Accommodations

The LGBTQ community continues to work toward full inclusion and protection in public spaces. Access to bathrooms, restaurants, and public transportation are all examples of the types of public spaces in question. At this time, there is no federal protection explicitly for sexual orientation or gender identity and expression. The states are left to decide how they will approach this issue. At the same time, states have differing laws regarding the deference to be given to religion. Though there is the Free Exercise Clause at the federal level, states have also passed state-level versions of the Religious Freedom Restoration Act. When a person believes providing services or access to public spaces is against their religion, there remains a question of how the courts will decide.

As mentioned previously, the Supreme Court recently decided *Masterpiece Cakeshop v. Colorado Civil Rights Commission.* The plaintiffs, two men, entered Masterpiece Cakeshop in search of a cake for their upcoming marriage. The owner, described by the court as a devout Christian, declined to provide a cake, stating that he did not make cakes for same-sex weddings. The Colorado Civil Rights Commission brought suit against the cake shop. The Court ultimately ruled that the Colorado rule, as applied to this case, violated the Free Exercise Clause. However, it is critical to note that the ruling was very fact-specific and the court specifically discussed the "hostile" language used towards the owner and his religion, which violated his right to have the law applied neutrally. Additionally, the court found that the baker viewed his cake making as an expressive statement, so using his art to make a cake for a same-sex wedding implicated his First Amendment right to freedom of speech. This case is limited in its general applicability but may provide insight on how courts will weigh competing interests when the state and the federal government remain silent on protections for LGBTQ persons in public accommodations.

## Employment Discrimination

Employment discrimination is a risk in the LGBTQ community. Studies have linked discrimination in the workplace to lower health outcomes. The LGBTQ population is in the position of having regional differences in workplace protections. Populations in the First, Sixth, Seventh, Ninth, and Eleventh Circuits have some protection under court precedents that interpret protection against gender discrimination as protecting LGBTQ populations on the basis of failing to conform to gender stereotypes. The other circuits do not have cases that interpret gender discrimination to protect the LGBTQ population. The U.S. Supreme Court is in the position at this point to make a decision that will provide clarification across the states. In the fall of 2019, the court heard *Bostock v. Clayton County, Georgia, Altitude Express, Inc. v. Zarda*, and *R.G. & G.R. Harris Funeral Homes v. EEOC*. In *Bostock* and *Altitude Express*, the court will answer the question: Does Title VII of the Civil Rights Act of 1964, which prohibits against employment discrimination "because of ... sex," encompass discrimination based on an individual's sexual orientation? Their answer will impact persons who bring employment discrimination cases on the basis of sexual orientation. At the same time, the Court heard the *R.G. & G.R. Harris Funeral Homes* case, which raises the question: Does Title VII of the Civil Rights Act of 1964 prohibit discrimination against transgender employees based on (a) their status as transgender or nonbinary, or (b) sex stereotyping under *Price Waterhouse v. Hopkins*, 490 U.S. 228 (1989)? The Court's decision will control subsequent cases brought for workplace discrimination against transgender and nonbinary employees. It is anticipated that the Court will release its decision in late spring 2020.

## CONCLUSION

The health inequities experienced by the LGBTQ community can be impacted by the public health approach. Current legislation and regulations too often leave protections for LGBTQ communities to the courts rather than explicitly provide protections for sexual orientation and gender identity and expression. Whether it is access to healthcare or public accommodations, it is unlikely that health outcomes for the LGBTQ community will improve if public health laws do not provide protection.

## CHAPTER REVIEW

### Review Questions

1. What kinds of discrimination are faced by the LGBTQ community?
2. Does federal antidiscrimination law protect all members of the LGBTQ community? Y/N
3. Choose two of the life domains or social determinants of health in which LGBTQ people experience discrimination (housing, public access/accommodations, employment, and healthcare) and for each, provide one policy example and describe how that policy can be used to discriminate against LGBTQ individuals (if a specific LGBTQ population, note which population).

| Life Domain | Policy Example | Possible Discrimination |
|---|---|---|
|  |  |  |
|  |  |  |

### Essay Questions

1. What considerations would you prioritize if you were to propose public health policy that directly impacted LGBTQ individuals and communities?
2. How can antidiscrimination policy help improve the well-being of LGBTQ individuals and communities?
3. How will you apply the information from this chapter in your work to promote health equity for LGBTQ individuals and communities?
4. Sam is a new public health graduate who has elected to work the public health liaison from the Department of Public Health with the Department of Housing in your state. Sam has already had two persons in his office who are experiencing difficulty in achieving housing stability. As Sam has been working with Tyne, it appears clear that each of the three times they have attempted to access state-subsidized housing, once the landlord discovered that they are transgender, something has "come up" to keep the landlord from renting to them.

    1. Is this a public health issue? If so, in what way? If not, why not?
    2. Using your state's law, is there a legal remedy?
    3. If there is not, what public health legal options might you pursue?

    Resources for Essay Question #4:

    1. Movement Advancement Project – Housing Laws: www.lgbtmap.org/equality-maps/non_discrimination_laws
    2. HUD (for federal law protections): www.hud.gov/program_offices/fair_housing_equal_opp/housing_discrimination_and_persons_identifying_lgbtq

3.  Urban Institute Article: www.urban.org/urban-wire/discrimination-limiting-lgbtq-peoples-access-rental-housing

5.  Kelly works as a public health educator in your state. They have noticed that the state has seen an increase in the rate of sexually transmitted infections in teens, which reflects the research that approximately two thirds of new syphilis cases are among young men who have sex with men (MSM; Centers for Disease Control and Prevention [CDC], 2016b) and 80% of new cases of HIV among youth ages 13 to 24 were among MSM (CDC, 2016a). These risks are even more heightened when considering the lack of LGBTQ-inclusive sexual health education, as well as the fact that research has found sexual minority youth are more likely to use internet-based resources for sexual health information (Mitchell et al., 2014). The increase is especially troubling in the sexual and gender minority adolescent population.

1.  Kelly understands that sexual health education in the state is primarily abstinence-only and, where the education includes birth control methods, there is no education in same-sex sexual experiences.
2.  What policy issues should Kelly explore before taking any action to work to impact the increase in infections?
3.  Based on what Kelly finds in the laws in your state, what are Kelly's next steps?

Resources for Essay Question #5:

■  GLSEN fact sheet: www.glsen.org/activity/inclusive-sexual-health-education-lesbian-gay-bisexual-transgender
■  HRC Fact Sheet: www.hrc.org/resources/a-call-to-action-lgbtq-youth-need-inclusive-sex-education
■  Trust for America's Health Report: www.tfah.org/wp-content/uploads/archive/assets/files/TFAH-2016-LGBTQ-SexEd-FINAL.pdf
■  Scarleteen: www.scarleteen.com
■  Also, check the laws on sex education in your state.

## Internet Activities

1.  How does your state treat medical transition for transgender persons? Does it provide any coverage for hormone therapy? Gender-affirming surgeries? Check out your state's Medicaid law.
2.  Go to the Movement Advancement Project website at www.lgbtmap.org/equality-maps/non_discrimination_laws Check out your state's coverage of nondiscrimination in public accommodations. Does your state provide protections based on sexual orientation? Gender identity? Both? Neither? While you are there, you can check on employment and housing discrimination laws as well.
3.  The U.S. Supreme Court has ruled that persons of the same sex can be married across the United States. Search your state statutes and see if the state's legal definition of "marriage" still is defined as between one man and one woman. If so, do you think that has an impact on (a) how the LGBTQ community feels they are accepted in the state or (b) the way others view marriage equality in that state? Why or why not?

## REFERENCES

Bierman, A. S., & Dunn, J. R. (2006). Swimming Upstream. *Journal of General Internal Medicine*, 21(1), 99–100. https://doi.org/10.1111/j.1525-1497.2005.00317.x

Blake, V. K., & Hatzenbuehler, M. L. (2019). Legal remedies to address stigma-based health inequalities in the United States: Challenges and opportunities. *The Milbank Quarterly, 97*(2), 480–504. https://doi.org/10.1111/1468-0009.12391

Brown, M. E., & Burill, D. (2018). *Challenging genders: Non-binary experiences of those assigned female at birth*. Boundless Endeavors.

Centers for Disease Control and Prevention. (2016a). *HIV among youth*. http://www.cdc.gov/hiv/group/age/youth/index.html

Centers for Disease Control and Prevention. (2016b). *Syphilis & MSM (men who have sex with men)—CDC fact sheet*. http://www.cdc.gov/std/Syphilis/STDFact-MSM-Syphilis.htm

*Covington, Vasquez, & One Iowa v. Reynolds*, 2020 WL 4514691, Iowa Ct. App.

Dastagir, A. E. (2016, April 28). The imaginary predator in America's transgender bathroom war. USA Today. http://www.usatoday.com/story/news/nation/2016/04/28/transgender-bathroom-bills-discrimination/32594395

Deitz, C. E. (2015). *Sexual orientation microaggressions and psychological well-being: A mediational model* (Doctoral dissertation). ProQuest Dissertations and Theses database. (Accession Order No. 3705170).

Drum, K. (2016, May 14). A very brief timeline of the bathroom wars. *Mother Jones*. http://www.motherjones.com/kevin-drum/2016/05/timeline-bathroom-wars

*Good v. Iowa Dep't. of Human Servs.*, 924 N.W.2d 853 (Iowa 2019).

Haas, A. P., Eliason, M., Mays, V. M., Mathy, R. M., Cochran, S. D., D'Augelli, A. R., Silverman, M. M., Fisher, P. W., Hughes, T., Rosario, M., Russell, S. T., Malley, E., Reed, J., Litts, D. A., Haller, E., Sell, R. L., Remafedi, G., Bradford, J., Beautrais, A. L., … Clayton, P. J. (2010). Suicide and suicide risk in lesbian, gay, bisexual, and transgender populations: Review and recommendations. *Journal of Homosexuality, 58*(1), 10–51. https://doi.org/10.1080/00918369.2011.534038

Hatzenbuehler, M. L., Bellatorre, A., Lee, Y., Finch, B. K., Muennig, P., & Fiscella, K. (2014). Structural stigma and all-cause mortality in sexual minority populations. *Social Science and Medicine, 103*, 33–41. https://doi.org/10.1016/j.socscimed.2013.06.005

Herman, J., Haas, A., & Rodgers, P. (2014). *Suicide attempts among transgender and gender nonconforming adults*. The Williams Institute, UCLA.

Iowa Civil Rights Act, Iowa Acts ch. 191, §§5, 6 (codified at Iowa Code §216.7[1][a] [2009]).

James, S. E., Herman, J. L., Rankin, S., Keisling, M., Mottet, L., & Anafi, M. (2016). *The report of the 2015 U.S. transgender survey*. National Center for Transgender Equality.

Johns, M. M., Lowry, R., Andrzejewski, J., Barrios, L. C., Demissie, Z., McManus, T., Rasberry, C. N., Robin, L., & Underwood, J. M. (2019). Transgender identity and experiences of violence victimization, substance use, suicide risk, and sexual risk behaviors among high school students—19 states and large urban school districts, 2017. *Morbidity and Mortality Weekly Report, 68*(3), 67–71. https://doi.org/10.15585/mmwr.mm6803a3

Kelleher, C. (2009). Minority stress and health: Implications for lesbian, gay, bisexual, transgender, and questioning (LGBTQ) young people. *Counselling Psychology Quarterly, 22*(4), 373–379. https://doi.org/10.1080/09515070903334995

Keuroghlian, A. S., Reisner, S. L., White, J. M., & Weiss, R. D. (2015). Substance use and treatment of substance use disorders in a community sample of transgender adults. *Drug and Alcohol Dependence, 152*, 139–146. https://doi.org/10.1016/j.drugalcdep.2015.04.008

Kralik, J. (2017, April 12). "Bathroom bill" legislative tracking. National Conference of State Legislators. http://www.ncsl.org/research/education/-bathroom-bill-legislative-tracking635951130.aspx

McLemore, K. A. (2018). A minority stress perspective on transgender individuals' experiences with misgendering. *Stigma and Health, 3*(1), 53–64. https://doi.org/10.1037/sah0000070

Meyer, I. H., & Frost, D. M. (2012). Minority stress and the health of sexual minorities. In C. J. Patterson & A. R. D'Augelli (Eds.), *Handbook of psychology and sexual orientation* (pp. 252–266). Oxford University Press. https://doi.org/10.1093/acprof:oso/9780199765218.003.0018

Meyer, I. H., & Northridge, M. E. (Eds.). (2007). *The health of sexual minorities: Public health perspectives on lesbian, gay, bisexual and transgender population*. Springer.

Mitchell, K. J., Ybarra, M. L., Korchmaros, J. D., & Kosciw, J. G. (2014). Accessing sexual health information online: Use, motivations and consequences for youth with different sexual orientations. *Health Education Research, 29*, 147–157. https://doi.org/10.1093/her/cyt071

Movement Advancement Project. (n.d.). *Nondiscrimination laws.* https://www.lgbtmap.org/equality
-maps/non_discrimination_laws

Nadal, K. L., Whitman, C. N., Davis, L. S., Erazo, T., & Davidoff, K. C. (2016). Microaggressions
toward lesbian, gay, bisexual, transgender, queer, and genderqueer people: A review of the
literature. *The Journal of Sex Research, 53*(4–5), 488–508. https://doi.org/10.1080/00224499.2016
.1142495

Office of Disease Prevention and Health Promotion. (n.d). *Lesbian, gay, bisexual, and transgender
health.* https://www.healthypeople.gov/2020/topics-objectives/topic/lesbian-gay-bisexual-and
-transgender-health

*Pinneke v. Preisser* 623 F.2d 546 (8th Cir. 1980).

Pitts, M. K., Couch, C., Mulcare, H., Croy, S., & Mitchell, A. (2009). Transgender people in Australia
and New Zealand: Health, well-being and access to health services. *Feminism and Psychology,
19*(4), 475–495. https://doi.org/10.1177/0959353509342771

Public Facilities Privacy & Security Act ("House Bill 2"), Sess. L. No. 2016-3, 2016 N.C. Sess. Laws 2d
Extra Sess. 12 (repealed 2017).

Ransom, M. (Ed.). (2016, April). *Public health law competency model: Version 1.0.* https://www.cdc
.gov/phlp/docs/phlcm-v1.pdf

*Smith v. Rasmussen* 249 F.3D 755 (8TH Cir. 2001).

Steinmetz, K. (2016, May 2). Why LGBT advocates say bathroom 'predators' argument is a red
herring. *Time.* http://time.com/4314896/transgender-bathroom-bill-male-predators-argument

Su, D., Irwin, J. A., Fisher, C., Ramos, A., Kelley, M., Mendoza, D. A. R., & Coleman, J. D. (2016).
Mental health disparities within the LGBT population: A comparison between transgender
and nontransgender individuals. *Transgender Health, 1*(1), 12–20. https://doi.org/10.1089/trgh
.2015.0001

Title VIII of the Civil Rights Act of 1968, 42 U.S.C. §§ 3601-3619

*Waterhouse v. Hopkins*, 490 U.S. 228 (1989).

U.S. Department of Housing and Urban Development. (n.d.). *Housing discrimination and person
identifying as LGBTQ.* https://www.hud.gov/program_offices/fair_housing_equal_opp/housing
_discrimination_and_persons_identifying_lgbtq

World Health Organization. (2008). *Commission on Social Determinants of Health: Closing the gap in a
generation: Health equity through action on the social determinants of health, final report of the commission
on social determinants of health.* http://www.who.int/social_determinants/final_report/en/
index.html

# 16

# Women's Health and the Law

## Exploring Reproductive and Sexual Health

Hayley Penan and Brianne Bostian Yassine

## Learning Objectives

By the end of this chapter, the reader will be able to:

- Analyze the impact of public health law on women's reproductive and sexual health.
- Discuss the legal concepts of the right to privacy and equal protection.
- Explain the legal frameworks for the right to birth control, the right to abortion, and access to reproductive and sexual healthcare.

## Key Terminology

**Federalism:** Describes the way in which government power is divided between the federal and state governments ("Federalism," n.d.).

**Health Equity:** The idea that everyone should have an equal opportunity to reach their maximum potential in terms of health. Achieving health equity requires removing barriers to achieving good health, especially for underserved and marginalized communities (Braveman et al., 2017).

**Life Course Approach:** The interaction of biological, behavioral, psychological, social, and environmental factors impact health outcomes throughout the course of an individual's life (Fine & Kottlechuck, 2010).

**Reproductive Health:** Defined as "a state of complete physical, mental and social wellbeing, not merely the absence of disease or infirmity, in all matters relating to the reproductive system and to its functions and processes" (United Nations, 2009, p. 18). Focused on the availability and accessibility of healthcare services, facilities, and research that impact reproductive and sexual health.

**Reproductive Justice:** "Reproductive justice links reproductive rights with the social, political and economic inequalities that affect a woman's ability to access reproductive health care services" (Ahmed & Gamble, 2017). It is focused on

---

"Women" is used throughout this chapter inclusively to encompass all those who identify as women as well as individuals who do not identify as women but who have female sex organs and thus may need similar reproductive and sexual healthcare to cisgendered women.

the ways in which persisting social inequalities mean that issues around access to reproductive healthcare have a greater impact on marginalized communities than privileged ones.

**Reproductive Rights:** The idea that there are certain rights, recognized in and protected by law, founded in protections of privacy, bodily integrity, and personal autonomy (United Nations, 2009). Focused on ensuring all people can exercise the right to make their own reproductive choices, including, but not limited to, decisions around contraception and abortion.

**SCOTUS:** Abbreviation for the Supreme Court of the United States. This is the highest federal court in the nation.

**Social Determinants of Health:** Factors that impact a person's health. These may include biological, socioeconomic, psychosocial, environmental, behavioral, or social characteristics (Centers for Disease Control and Prevention, n.d.-b).

## Public Health Law Competencies

This chapter addresses the following competencies from the Public Health Law Competency Model (PHLCM; Ransom, 2016).

**1.1** Define basic constitutional concepts and legal principles framing the practice of public health across relevant jurisdictions.

**1.2** Identify and apply public health laws (e.g., statutes, regulations, ordinances, and court rulings) pertinent to practitioner's jurisdiction, agency, program, and profession.

**2.3** Recognize the legal authority and limits of critical system partners and others who influence health outcomes.

---

### Spark Questions

1. How do women's reproductive and sexual health needs change during critical periods of the life course? How might law be a tool or a barrier during these critical periods?

2. For example, how might an individual's reproductive and sexual health needs be different for adolescents as compared to aging populations or women of childbearing age who are actively trying to get pregnant? Think about some ways these changes are reflected in existing laws and government programs impacting access to reproductive healthcare.

---

## INTRODUCTION

Reproductive and sexual health is imperative to overall health and well-being. Issues surrounding this aspect of public health have a long history and have often been at the forefront of national discussions, social movements, policy, and law. Like all public health issues, there are also significant **health equity** concerns, as highlighted in Box 16.1.

United States law has regularly impacted women's health and has had two main functions. First, the law establishes the foundation for health practices, such as by providing funding for agencies and activities. Second, the law acts as an intervention for reproductive and sexual healthcare, both enabling and prohibiting certain services.

According to the World Health Organization (WHO, n.d.), reproductive and sexual health encompasses physical, emotional, mental, and social well-being. In the public health discourse around women's health, the primary framework through which physical, emotional, mental, and social issues are viewed and addressed is the **life course approach**. A hybrid theory combining the **social determinants of health** with an emphasis on **health equity**, the life course approach is used to conceptualize health in the context of the greater environment throughout individuals' lives (Fine & Kottlechuck, 2010; Halfon et al., 2014).

## BOX 16.1 HEALTH EQUITY IN REPRODUCTIVE AND SEXUAL HEALTH

Access to reproductive and sexual health services can vary greatly from person to person, and factors like race, sexual orientation, socioeconomic status, immigration status, education, age, and geography can greatly impact the likelihood someone will experience issues needing care. The ways these different characteristics intersect can cause even greater disparities for some individuals. Thus, it is important to think broadly about who needs reproductive and sexual healthcare, and why it may be more difficult for some to access care than others. For example, trans men need **reproductive health** services and should be receiving regular preventive care, but often experience barriers to accessing proper care (Mamone, 2019). These barriers can arise from provider ignorance and outright discrimination, among other issues. This can be compounded by the fact that transgender individuals face higher rates of being uninsured and in poverty than cisgendered individuals. And according to the 2015 U.S. Transgender Survey, if the individual is also a person of color, they are likely to experience "deeper and broader patterns of discrimination than White respondents and the U.S. population" and greater health disparities (James et al., 2016).

## BOX 16.2 LIFE COURSE APPROACH

*Life course* highlights the importance of access to healthcare services during critical periods of life, as this can impact health trajectories. For example, nearly half of pregnancies in the United States are unplanned, and 20% of those are among youths aged 15 to 19. Teen mothers are 50% less likely to graduate from high school or get a General Education Development (GED) degree than their peers. Not graduating from high school affects earning potential, and reduced income can be a barrier to accessing care. Further, children of teen mothers are more likely to have health problems, drop out of school, and become teen parents themselves (Fine & Kottlechuck, 2010; James et al., 2016; Rosenzweig et al., 2018).

Life course, as described in Box 16.2, is important to keep in mind when considering laws that impact reproductive and sexual health. Life course considers the social, physical, political, and economic context of public health on societal and individual levels, and views health as an interactive process involving risk and protective factors within and across generations. In the United States, our government has long recognized the impact of law on reproductive and sexual health over the life course. Public health law facilitates access to healthcare services and education. Many laws are designed to target populations during critical periods, such as during adolescence or pregnancy, and for underserved populations.

## LEGAL FRAMEWORKS

Many legal frameworks and legally protected rights impact reproductive and sexual health in the United States, several of which are covered in this chapter: the legal right to birth control, the legal right to abortion, and access to reproductive healthcare services. While these areas of reproductive and sexual health provide a foundation for understanding the impact of law on this aspect of public health, it is important to note that this chapter is not exhaustive of all the potential legal and social issues impacting access to reproductive and sexual healthcare.

Nationally, reproductive rights are protected by two concepts from the U.S. Constitution: the *right to privacy* and the *right to equal protection* under the laws. (See Boxes 16.3 and 16.4.) These rights have not always been protected as they are today, and there is a long history of government regulation of *reproductive health* at both the federal and state levels. At times, government

---

### BOX 16.3  RIGHT TO PRIVACY

The right to privacy is a foundational aspect of **reproductive rights** in the United States and protects the right to contraception and abortion. The right to privacy stems from a "penumbra," or zone of rights, from the Bill of Rights and the First, Third, Fourth, and Fifth Amendments of the U.S. Constitution. This constitutional privacy right has also been solidified and expanded through federal and state statutory law. For example, Congress created the Health Insurance Portability and Accountability Act (HIPAA) in 2000, which includes privacy protections that apply to personally identifying health information. There are also numerous state regulations that expand privacy protections as they relate to reproductive health. For example, in California, there is a state law that protects the home addresses of reproductive healthcare providers, volunteers, employees, and patients (2 Cal. Code Regs. § 22100).

---

regulation has restricted reproductive healthcare and at other times facilitated greater access. (See Table 16.1 for a Timeline of Women's Reproductive and Sexual Health Law.) Over time, Supreme Court of the United States **(SCOTUS)** has held that the Constitution provides a base level of protections that must be afforded to individuals seeking reproductive healthcare services.

## Structure of U.S. Government and Federalism

Government regulation of healthcare can occur at the state, federal, or local levels. At the federal level, there are three branches of government: executive branch (the president and federal administrative agencies), legislative branch (the House and Senate in Congress), and judicial branch (SCOTUS and lower federal courts). Congress has the power to pass laws that affect interstate commerce or require the use of federal funds (tax and spend power), and can delegate some of its powers to administrative agencies. The president can pass executive orders, but this power is limited in scope by the separation of powers set out in the Constitution. Administrative agencies enact rules and regulations providing guidance and parameters for programs and laws created by Congress. The judiciary, among other roles, adjudicates claims between the government and the people of the United States, often assessing the constitutionality of laws passed by Congress or regulations and rules from administrative agencies. The judiciary also resolves questions of law where there have been conflicting decisions from lower courts in different parts of the country.

   Under the 10th Amendment of the Constitution, all powers not explicitly granted to the federal government are reserved by the states. States likewise have their own executive, legislative, and judicial branches of government with distinct responsibilities. Government actions impacting women's health can occur within all three branches at the federal and state levels, as well as in local governments. For example, Congress (legislative branch) enacted the Patient Protection and Affordable Care Act (ACA), which included a mandate requiring specified insurance plans to cover contraception without cost-sharing; the executive branch (through administrative agencies) has promulgated regulations governing the application of employer exemptions from the ACA's contraceptive mandate; and the judiciary has weighed in on challenges to these legislative actions and regulations, such as in the case of *Burwell v. Hobby Lobby*, where it expanded the exemption to apply to closely held for-profit companies (Moran, 2018). States and localities have also taken recent actions that impact contraception access. California enacted a state law allowing pharmacists to provide birth control pills without a prescription in 2016 (Kritz, 2019) and San Francisco passed an ordinance prohibiting crisis pregnancy centers that do not provide abortion and contraception services from putting out false or misleading advertising that gives the impression that they offer such services (City Attorney of San Francisco, 2018). It is important to think about the interplay between federal and state law, as well as between the different branches of government at the federal and state levels.

The 14th Amendment of the Constitution prohibits states from "deny[ing] to any person within its jurisdiction the equal protection of the laws." This also applies to the federal government through the due process clause of the Fifth Amendment. Essentially, equal protection prohibits the government from discriminating between classes of people without a justification for doing so. Equal protection applies to a set of specific protected classes, which includes discrimination on the basis of gender.

In assessing whether the government has violated the equal protection clause, courts apply different levels of scrutiny depending on whether a protected class[1] is involved. If there is no protected class, the government need have only a rational basis for discriminating (*Williamson v. Lee Optical Co.*, 1954). If a protected class is involved, the government's reasoning must pass either strict scrutiny or intermediate scrutiny. Strict scrutiny means there must be a compelling government purpose and the government conduct must be narrowly tailored to achieve that purpose (*Korematsu v. U.S.*, 1944). Under intermediate scrutiny, which is the classification that applies to gender discrimination, courts assess whether the government is discriminating for an important government purpose and whether its actions are substantially related to that purpose (*Craig v. Borden*, 1976).

## Legal Right to Birth Control

While birth control comes in many forms and can be used to manage a variety of health issues, the primary use is to prevent unintended pregnancy. It allows for control over timing and spacing of pregnancies, which is particularly important to low-income individuals and others who experience barriers to accessing care. Pregnancy spacing allows a level of autonomy over the life course and significantly increases economic and social opportunities and overall well-being. Increasing spacing between pregnancies has led to a decrease in maternal morbidity and mortality and improved social and economic conditions (Stover et al., 2016). Access to birth control has been regulated in different ways over time, with the legal landscape changing to reflect public health demands.

In 1873, Congress passed the Comstock Act, which criminalized publishing, distributing, and possessing devices or medications, or information related to devices and medications, that could be used for "unlawful" contraception or abortion. The key here is "unlawful": the Comstock Act applied only to these practices as they related to prohibited contraception and abortion services. Generally, these kinds of prohibitions and restrictions are found in state law. In 1960, 30 states had laws on the books that restricted advertising and sale of contraceptives, including, in some cases, outright prohibitions on the use of birth control.

This changed in 1965, with the decision of SCOTUS in *Griswold v. Connecticut* (1964). Connecticut had a state law that prohibited using contraception and criminalized aiding in obtaining or using birth control. This law, enacted in the 1800s, was almost never enforced, but in 1961, the Executive Director of Planned Parenthood of Connecticut and a professor at Yale Medical School opened a birth control clinic to challenge the ban's constitutionality. The clinic provided information and prescriptions for contraception to married people. The doors were open for 10 days before the clinic's founders were arrested, prosecuted, and found guilty of violating the law. They appealed their convictions and their case found its way up to SCOTUS.

---

[1] This describes a group of individuals that share a common characteristic, such as race, gender, national origin, age, etc., which the law protects from discrimination of the basis of their shared characteristic.

## TABLE 16.1 Timeline of Women's Reproductive and Sexual Health Law

| PUBLIC HEALTH LAW EVENT | YEAR | BACKGROUND AND EFFECTS |
|---|---|---|
| Comstock Act passed by the Congress | 1873 | ■ Criminalized publishing, distributing, and possessing information about, or devices or medications that could be used for, unlawful contraception or abortion.<br>■ 45 states enacted or amended antiobscenity statutes mentioning contraception.<br>■ The medical community was not trained in contraceptive methods.<br>■ Resulted in the spread of information and misinformation, through informal networks like families and friends (Bailey, 2013). |
| Margaret Sanger, birth control activist, indicted in New York | 1914 | ■ Sanger was arrested for nine violations of the Comstock Act for using the words "birth control" in a publication.<br>■ Sanger's arrest catalyzed the birth control movement (Bailey, 2013). |
| National Birth Registry established by the U.S. Bureau of the Census | 1915 | ■ Improved vital statistics data collection.<br>■ Established first evidence of relationships between social causes and infant mortality.<br>■ By 1933, all states participated in registering live births and deaths and providing the required data to the Bureau of the Census.<br>■ Data highlighted the connection between poverty and health. |
| American Birth Control League established by Margaret Sanger | 1921 | ■ Worked to educate women on reproductive and sexual health.<br>■ Sanger's advocacy laid the groundwork for organizations like Planned Parenthood. |
| Sheppard-Towner Maternity and Infancy Protection Act enacted by Congress to fund health clinics and programs | 1921 | ■ Set the precedent for federal grants to states for Maternal and Child Health (MCH) services (Title V).<br>■ Repealed in 1929: all states but one had adopted it, and upon repeal, continued efforts to provide nurse training. |
| Social Security Act (SSA) established by Congress, funding Title V MCH Block Grant Program | 1935 | ■ MCH Block Grant Program funds states to provide maternity, infant, and child care, specifically targeting vulnerable populations.<br>■ Longest standing U.S. public health legislation.<br>■ Aftermath of Great Depression (MCH, n.d.). |
| Congress created the Emergency Maternity and Infant Care (EMIC) Program | 1943 | ■ Enabled funds for MCH care for families of servicemen in the four lowest pay grades.<br>■ Largest federally funded medical care program undertaken to date.<br>■ Supported in part because of affiliation with WWII. |
| The U.S. Food and Drug Administration (FDA), a federal administrative agency, approved oral contraception | 1960 | ■ Comstock laws, although outdated at this point, were still in effect.<br>■ Physicians were prohibited from prescribing oral contraception, and pharmacists were unable to sell it.<br>■ Comstock laws were difficult to enforce, and within 2 years, 1.2 million U.S. women were using oral contraception (Bailey, 2013; MCH, n.d.). |
| Griswold v. Connecticut | 1965 | ■ SCOTUS determined that banning sale of birth control in CT violated due process and the right to privacy, reversing the 1873 Comstock Act.<br>■ This decision allowed married couples to make their own choices regarding birth control.<br>■ By 1970, the federal government and all states permitted contraceptive sales to married individuals (Bailey, 2013; MCH, n.d.). |

**TABLE 16.1  Timeline of Women's Reproductive and Sexual Health Law (*continued*)**

| PUBLIC HEALTH LAW EVENT | YEAR | BACKGROUND AND EFFECTS |
|---|---|---|
| Medicaid, Title XIX of the Social Security Act (SSA) enacted by Congress | 1965 | ■ Established as part of national efforts in the War on Poverty.<br>■ Pays for medical assistance to both "categorically" and "medically" eligible groups with limited resources.<br>■ Provides physical and mental healthcare coverage for children and families with low incomes.<br>■ Provides care to low-income children. |
| Family Planning Act, authorized under Title X of the Public Health Service Act, enacted by Congress | 1970 | ■ First U.S. statute that provided authority and funds for family planning services.<br>■ Passed with bipartisan support.<br>■ Serves over 4 million women today in family planning services and positive birth outcomes  (Bailey, 2013; MCH, n.d.). |
| *Eisenstadt v. Baird* | 1971 | ■ SCOTUS expanded protections in *Griswold* to unmarried persons. |
| Comstock Act revised by Congress | 1971 | ■ Language applying the Comstock Act to contraception was removed, leaving it to apply only to unlawful abortions. |
| *Roe v. Wade* | 1973 | ■ SCOTUS determined laws prohibiting abortion were a violation of the constitutional right to privacy.<br>■ This decision establishes the constitutionally protected fundamental right to an abortion. |
| Church Amendment enacted by Congress | 1973 | ■ Passed in reaction to the controversy resulting from the passing of *Roe v. Wade* (*Eisenstadt*, 2003).<br>■ Permits providers and institutions receiving federal funding to opt out of providing abortions or sterilizations if it is against their "religious beliefs or moral convictions" (U.S. Department of Health and Human Services, n.d.). |
| *Bellotti v. Baird* | 1978 | ■ SCOTUS ruled that parental consent is not needed for minors seeking abortion services. |
| *Planned Parenthood v. Casey* | 1991 | ■ SCOTUS reaffirmed the right to abortion, finding that a Pennsylvania law requiring spousal notification placed an undue burden on married women.<br>■ In this case, SCOTUS changed the framework for the court's analysis from a trimester framework (established in *Roe*) to a "viability" framework. |
| Title V Abstinence-Only-Until-Marriage enacted by Congress, funding states to implement abstinence-only sexual education programs | 1996 | ■ Abstinence-only education was subsequently found to be less effective than comprehensive sex education and to contribute to teen pregnancy rates.<br>■ States began to turn down federal funding; support shifted to comprehensive, age-appropriate pregnancy prevention programs (MCH timeline, n.d.; Stanger-Hall & Hall, 2011).<br>■ Today, 18 states and Washington, D.C., require contraception education to be part of sex education (Kaiser Family Foundation, 2018). |

(*continued*)

TABLE 16.1  Timeline of Women's Reproductive and Sexual Health Law (*continued*)

| PUBLIC HEALTH LAW EVENT | YEAR | BACKGROUND AND EFFECTS |
|---|---|---|
| FDA approved Plan B | 1999 | ■ Authorized emergency contraception to be more readily available.<br>■ 2006: Approved for over-the-counter sale to ages 18+.<br>■ 2009: Approved for over-the-counter sale to ages 17+, and by prescription to individuals 16 and younger.<br>■ This was later reversed, until 2013. |
| Patient Protection and Affordable Care Act (ACA) enacted by Congress | 2010 | ■ Limits cost-sharing requirements for women's preventive services: mammograms, annual check-ups, cervical cancer screenings, prenatal care, etc. |
| *Tummino v. Hamburg* | 2013 | ■ SCOTUS determined the FDA's limitations on Plan B to those over 18 had no scientific basis.<br>■ Plan B became available over the counter for all individuals. |
| *Whole Woman's Health v. Hellerstedt* | 2015 | ■ SCOTUS determined that Targeted Regulation of Abortion Providers (TRAP) laws were unconstitutional. |
| Conscience clause regulations extended by the U.S. Department of Health and Human Services | 2019 | ■ Expanded the ability of individuals and organizations to refuse to provide abortion information, services, and referrals based on religious and moral objections. |
| Medical deferred action program cancelled by U.S. Citizenship and Immigration Services | 2019 | ■ The program allowed people to remain in the United States for up to 2 years to receive medical treatment. |

In 1965, SCOTUS overturned their convictions, finding the Connecticut law violated the 14th Amendment of the Constitution, which prohibits states from "depriv[ing] any person of life, liberty, or property, without due process of law." SCOTUS also determined that the law violated the constitutional right to privacy, which it determined protects the rights of married couples to make their own choices about birth control.

Seven years after *Griswold*, SCOTUS decided another case about contraception: *Eisenstadt v. Baird* (1971). In *Eisenstadt*, SCOTUS expanded the protections in *Griswold* to unmarried individuals, finding a Massachusetts law that prohibited providing contraceptives to unmarried individuals unconstitutional. SCOTUS's decision reasoned that the same privacy protections applied to unmarried and married individuals, and that the Massachusetts law's distinction based on marriage status violated the Equal Protection Clause of the 14th Amendment. The Court determined that the Massachusetts law's distinction between married and unmarried individuals lacked any *rational basis* and was thus unconstitutional.

Recent cases have questioned, and in some contexts expanded, our understanding of the right to accessing contraception. In 2013, SCOTUS decided in *Tummino v. Hamburg* that the decision of the U.S. Food and Drug Administration (FDA) to limit over-the-counter access to emergency contraception ("Plan B") to women 18 years and older was baseless and held that emergency contraception must be made available over the counter for all individuals (*Tummino v. Hamburg*, 2013).[2]

---

[2] The FDA was still left with some discretion on the issue of which formulation is made available over the counter (OTC), and decided that only the one pill formulation would be available OTC (Plan B One-Step and its generic alternatives). Those wishing to obtain the two-pill formulation must be at least 17 years old and provide valid identification to prove their age to a local pharmacist as the FDA has not allowed it to be provided OTC. Those under 17 will need a prescription for this and alternative formulations.

## Legal Right to Abortion

Although abortion rates are at their lowest in United States history, abortions are common procedures, with nearly one in four American women seeking these services in their lifetime (Jones & Jerman, 2017). Individuals have abortions for a variety of reasons ranging from financial considerations to concerns over other responsibilities such as education, work, or dependents (Finer et al., 2005). Women in poverty are at the greatest risk of inadequate access to reproductive healthcare services, and are the largest segment of the population seeking abortion services (Jones & Jerman, 2017). Abortion rights have had a long, contentious legal history that has played out in several key cases.

In 1971, Congress removed the language of the Comstock Act that applied to contraception, instead leaving only the language related to "unlawful abortion." Previously, until 1973, it was entirely left to the states to determine the legality of abortion in their state. California, for example, passed a state law legalizing abortion in 1967. But in 1973, in the seminal case of *Roe v. Wade*, SCOTUS decided that the 14th Amendment's protections extend to the right to abortion (*Roe v. Wade*, 1973). SCOTUS struck down a Texas law criminalizing abortion as an unconstitutional infringement on the fundamental right to decide whether or not to terminate a pregnancy. Under *Roe*, this right was subject to strict scrutiny, and thus any infringement must be narrowly tailored to serve a compelling government interest, using a trimester framework to determine when state interests in protecting fetal life become compelling. To be narrowly tailored, the infringement must not be over- or under-inclusive, and must be the least restrictive way to achieve the government's objective.

SCOTUS has reaffirmed the right to abortion in a number of subsequent cases, the most notable of which is *Planned Parenthood v. Casey* (*Planned Parenthood of Southeastern Pennsylvania v. Casey*, 1991). In *Casey*, the Court shifted away from the trimester framework to a viability framework and away from strict scrutiny to an *undue burden analysis* where an "undue burden exists, and therefore the provision of law is invalid, if its purpose or effect is to place a substantial obstacle in the path of a woman seeking an abortion before the fetus attains viability" (*Planned Parenthood of Southeastern Pennsylvania v. Casey*, 1991). The issue of when a fetus obtains viability is still hotly debated.

Since *Casey*, states have passed hundreds of laws containing various restrictions on abortion. Recently, in *Whole Woman's Health v. Hellerstedt*, SCOTUS weighed in on a case challenging a Texas law that placed restrictions on abortion providers (commonly referred to as "Targeted Regulation of Abortion Providers," or "TRAP" laws), striking down as unconstitutional the law's requirement that abortion providers in the state have admitting privileges at a local hospital and clinics that provide abortions meet the standards required for ambulatory surgical centers (*Whole Woman's Health v. Hellerstedt*, 2015). In *Hellerstedt*, the Court recognized that without access to abortion services, the right to abortion becomes meaningless.

## ACCESSING REPRODUCTIVE AND SEXUAL HEALTHCARE SERVICES

The right to make one's own reproductive and sexual healthcare decisions does not necessarily mean that all those that want contraception and abortion services are able to access them easily. One in five sexually active women do not use contraception, and this percentage is disproportionately made up of women in poverty (Rosenzweig et al., 2018). Several government programs and structures exist to increase access to reproductive and sexual healthcare. There are several considerations that come into play when thinking about constraints on access, but this chapter focuses on cost and insurance coverage concerns as well as limitations on the scope of reproductive rights.

## Cost, Coverage, and Government Programs Facilitating Access

Many reproductive healthcare services are covered by health insurance plans. See Box 16.5 for a list of the primary types of insurance plans. There is a wide range of different types of insurance plans, including, but not limited to, private employer-sponsored insurance, Patient Protection and Affordable Care Act (ACA) federal and state marketplace plans, Medicaid, and Medicare. This chapter focuses on the protections afforded to plans governed by the ACA and Medicaid plans because they offer the greatest protections for reproductive and sexual healthcare services. However, there are some limitations on abortion in federally funded health insurance programs.

### Reproductive Healthcare in ACA Plans/Protections

The ACA included protections for preventive reproductive and sexual health services by adding Section 2713 to the Public Health Service Act. Section 2713 requires that plans subject to the ACA provide coverage for certain preventive health services without cost sharing (42 U.S.C. § 300gg-13[a][4]). The required services are those promulgated by the Health Resources and Services Administration (HRSA) guidelines, which include "[a]ll [18] Food and Drug Administration approved contraceptive methods, sterilization procedures, and patient education and counseling for all women with reproductive capacity."

### Reproductive Healthcare in Medicaid

The Social Security Amendments of 1965 created the Medicaid program, adding Title XIX to the Social Security Act (42 U.S.C. §§ 1396 et seq.). Medicaid is a federal-state partnership in which the federal government provides matching funds to states to help them pay for healthcare for qualifying indigent individuals. As of 1982, all states participate in the Medicaid program (they are not required to participate but must comply with federal Medicaid law and its protections if they do participate) and administer Medicaid to low-income residents in their states. Some benefits and eligibility standards under the Medicaid program vary from state to state.

---

### BOX 16.5  PRIMARY TYPES OF INSURANCE PLANS

- Employer plans
  - Small group market plans
  - Employee Retirement Income Security Act (ERISA) plans
  - Consolidated Omnibus Budget Reconciliation Act (COBRA)
  - Federal Employees Health Benefit Plan (FEHBP)

- Association Health Plans
- ACA Marketplace plans
  - Federal marketplace plans
  - State exchange plans

- Medicaid
  - Children's Health Insurance Program (CHIP)

- Medicare
  - Medicare Advantage
  - Medicare Parts A, B, C, and D

States participating in the Medicaid program must provide "family planning services and supplies to beneficiaries of childbearing age" (42 U.S.C. § 1396[a][4][C]). Federal law does not define the exact scope of services that must be provided, so there is variation in services covered from state to state. Recognizing the importance of family planning to public health, the federal government provides an increased match rate, paying for 90% of these services in Medicaid (as compared to the 50% match rate for many other services). Under federal law, states, Medicaid providers, and Medicaid insurance plans cannot impose any co-payments or other cost sharing on family planning services and supplies (42 C.F.R. § 447.53[b] [5]; 42 U.S.C. § 1396o[a][2]).

Medicaid law also requires that Medicaid beneficiaries have *freedom of choice* of providers. This means that they can obtain family planning services and supplies from any qualified Medicaid provider, whether the provider is inside their managed care network or not (42 C.F.R. § 431.51).

For abortion services, there is significant variation between states as to what is covered under Medicaid. Disagreements about abortion have led to compromises that have placed limitations on federal spending for abortion, including through the Hyde Amendment. Under the Hyde Amendment, federal funds can be used for abortion services only if the abortion is necessary to protect the life of the pregnant person or if the pregnancy was the result of rape or incest (Pub. L. 111-17 § 507-08, 2010). Some states have chosen to use state funds to cover abortion services outside these limited exceptions, while others have not. For example, California covers all abortion services for Medi-Cal (the state Medicaid program) enrollees (California Department of Health Care Services, 2020). However, even where abortion is not covered, prenatal care prior to an abortion, treatment of complications resulting from an abortion, and treatment of ectopic pregnancies are all covered services in Medicaid (State Medicaid Manual §§ 441.208, 4432.B.2, 2005).

## Potential Limitations on Reproductive Healthcare Access

There are some categories of persons and situations where United States law continues to allow certain limitations on reproductive rights, and thus reproductive healthcare access. Two major areas of limitations surround minors and parental consent or notification, and the balance of religious freedom in certain situations. When it comes to minors, parents' rights to make decisions for their children are often weighed against the ways in which parental consent or notification requirements can pose barriers for minors who need access to care during a critical period of their lives. When it comes to religious freedom of providers, states have weighed these competing rights and applied laws in different ways, as discussed in the following.

---

### HYPOTHETICAL CASE STUDY #1: ADOLESCENT CONFIDENTIALITY IN ACCESSING REPRODUCTIVE HEALTHCARE

Edriss is a policy analyst in his state health department's Division of Maternal and Child Health. Over the past 10 years, state epidemiologists have reported consistent increases in sexually transmitted infections (STIs)/sexually transmitted diseases (STDs) among youth ages 15 to 24 in his jurisdiction. Half of all new STIs each year are among youth (CDC, n.d.-a). The current incident rate is 35 out of 100 youth, approximately 10% higher than the national average. Edriss's state has ambivalent language in a state statute addressing the confidentiality of youth reproductive health services. His director has recently assigned him to a task force with a goal of developing an updated policy to address the issue. Edriss understands this is a sensitive topic with competing interests. On one side, confidentiality is a major barrier to accessing needed services that are critical for long-term health and well-being (Brindis & Moore, 2014; Leichliter et al., 2017). On the other side, parents and caregivers may have a right to know the health issues of their children and may be the best situated to help their children make the best decision for their situation. As discussed in what follows, there are also baseline legal requirements from SCOTUS around minor consent and confidentiality with respect to reproductive and sexual healthcare.

- What are the facts of the public health issue at hand?
- What are the competing rights in this scenario? Are there any others aside from the rights of the minor and their parents/guardian?
- What state laws surrounding minors' confidentiality already exist, in your state or others? Where can you find this information?
- At what age does your state allow individuals to consent to reproductive services without parental involvement or court approval?
- What requirements for minors' confidentiality and parental notification of minors' services will you recommend to the task force?
- What ethical concerns may arise and need to be addressed?
- What other considerations might inform your task force in developing this new law? Consider the political and social landscape in your state and how it might be different from the context in another state.
- Based on the seminal cases addressing parental consent and notification discussed in what follows, what standard has SCOTUS set for the base level of protection for minors' rights when seeking an abortion?

## Minors and Parental Consent or Notification Requirements

Courts have found that minors have the same reproductive rights as adults. However, there are some limitations on minors' ability to exercise their rights in certain situations. SCOTUS has found that minors under age 18 have a right to access contraceptives (*Carey v. Population Services International*, 1976). However, there is variation among states as to whether and to what extent parental consent is required. No states have enacted blanket requirements that minors must obtain parental consent for contraceptive services, but 26 states allow minors to consent to contraceptive services at a specified age (usually 12 or 14 years old) and 20 states allow only certain groups of minors to consent without parental notification or consent, such as minors who are married, are pregnant, or already have children. The remaining four states have no formal policy or pertinent case law, and generally in these states, health professionals will provide contraceptive services without parental consent if they think the minors are mature enough to make their own decisions about contraception (Guttmacher Institute, 2019).

With respect to abortion, in 1979, SCOTUS decided *Belotti v. Baird,* striking down a Massachusetts law requiring minors to gain parental consent before obtaining an abortion (*Bellotti v. Baird*, 1978). Under the Massachusetts law, if either parent refused to consent, the minor could then seek approval from the courts. SCOTUS found the law unconstitutional because it required parental notification in all cases and could have resulted in an abortion being denied to a minor who was competent and mature enough to make their own independent decision. But in *Ohio v. Akron Center for Reproductive Health,* SCOTUS upheld an Ohio law requiring one parent to be notified because the law contained a procedure by which the minor could seek judicial bypass of the notification requirement (*Ohio v. Akron Center*, 1989). Then, in *Hodgson v. Minnesota,* SCOTUS found a Minnesota state law that required minors to notify both parents and did not have a judicial bypass option unconstitutional (*Hodgson v. Minnesota*, 1989).

In all states, minors can consent to sexually transmitted infections (STIs) services. Thirty-nine states and the District of Columbia allow minors of any age to consent to STI and HIV services without parental consent, with the remaining states allowing limited categories (e.g., minors who are age 12 or older) to independently consent to this care. In 18 states, physicians are allowed, though not required, to inform a minor's parents that they are seeking STI services when the provider believes it is in the minor's best interest to do so (Guttmacher Institute, 2019).

---

### HYPOTHETHICAL CASE STUDY #2: REPRODUCTIVE RIGHTS AND REFUSALS

Baylee is a program manager at a reproductive health clinic in the state of "Caledonia" and she has been seeing many clients who have been turned away when seeking contraception and abortion services from other health clinics affiliated with a local religious hospital. The only local hospitals and clinics besides hers are religiously affiliated. Often, by the time these clients get to the clinic, significant time has passed from when they first sought care. Many, including at least one transgender patient, have expressed that these refusals were traumatic experiences and caused them to delay seeking follow-up care. Baylee's clinic is the only provider in the area that will provide abortions, and the staff physician is booked up for a couple of months. Baylee's state offers no additional protections for reproductive health services or religious refusals than what is provided in federal law, but also does not have further restrictions that would impede access to care. There are a couple of hospitals a couple of hours away that provide abortions, but Baylee's clients are often unable to afford to travel that distance.

First trimester abortions are less expensive. About 75% of patients seeking abortion are low-income, and 51% pay out of pocket (Kennedy & Baker, 2005). With each week of gestation, the risk of abortion-related maternal mortality increases. Other risks include infection, hemorrhage, and uterine perforation (American College of Obstetricians and Gynecologists, 2013). Patients denied abortions are more likely to face economic insecurity that lasts for approximately five years. Public assistance is not sufficient to alleviate poverty among these individuals (Greene Foster et al., 2018).

- What are some strategies Baylee could use to try to facilitate access for these patients, given her clinic's wait time and limited capacity?
- Think about strategies to get them the care they need locally, including through Medicaid or other insurance, different types and locations of providers, and so forth.
- Are there changes Baylee could make to clinic operations to increase capacity? What potential role could technological advances like telehealth play?
- What issues should Baylee consider in advocating for changes in state law to increase access to abortion?
- How might your approach be different if Baylee were in Texas, where there are additional restrictions on abortion and limited state spending in the Medicaid program rather than Caledonia? What if she were instead in California, where there are expanded protections and state funding for abortion?
- What are the competing rights at stake in this scenario?

---

## Balancing Reproductive Rights With Religious Rights of Providers/Private Plans/Others

Shortly after the *Roe v. Wade* decision, "conscience clauses" began to appear in laws, balancing the free exercise of religious beliefs against reproductive rights. The first such federal provision was the Church Amendment, which allows individuals and institutions receiving federal funding to opt out of providing abortions or sterilizations if it is against their "religious beliefs or moral convictions" (2006). It also prohibits institutions from discriminating against providers who *do* perform abortion or sterilization procedures. The Weldon Amendment was added (first in 2005) as an annual rider to the Federal Appropriations Act, prohibiting "discrimination" by a state (or local) or federal agency against an individual or institution refusing to pay for, or provide coverage or referrals for, abortion services.[3]

Many states have also enacted their own refusal or conscience clauses. Some allow providers to refuse to perform or participate in abortion or sterilization services, some allow pharmacists to refuse to fill prescriptions for contraception, and some states allow providers to refuse to provide referrals or information related to abortion or contraceptive services if it conflicts with a provider's religious or moral beliefs (Guttmacher Institute, 2019).

These conscience clauses have also been applied to the contraceptive mandate in the ACA. Through the enacting regulations, the Department of Health and Human Services (DHHS) exempt certain religious employers from complying with this mandate. Further, in *Burwell v. Hobby Lobby*, SCOTUS found the initial DHHS regulations requiring all employers to provide contraceptive coverage to their female employees without cost sharing violated the Religious Freedom Restoration Act, as applied to closely held corporations that did not fall into the religious employers exemption (*Burwell v. Hobby Lobby*, 2013). The Trump Administration made changes to these regulations to expand the exemptions to those with religious or moral objections, among other changes. There have been court challenges to these expansions, but none had yet reached SCOTUS review when this chapter was written (*Commonwealth of Massachusetts v. U.S Department of Health and Human Services*, 2012).

## CONCLUSION

Reproductive and sexual health relies heavily on law, from allocating agency funding to regulating rights to access to services. Recognition of reproductive and sexual health rights has resulted in important benefits to individual, family, and community public health and well-being. While laws have both restricted and facilitated greater access over time and across different jurisdictions, it is clear that law remains one of the most critical factors in reproductive and sexual health throughout the life course.

## CHAPTER REVIEW

### Review Questions

1.  How has the Patient Protection and Affordable Care Act (ACA) impacted access to reproductive and sexual healthcare?
2.  What legal limitations might minors experience in accessing reproductive and sexual healthcare?
3.  How are reproductive rights balanced against the religious rights of providers and private health insurance plans? How might this balancing of rights impact access to reproductive and sexual healthcare?
4.  Which level of scrutiny applies when a court reviews an assertion of an equal protection violation on the basis of gender? What is the standard used to evaluate these claims?
5.  Which SCOTUS case changed the standard for reviewing whether an unconstitutional infringement on the right to abortion has occurred from the trimester framework to an undue burden analysis?
6.  From which parts of the Constitution does the right to privacy originate?

---

[3] Consolidated Appropriations Act, 2005, Pub. L. No. 108-447 § 508(d)(1), 118 Stat. 2809, 3163 (2004); Consolidated Appropriations Act, 2008, H.R. 2764 110th Cong. § 508(d)(1) (2007); Departments of Labor, Health and Human Services, Education, and Related Agencies Appropriations Act, 2006, Pub. L. No. 109-149, 119 Stat. 2833, 2851 (2006).

## Essay Question

Discuss how courts have struck a balance between protecting an individual's fundamental right to make their own reproductive health decisions and the rights of others involved in the decision-making process, such as parents or spouses. How is this different from the ways courts have approached the balance between an individual's fundamental right to make their own reproductive health decisions and the religious and moral objections of providers and other healthcare workers? Consider both the privacy and equal protection lines of cases in your analysis.

## Internet Activities

7.  Contraceptive Equity: State Comparisons and Advocacy Opportunities

    ■ Visit the Guttmacher Institute website. Find the publication on insurance coverage of contraception in each state. Compare your state's coverage to neighboring states. The National Health Law Program has put out a toolkit on Model Contraceptive Equity Acts for state advocates. Look at this publication. Compare the states you examined on Guttmacher's website with whether they have passed some kind of Contraceptive Equity legislation.
    ■ Guttmacher Institute: https://www.guttmacher.org
    ■ National Health Law Program, Contraceptive Equity Toolkit: https://healthlaw.org/resource/contraceptive-equity-in-action-a-toolkit-for-state-implementation

        □ Are there major differences in coverage and requirements between the states you examined?
        □ If you were to pick one state of those you looked at to improve coverage, which would you select and why?

8.  Youth Behavior Data

    ■ Go to the national Youth Risk Behavior Surveillance System and access the "Youth Online Data Analysis Tool." Examine variations in statistics for high school sexual health behavior across a few states.
    ■ CDC Youth Risk Behavior Surveillance System: https://www.cdc.gov/healthyyouth/data/yrbs/index.htm

        □ Develop a research question with a legal focus that you might want to investigate. For example: What legal factors might help explain the variations you see in state statistics?

## REFERENCES

42 C.F.R. § 431.51. https://doi.org/10.1017/CBO9781107415324.004
42 C.F.R. § 447.53(b)(5).
42 U.S.C. § 1396 et seq.
42 U.S.C. §§ 1396o(a)(2).
42 U.S.C. § 1396(a)(4)(C).
42 U.S.C. § 300a-7.
42 U.S.C. § 300gg-13(a)(4).
Ahmed, O., & Gamble, C. (2017). *Reproductive justice: What it means and why it matters (now, more than ever)*. https://www.publichealthpost.org/viewpoints/reproductive-justice

American College of Obstetricians and Gynecologists. (2013). Practice Bulletin No. 135: Second-trimester abortion. *Obstetrics and Gynecology, 121,* 1394–1406. https://doi.org/10.1097/01.AOG.0000431056.79334.cc

Bailey, M. J. (2013). Fifty years of family planning: New evidence on the long-run effects of increasing access to contraception. *Brookings Papers on Economic Activities, 2013,* 341–409. https://doi.org/10.1353/eca.2013.0001

*Bellotti v. Baird,* 443 U.S. 622 (1978). https://cdn.loc.gov/service/ll/usrep/usrep443/usrep443622/usrep443622.pdf

Braveman, P., Arkin, E., Orleans, T., Proctor, D., & Plough, A. (2017). *What is health equity?* https://www.rwjf.org/en/library/research/2017/05/what-is-health-equity-.html

Brindis, C. D., & Moore, K. (2014). Improving adolescent health policy: Incorporating a framework for assessing state-level policies. *Annual Review of Public Health, 35,* 343–361. https://doi.org/10.1146/annurev-publhealth-032013-182455

*Burwell v. Hobby Lobby* (2013). https://www.supremecourt.gov/opinions/13pdf/13-354_olp1.pdf

California Code Regs. § 22100. https://www.sos.ca.gov/administration/regulations/current-regulations/registries/safe-home-confidential-address-program/#22100

California Department of Health Care Services. (2020). *Abortions: Medi-Cal provider manual.* https://files.medi-cal.ca.gov/pubsdoco/Publications/masters-MTP/Part2/abort.pdf

*Carey v. Population Services International,* 431 U.S. 678 (1976). https://cdn.loc.gov/service/ll/usrep/usrep431/usrep431678/usrep431678.pdf

Centers for Disease Control and Prevention. (n.d.-a). *Sexually transmitted diseases surveillance 2018: STDs in adolescents and young adults.* https://www.cdc.gov/std/stats17/adolescents.htm

Centers for Disease Control and Prevention. (n.d.-b). Social determinants of health: Know what affects health. https://www.cdc.gov/socialdeterminants/index.htm

City Attorney of San Francisco. (2018). U.S. Supreme Court denies review of SF crisis pregnancy law, ordinance stands. https://www.sfcityattorney.org/2018/06/28/u-s-supreme-court-denies-review-sf-crisis-pregnancy-law-ordinance-stands

*Commonwealth of Massachusetts v. United States Department of Health and Human Services* 682 F.3d 1 (2012). https://www.leagle.com/decision/infco20120531000t

Consolidated Appropriations Act, 2005, Pub. L. No. 108-447 § 508(d)(1), 118 Stat. 2809, 3163 (2004).

Consolidated Appropriations Act, 2008, H.R. 2764 110th Cong. § 508(d)(1) (2007).

*Craig v. Borden,* 429 U.S. 190 (1976). https://cdn.loc.gov/service/ll/usrep/usrep429/usrep429190/usrep429190.pdf

Eisenstadt, L. (2003). Separation of church and hospital: Strategies to protect pro-choice physicians in religiously affiliated hospitals. *Yale Journal of Law and Feminism, 15.* https://digitalcommons.law.yale.edu/yjlf/vol15/iss2/2/

*Eisenstadt v. Baird,* 405 U.S. 438 (1972). (1971). https://cdn.loc.gov/service/ll/usrep/usrep405/usrep405438/usrep405438.pdf

Federalism. (n.d.). In *Wex Legal Dictionary.* Legal Information Institute. https://www.law.cornell.edu/wex/federalism

Fine, A., & Kottlechuck, M. (2010). *Rethinking MCH: The life course model as an organizing framework.* U.S. Department of Health and Human Services. https://www.hrsa.gov/sites/default/files/ourstories/mchb75th/images/rethinkingmch.pdf

Finer, L. B., Frohwirth, L. F., Dauphinee, L. A., Singh, S., & Moore, A. M. (2005). Reasons U.S. women have abortions: Quantitative and qualitative perspectives. *Perspectives on Sexual and Reproductive Health, 37*(3), 110–118. https://doi.org/10.1363/psrh.37.110.05

Greene Foster, D., Antonia Biggs, M., Ralph, L., Gerdts, C., Roberts, S., & Maria Glymour, M. (2018). Socioeconomic outcomes of women who receive and women who are denied wanted abortions in the United States. *Public Health, 108,* 407–413. https://doi.org/10.2105/AJPH.2017

*Griswold v. Connecticut,* 381 U.S. 479 (1965). (1964). https://cdn.loc.gov/service/ll/usrep/usrep381/usrep381479/usrep381479.pdf

Guttmacher Institute. (2019). *An overview of consent to reproductive health services by young people.* https://www.guttmacher.org/state-policy/explore/overview-minors-consent-law

Guttmacher Institute. (n.d.). *Refusing to provide health services.* https://www.guttmacher.org/state-policy/explore/refusing-provide-health-services

Halfon, N., Larson, K., Lu, M., Tullis, E., & Russ, S. (2014). Lifecourse health development: Past, present and future. *Maternal and Child Health Journal, 18,* 344–365. https://doi.org/10.1007/s10995 -013-1346-2

Health Resources & Services Administration. (2017). *Women's preventive services guidelines.* https:// www.hrsa.gov/womens-guidelines-2016/index.html

*Hodgson v. Minnesota,* 497 U.S. 417 (1989). https://cdn.loc.gov/service/ll/usrep/usrep497/usrep 497417/usrep497417.pdf

James, S. E., Herman, J. L., Rankin, S., Keisling, M., Mottet, L., & Anafi, M. (2016). *The report of the 2015 U.S. transgender survey.* https://transequality.org/sites/default/files/docs/usts/USTS-Full -Report-Dec17.pdf

Jones, R. K., & Jerman, J. (2017). Population group abortion rates and lifetime incidence of abortion: United States, 2008–2014. *American Journal of Public Health, 107*(12), 1904–1909. https:// doi.org/10.2105/AJPH.2017.304042

Kaiser Family Foundation. (2018). *Abstinence education programs: Definition, funding, and impact on teen sexual behavior.* https://www.kff.org/womens-health-policy/fact-sheet/abstinence-education -programs-definition-funding-and-impact-on-teen-sexual-behavior

Kennedy, C., & Baker, T. (2005). Changing demographics of public health graduates: Potential implications for the public health workforce. *Public Health Reports, 120*(3), 355–357. https://www .guttmacher.org/report/delays-in-accessing-care-among-us-abortion-patients

*Korematsu v. United States,* 323 U.S. 214 (1944). https://cdn.loc.gov/service/ll/usrep/usrep323 /usrep323214/usrep323214.pdf

Kritz, F. (2019). *Pharmacists can now prescribe birth control, but few do.* https://www.calhealthreport .org/2019/02/15/pharmacists-can-now-prescribe-birth-control-but-few-do-

Leichliter, J. S., Copen, C., & Dittus, P. J. (2017). Confidentiality issues and use of sexually transmitted disease services among sexually experienced persons aged 15–25 years—United States, 2013–2015. *Morbidity and Mortality Weekly Report, 66*(9), 237–241. https://doi.org/10.15585/mmwr.mm6609a1

Mamone, T., (2019, July 3). For trans men seeking reproductive health care: There are barriers every step of the way. *Rewire.* https://rewirenewsgroup.com/article/2019/07/03/trans-men -reproductive-health-care/

Maternal and Child Health Bureau. (n. d.) *MCH timeline.* https://mchb.hrsa.gov/about/timeline/ timeline-scrn-rdrs.html

Moran, P. (2018). *The Affordable Care Act's contraceptive mandate: A loss in Massachusetts and other current events.* https://www.mintz.com/insights-center/viewpoints/2226/2018-03-affordable -care-acts-contraceptive-mandate-loss

*Ohio v. Akron Center,* 497 U.S. 502 (1989). https://cdn.loc.gov/service/ll/usrep/usrep497/usrep497502 /usrep497502.pdf

*Planned Parenthood of Southeastern Pennsylvania v. Casey,* 505 U.S. 833 (1991). https://cdn .loc.gov/service/ll/usrep/usrep505/usrep505833/usrep505833.pdf

Public Law 111-17 § 507-08. (2010).

Ransom, M. M. (Ed.). (2016). *Public health law competency model: Version 1.0.* https://www.cdc.gov/ phlp/docs/phlcm-v1.pdf

*Roe v. Wade,* 410 U.S. 113 (1973). https://cdn.loc.gov/service/ll/usrep/usrep410/usrep410113/ usrep410113.pdf

Rosenzweig, C., Ranji, U., & Salganicoff, A. (2018). *Women's sexual and reproductive health services: Key findings from the 2017 Kaiser Women's Health Survey.* https://www.kff.org/womens-health -policy/issue-brief/womens-sexual-and-reproductive-health-services-key-findings-from-the -2017-kaiser-womens-health-survey

Stanger-Hall, K. F., & Hall, D. W. (2011). Abstinence-only education and teen pregnancy rates: Why we need comprehensive sex education in the U.S. *PLOS One, 6*(10), e24658. https://doi.org/ 10.1371/journal.pone.0024658

State Medicaid Manual §§ 441.208, 4432.B.2. (2005).

Stover, J., Hardee, K., Ganatra, B., García Moreno, C., & Horton, S. (2016). *Interventions to improve reproductive health. Reproductive, maternal, newborn, and child health: Disease control priorities, Third Edition (Volume 2).* The International Bank for Reconstruction and Development/The World Bank. https://doi.org/10.1596/978-1-4648-0348-2_CH6

*Tummino v. Hamburg* 936 F. Supp. 2d 162 (2013). https://www.leagle.com/decision/infdco20130408a25

United Nations. (2009). *Reproductive rights are human rights.* https://www.unfpa.org/sites/default/files/pub-pdf/NHRIHandbook.pdf

U.S. Department of Health and Human Services. (n.d.). *Conscience protections for health care providers.* https://www.hhs.gov/conscience/conscience-protections/index.html

*Whole Women's Health v. Hellerstedt,* 136 S. Ct. 2292 (2015). https://www.supremecourt.gov/opinions/15pdf/15-274_new_e18f.pdf

*Williamson v. Lee Optical Co.,* 348 U.S. 483 (1954). https://cdn.loc.gov/service/ll/usrep/usrep348/usrep348483/usrep348483.pdf

World Health Organization. Sexual and reproductive health. (n.d.). https://www.who.int/reproductivehealth/topics/engender_rights/sexual_health/en

## Additional Resources

- **National LGBT Health Education Center**
  - https://www.lgbthealtheducation.org/lgbt-education/webinars
- **Bixby Center for Global Reproductive Health**
  - https://bixbycenter.ucsf.edu/education-and-training
- **Centers for Disease Control and Prevention**
  - Women's Reproductive Health
    https://www.cdc.gov/reproductivehealth/womensrh/index.htm
  - Contraceptive and Reproductive Health Services for Teens
    https://www.cdc.gov/teenpregnancy/practitioner-tools-resources/contraceptive-reproductive-services.html
- **Health Resources Services Administration**
  - Maternal and Child Health Bureau
    https://mchb.hrsa.gov
- **Center for Reproductive Rights**
  - https://reproductiverights.org/resources
- **National Women's Law Center**
  - Health Care and Reproductive Rights
    https://nwlc.org/issue/health-care-reproductive-rights
- **Guttmacher Institute**
  - https://www.guttmacher.org
- **World Health Organization**
  - Reproductive Health https://www.who.int/reproductivehealth/en

# LAW: A TRANSDISCIPLINARY PUBLIC HEALTH TOOL

# 17

# Law as a Social Determinant of Health

Jason A. Smith

## Learning Objectives

By the end of this chapter, the reader will be able to:

- Define health as a social phenomenon.
- Describe the social determinants of health.
- Distinguish between intermediate social determinants of health and structural determinants.
- Define health inequities.
- Describe the influence of racism in understanding health disparities.

## Key Terminology

**Health inequities:** differences in health that are socially produced, systemic, and unfair.
**Intermediate determinants of health:** the places where people live and work.
**Social determinants of health:** the factors that affect the health of communities and populations.
**Socioeconomic position:** description of the access to resources and to power based on an individual's social position.
**Structural determinants of health:** the context, socioeconomic position of individuals, and the institutions and mechanisms that create and maintain stratifications that affect health.

## Public Health Law Competencies

This chapter addresses the following competencies from the Public Health Law Competency Model (PHLCM; Ransom, 2016):

**1.1** Define basic constitutional concepts and legal principles framing the practice of public health across relevant jurisdictions.
**2.3** Recognize the legal authority and limits of critical system partners and others who influence health outcomes.

**Spark Questions**

1. What is an example of a law that affects where people live and work and their health?
2. What is an example of a law that creates social stratification that underlies health inequity?
3. How do laws relate to health outcomes, including how they relate to health disparities and health equity?
4. What are some examples of the relationship between law and the determinants of health?
5. What are some ways in which law might be understood as a determinant of health?

## INTRODUCTION

This chapter discusses human health and the role that social and environmental factors have in either supporting or weakening health for individuals, communities, and society. Individual choices about health matter less than the larger forces setting the context for our lives. This is followed by discussing the law's role as the primary force in shaping that context. The chapter also discusses the role that racism has played in understanding the law and **social determinants of health.**

## SOCIAL DETERMINANTS OF HEALTH AND HEALTH EQUITY

### Defining Health

Before discussing the social and structural determinants, it is essential to review what we mean by "health". Health itself is difficult to define in a clear and measurable way upon which we can all agree. The definition of health provided by the World Health Organization (WHO) has remained a standard definition, "Health is a state of complete physical, mental and social well-being and not merely the absence of disease or infirmity" (WHO, 1948, p. 100). This definition of health situates health clearly in the domain of the social. *Social* simply signals that individuals' interactions with others define individual human life and experience. These interactions and interactions with the environment impact the health of individuals and the health of populations.

Sean Valles, a scholar of population health, has described how our shared definition of health is social in four important ways: *metaphysically, empirically, ethically,* and *methodologically*. That health is not merely defined using a biomedical approach and that it includes our mental and social well-being is *metaphysically social*. That health is affected by social determinants and can be measured is *empirically social*. That health is related to empowerment and social justice is *ethically social*. Finally, the relationship between health and social structures can be measured, making health *methodologically social*.

Given that human health is firmly rooted in the social, what then are the social factors that determine individuals' and populations' health?

### Social Determinants of Health

The social determinants of health are factors that determine the health of individuals and populations. The simplest definition of "social determinants of health" are the "conditions in the environments where people are born, live, learn, work, play, worship, and age that affect a wide range of health, functioning, and quality-of-life outcomes and risks" (Office of Disease Prevention and Health Promotion, n.d., para. 1) This definition of the social determinants of health asks us to look beyond the individual and to ask questions about the environment in which that person lives. The physical environment and neighborhood can affect health outcomes depending on pollution, crime, housing policy, and many other factors—place matters. Differences in where people live and work and differences from social stratification affect the health and welfare of individuals more powerfully than individual factors alone. Some estimates suggest that the provision of individual medical care can account for at most 20% of population health. Environmental and social determinants provide the remaining 80% in affecting human health. Daniel Dawes points out in his work that additional life expectancy in the United States cannot be achieved by relying on biomedical approaches alone. The key to health equity and improving population health is addressing the social determinants of health upstream, and law is key to that project.

This definition is only a starting point. We must also be more specific in our inquiry. Are the conditions in which people live random? Do they improve health or worsen it? How did these conditions come to be? These questions ask us to evaluate the differences among environments and populations. This evaluation of differences in social stratification and environments is the basis of health equity. Health equity is subsistent in the social determinants of health.

## Health Equity and Systems

There are differences in health among individuals, groups, and societies. When those differences are socially produced, systematic, and unfair, they are **health inequities**. Differences that are socially made are differences that derive from the operating social context. For example, suppose I cycle and my neighbor does not and does not wish to. In that case, my knee-related pain associated with poor bike fit is a health difference but not a health disparity or health inequity because it is not related to socioeconomic context but only different preferences about exercise. These health differences must also be systematic—driven by the interactions of other parts, working together, for a purpose or result. For this discussion, a systemic difference is one that is the result of interactions in a system rather than a random phenomenon. Donna Meadows offers an outstanding, entry level overview of systems, their operation, characteristics, and changing them. (See Meadows, 2008). That a system has a particular purpose or intention in its actions does not mean that the participants in that system necessarily intend that purpose. Finally, the differences in health must be unfair or based on divisions and circumstances and conditions that are unjust or biased in their origins. Focusing on health equity in evaluating the social determinants of health means that we must evaluate differences between individuals, groups, and societies based on this three-part test. If the differences meet this test, they represent a health inequity and should be remedied.

## SOCIAL DETERMINANTS OF HEALTH AND STRUCTURAL DETERMINANTS OF HEALTH

In the previous discussion, the social determinants of health were defined as the conditions and environments where people live their lives. Relying on this definition alone, the effect of larger systems, structures, and decisions are hidden and can appear natural or ahistorical. What are the factors that affect these environmental factors and social conditions? To answer this more important question, it is better to rely on the WHO conceptual framework of social determinants of health as it provides a greater depth of analysis than the version discussed previously. In the WHO framework, the conditions in which people live and work are their intermediary social determinants. These intermediary social determinants operate as downstream factors affecting health. These intermediate determinants are created by the socioeconomic and political context and by structural mechanisms. The context refers to the institutions, values, and systems that "generate, configure and maintain social hierarchies"

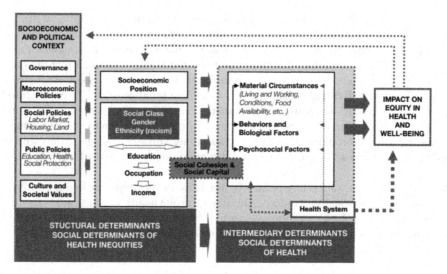

**FIGURE 17.1** Framework developed by the WHO Commission on Social Determinants of Health.

(WHO, 2010, p. 5). This context employs structural mechanisms such as law, policy, and power to create the socioeconomic context which produces the intermediary social determinants. (See Figure 17.1.) The context, structural mechanisms, socioeconomic and environmental positions, and their interactions are the structural determinants (WHO, 2010, p. 28). These structural determinants "generate or reinforce stratification in the society and … define individual socioeconomic position" (WHO, 2010, p. 34). The WHO framework allows the examination of not only the environments and conditions in which people live, work, and play but also the examination of the larger structural forces and conditions that produce those environments. Discussions of the social determinants of health must not focus only on the intermediary determinants of health—the conditions of living—but must also include the structural determinants of health that produce these intermediate conditions and that are created, supported, and impacted by law.

## LAW AS A DETERMINANT OF HEALTH

The law is a determinant of health and operates in four ways. First, the law can be a set of commands, requirements, or prohibitions on action. Traffic safety laws are a clear example. The law requires helmets and seat belts for operating motorcycles and automobiles respectively. These commands require action and are linked to a punishment—usually a fine—for noncompliance. These requirements—helmet laws—change the environment in which individuals ride and drive and have reduced death and injuries in accidents. The Highway Safety Act of 1966 allowed the federal government to withhold up to 10% of funds from states without a motorcycle helmet requirement. This led to 47 states having required motorcycle helmet laws. In the 1990s, those federal requirements were lifted with a number of states repealing their helmet requirements. States that did so saw an increase in fatalities related to motorcycle use.

Second, law creates processes and procedures for making decisions, creating new laws, and for interpreting existing laws. As discussed in Chapter 2, the Constitutional framework in the United States assigns power for public health primarily to the state governments, not federal. The law also structures the values and processes applied to resolving controversies. *San Antonio Independent School District v. Rodriquez* provides a good example. In this Supreme Court case, parents brought suit alleging that the school financing system in Texas, relying on property tax, was discriminatory and interfered with a fundamental right to education. The Supreme Court found that wealth was not a suspect classification and rejected the claims. The Court's analysis was based on a history of interpretation and analysis that framed the question in a way that disregarded the history of housing and educational segregation and the relationship of socioeconomic status to race and a history of racism. The rules of interpretation did not have a *direct* impact on health in the way that the motorcycle helmet law might but have a more distal and more profound effect at a systemic level by foreclosing a right to education in the U.S. Constitution.

Third, law represents a set of norms and expectations that can influence behavior, even in the absence of a command, prohibition, or requirement. The perception of medical malpractice liability under the system of torts, for example, can alter the practice of medicine. While the actual relationship of tort litigation to healthcare costs is contentious, the idea of defensive medicine rooted in norms and expectations, valid or not, associated with tort liability in the United States is a powerful one that impacts clinical behavior and thus impacts health policy and regulation.

Finally, law organizes rights and obligations that individuals have. At its core, law structures and outlines the power relationships in society and the political context which are fundamental to human health and flourishing. This aspect of law can also be described as the political determinants of health. "Political determinants of health involve the systematic processes of structuring relationships, distributing resources, and administering power, operating simultaneously in ways that mutually reinforce or influence one another to shape opportunities that either advance health equity or exacerbate health inequities" (Dawes, 2020, p. 44)

For this chapter, the discussion focuses on how the law creates, ameliorates, and intensifies health inequities and acts as a powerful determinant of health. At the structural level, law sets the policies and values that have widespread effect creating the environments in which people live, the intermediary determinants of health. The effects of law and the use of law as a tool to address the social determinants of health and health inequity can be grouped based on the structure discussed. At the most immediate and proximate level, the law can be used to reduce the impact of health inequities. At the intermediary level, the law can be used to reduce exposures to conditions that impact health. At the structural level, law can be used to both create inequities in **socioeconomic positions** as well as be used as a tool to address those inequities. The opioid epidemic provides a useful example to explore the role of law as a social determinant of health.

## Example: The Opioid Epidemic

The opioid epidemic has grown over the past three decades to become a major public health concern in the United States. In 2019, there were 70,360 overdose deaths with 70.6% of those death involving opioids and 51.5% involving synthetic opioids (Mattson et al., 2021). Since 1999, over 400,000 people have died from overdose (Centers for Disease Control and Prevention, n.d.). This epidemic is complex in its origin and is profoundly influenced by the law.

The epidemic has three phases. In the first phase beginning in 1999, an increase in opioid prescriptions led to an increase in opioid use and overdose deaths. In the second phase, beginning in 2010, heroin use increased with an increase in overdose deaths related to heroin. In the third phase, beginning in 2013, the use of synthetic opioids increased, particularly illegally made fentanyl. The use of fentanyl along with the inclusion of fentanyl in other illicit drugs—often without the knowledge of the user—has further driven overdose deaths. The epidemic of overdose deaths has been intertwined with the law which has had a profound effect.

The initial phase of the epidemic was driven by an increase in prescriptions of opioids for pain management. As the number of people using opioids increased along with an increase in dependence, the number of overdose deaths began to also increase. Governments sought a legal and policy solution to this problem and tried to restrict access to prescription opioids using prescription drug–monitoring programs (PDMP). These programs allow healthcare providers and systems to monitor and share information about opioid prescriptions and increase oversight of prescriptions, making it more difficult to obtain prescription opioids. The legal intervention was designed to address an intermediary social determinant of health—the relative ease of access to prescription opioids—and present the use of the law as a command or requirement. The intervention itself then became a structural determinant of the second wave of the epidemic. As it became more difficult to obtain prescription opioids, more people who used drugs switched to heroin, "which became more easily available at a lower cost" (Park et al., 2020). This second wave of the epidemic resulted in additional law enforcement action to restrict heroin supply. This led to users turning toward synthetic opioids like fentanyl which is "50 times more potent than heroin and accounts for 40% of overdose deaths" (Park et al., 2020, p. 8). These legal interventions were altering the environment making the opioids that were available for new drug users more dangerous than previous environments.

The law also drives the opioid epidemic in more structural and significant ways. Drug initiation is associated with structural racism and inequality as well as with a lack of affordable housing. These same factors as well as homelessness are associated with addiction and with overdose risk. The law is a driver in each of these areas. For example, a number of practices using law as a tool have been employed to enforce housing segregation. The law has been used to enforce explicit zoning exclusions based on race, to enact exclusionary zoning practices such as single-family zoning, and to support predatory and exploitative lending practices. During the New Deal, the Public Works Administration specifically segregated housing projects between Black and White. This policy of segregation continued into the construction of worker housing for World War II as well as in federal public housing projects through the mid-20th century. These policies by the federal government had the effect of introducing Jim Crow practices into regions where it did not exist (Rothstein, 2018). These policies, and others, created an environment in many areas that exacerbated problems of housing affordability, homelessness, racial segregation, and mobility. All were associated with health risk in the opioid epidemic, and, in many ways, root causes to that epidemic.

### Targeting Inequality Structurally

It is possible to use the law to target inequality at a structural level and to achieve health equity. Park et. al outline a number of actions that can be taken in law to address the opioid crisis. Laws currently in place often politically disenfranchise people who have been incarcerated. Drug convictions can be used to prevent individuals from obtaining student financial aid, employment, access to housing, and from participating in the political process. Changing these legal policies can be a powerful step in empowering communities in the political process. Focusing on structural laws, such as exclusionary zoning, that maintain segregation in housing can be used to support efforts to reduce overdose deaths. Removing legal barriers to overdose prevention sites (OPS) is another legal tool that can be used to target health inequities structurally. Overdose prevention sites are sites that provide a space for users to safely use drugs with supervision. OPS can reduce risks of overdose and help reduce infectious diseases associated with injection drug use. Finally, focusing on poverty, homelessness, systemic racism, and the root causes of these processes provides a way to focus on structural solutions.

## RACISM AS A PUBLIC HEALTH ISSUE

Racism has been and continues to be a powerful force affecting public health in the United States. The long-standing structures rooted in racial bias have had on-going effects on the health of individuals and of communities. In the United States, racism has been enacted, enforced, and supported by law. Racism is a complex and multifaceted reality. Byrd and Clayton's discussion of racism and the history of the healthcare system in the United States outlines some of the core features of racism. First, racism is the intentional and unintentional distribution of power and resources in society and the ongoing enforcement of the inequity based on an imposed ethnocentrism that justifies that ethnocentrism for the benefit of the other group or by blaming the other group (Byrd & Clayton, 2000, p. 36). The law has been used repeatedly to enforce and enact this type of racism. The imposition of chattel slavery in the United States is the most explicit example. Other, more modern examples include the Chinese Exclusion Act which specifically excluded Chinese immigration to the United States from 1882–1943 and the imposition of segregation across the United States in the 20th century. Second, racism is the belief in race as a determinative factor in human traits, capabilities, and behaviors. The law has also been used to enforce this racist belief. The widespread use of theories of eugenics were influential in legal decision-making with *Buck v. Bell* being the most well-known example. Third, racism can refer to structural inequities based on race that are no longer rooted in explicit animus and that operate in the background. Ongoing segregation in housing in the United States reflects this aspect of racism.

Chattel slavery and its legacy continue to impact public health and the healthcare system today. The system of chattel slavery in the United States was protected by law from the founding of the Republic through the Civil War. Chattel slavery and the slave trade together with a ubiquitous rhetoric of White supremacy laid the foundations of mistrust and exploitation that are still experienced today. From the widespread medical experimentation on enslaved peoples to ongoing exploitation of African American communities in biomedical research in the United States, this intentional exploitation has moved from intentional racism to structural racism and set the foundation for ongoing mistrust and skepticism that is evident today. The use of law was used to stratify U.S. society by race and class following the Civil War with the failure of Reconstruction; the resurgence of the Southern plantation system through sharecropping, the restriction of African American civil rights and ongoing exploitation, and federal housing policy. The resurgence of domestic terrorism and rising fundamentalism also exacerbated this stratification. These ongoing systemic actions throughout the 20th century have resulted in a highly stratified society and a healthcare and public health system that reflects that stratification. These stratifications and their maintenance were also key to blocking efforts to reform the United States healthcare system.

The role of racism and these different manifestations in the history and development of the public health and healthcare systems is profound and impossible to fully explore in this short chapter. Racism and social stratification are deeply entangled with the history of the public health system, and law has played a key role in creating and enforcing that stratification. This very brief section is only to highlight the importance of understanding the historical socioeconomic context and the outsized role of racism in U.S. history in order to understand health equity and the social determinants of health today. The profound racial disparities in the COVID-19 pandemic have surfaced how profound these inequities remain in U.S. society. As Chowkwanyun and Reed argue persuasively, it is critical to understand this historical context to avoid perpetrating racist stereotypes and analysis in trying to understand health disparities. It is also critical to equally link historical context of racism and discrimination to socioeconomic status, stress, and place-based discrimination (Chowkwanyun & Reed, 2020). These differences between socioeconomic status, stress, and place have roots in a history of discrimination.

## CONCLUSION

Law is the fundamental determinant of health. It makes possible and prohibits. It can create differences and erase them. It allocates resources and political and economic power. This fundamental role of law makes it ubiquitous. Given its ubiquity and fundamental nature, this chapter has sought to provide only a framework and to point toward the role of law. A brief investigation of any persistent health inequity and health disparity will uncover the role that law has in creating the environment that makes that disparity possible. Finally, to focus on health disparities without addressing their root causes is to fundamentally avoid addressing them. Law provides not only the tools to improve the experience of intermediate health disparities, but also to remedy them structurally. No other health intervention has this power and flexibility.

# CHAPTER REVIEW

## Review Questions

1. What makes motorcycle helmet law a unique example for studying how laws determine health outcomes?
2. What is an example of how a law relates to the social determinants of health in your community?
3. What makes zoning a unique example for studying how laws are related to health outcomes?
4. How has the law shaped and exacerbated the opioid epidemic in the United States?

## Essay Question

Read the sentence below and identify all the possible determinants of health that are related to this health outcome. Why do these determinants exist? How might law relate to this health outcome?

Minorities, foreign-born persons, and persons who speak Spanish or another non-English language at home were more likely to be living near major highways in 2010, suggesting increased exposure to traffic-related air pollution and elevated risk for adverse health outcomes.

## Internet Activities

1. Watch the video entitled Housing Segregation and Redlining in America: A Short History https://www.youtube.com/watch?v=O5FBJyqfoLM, and write a one-page paper offering your reflections on the following:
   - What is redlining? Where does the word come from?
   - What policies led to the practice of redlining?
   - In what ways are the racial health inequities we see today a consequence of redlining?

## REFERENCES

Braveman, P. A. (2003). Monitoring equity in health and healthcare: A conceptual framework. Journal of Health, Population and Nutrition, 21(3), 181–192. https://www.jstor.org/stable/23499216

Byrd, W. M., & Clayton, L. A. (2000). An American health dilemma: A medical history of African Americans and the problem of race: Beginnings to 1900. Taylor & Francis Group.

Centers for Disease Control and Prevention. (n.d.). Understanding the epidemic. https://www.cdc.gov/drugoverdose/epidemic/index.html

Chowkwanyun, M., & Reed, A. L. (2020). Racial health disparities and COVID-19—Caution and context. New England Journal of Medicine, 383(3), 201–203. https://doi.org/10.1056/NEJMp2012910

Dawes, D. E. (2020). The political determinants of health. Johns Hopkins University Press.

Mattson, C. L., Tanz, L. J., Quinn, K., Kariisa, M., Patel, P., & Davis, N. L. (2021). Trends and geographic patterns in drug and synthetic opioid overdose deaths—United States, 2013–2019. Mortality and Morbidity Weekly Report, 70, 202–207. http://dx.doi.org/10.15585/mmwr.mm7006a4

Meadows, D. H. (2008). Thinking in systems: A primer. Chelsea Green Publishing.

Office of Disease Prevention and Health Promotion. (n.d.). Social determinants of health. https://health.gov/healthypeople/objectives-and-data/social-determinants-health

Park, J. N., Rouhani, S., Beletsky, L., Vincent, L., Saloner, B., & Sherman, S. G. (2020). Situating the continuum of overdose risk in the social determinants of health: A new conceptual framework. The Milbank Quarterly, 98(3), 700–746. https://doi.org/10.1111/1468-0009.12470

Ransom, M. M. (2016). Public health law competency model: Version 1.0. CDC. https://www.cdc.gov/phlp/docs/phlcm-v1.pdf

Rothstein, R. (2018). *The color of law: A forgotten history of how our government segregated America.* Liveright.

World Health Organization. (1948). Preamble to the Constitution of WHO as adopted by the International Health Conference, New York, 19 June–22 July 1946; signed on 22 July 1946 by the representatives of 61 States (Official Records of WHO, no. 2, p. 100) and entered into force on 7 April 1948.

World Health Organization. (2010). *A conceptual framework for action on the social determinants of health: Debates, policy & practice, case studies.* http://apps.who.int/iris/bitstream/10665/44489/1/9789241500852_eng.pdf

## Additional Resources

- **Guest Chair's Column: Dying to Belong: Racism as a Public Health Issue**
    - https://www.americanbar.org/groups/health_law/publications/health_lawyer_home/2020-june/chair/
- **A Pitt Law moderated the virtual Town Hall, Law as a Social Determinant of Health, in response to the COVID-19 pandemic.**
    - https://www.youtube.com/watch?v=tnccr7oNvNM
- **From Health Care Law to the Social Determinants of Health: A Public Health Law Research Perspective**
    - https://scholarship.law.upenn.edu/penn_law_review/vol159/iss6/3/

# 18

# Health in All Policies

Maxim Gakh and Rosa Abraha

## Learning Objectives

By the end of this chapter, the reader will be able to:

- Analyze the approach of Health in All Policies (HiAP) and its potential to address the social determinants of health to promote health equity.
- Compare law-based and non-law-based HiAP initiatives and appraise the advantages and disadvantages of each.
- Formulate a law-based HiAP strategy and assess its potential strengths and challenges.
- Identify examples of HiAP in action at the state, local, and national levels.
- Recognize the role of law in promoting a HiAP strategy.

## Key Terminology

**Health in All Policies (HiAP):** A systematic approach to incorporate health concerns across decisions that normally do not consider health but nevertheless have health consequences (Institute of Medicine [IOM], 2011).

**Health Equity:** When all have a fair chance to reach their health potential and when health potential is not impeded by social factors or positions (Braveman, 2003).

**Health Impact Assessment (HIA):** A systematic process that uses research, data, analysis, and stakeholder feedback to determine the possible health effects and their distribution of a policy, project, or plan and to recommend ways to maximize health (National Research Council [NRC], 2011).

**Social Determinants of Health:** Social factors, systems, and conditions created through choices that shape how resources and power are distributed and that affect health outcomes and can impede health equity (Marmot et al., 2008).

## Public Health Law Competencies

This chapter addresses the following competencies from the Public Health Law Competency Model (PHLCM; Ransom, 2016).

**1.1** Describe the public health laws and regulations governing public health programs and related practices.

**2.2** Describe how law and legal practices contribute to the current health status of the population.

267

2.3 Distinguish public health agency powers and responsibilities from those of other governmental agencies, executive offices, police, legislatures, and courts.

---

### Spark Questions

1. What is one way that law contributes to health inequity in your community?
2. What organizations or entities in your community can have an impact on health?

---

## INTRODUCTION

## Health in All Policies (HiAP) in the Context of the Social Determinants of Health and Health Equity

Clinical care is vital for both prevention and treatment but is a comparatively weak health determinant (Artiga & Hinton, 2018). Public health recognizes that social factors are critical in shaping health outcomes and **health equity** realities. Collectively, health behaviors, physical environments, and social and economic factors are responsible for the vast majority of community health outcomes and their too-often inequitable distributions (County Health Rankings & Roadmaps, University of Wisconsin School of Medicine and Public Health, Wisconsin Population Health Institute, n.d.).

Public health models and frameworks try to capture how and why this is the case. For example, the Social-Ecological Model posits that factors at the individual, interpersonal, community,

---

### BOX 18.1 NON-HEALTH SECTORS SHAPE HEALTH OUTCOMES AND INEQUITIES

Many factors impact health outcomes and can impede health equity. One model often employed in public health attributes 20% of health outcomes to clinical care and the remainder to other factors—10% to the physical environment, 30% to health-related behaviors, and 40% to social and economic factors (County Health Rankings & Roadmaps, n.d.). HiAP tries to integrate health concerns across decisions so that all factors that shape health outcomes consider it.

---

### BOX 18.2 RELEVANT LEGAL PRINCIPLES AND FRAMEWORKS

1. Government's legal duty—a requirement that necessitates specific action by a governmental entity, or what a governmental entity must do. Legal duties may lead to actions with health implications.
2. Government's legal power—the authority of a governmental entity to engage in specific actions, or what a governmental entity may do. Legal powers may be exercised in ways that have health implications.
3. Legal mechanism—a constitutional provision, ballot initiative or referendum, statute or ordinance, rule or regulation, decision of a judicial or administrative body, enforceable agreement, or other law-based instrument that establishes or implements governmental policy.
4. Public laws—laws that target relationships among governmental entities and between governmental entities and private parties (Garner, 2001).

institutional, and policy levels all affect health outcomes and inequities (Max et al., 2015) and that public health interventions are most effective when they can simultaneously target multiple levels (DiClemente et al., 2007). Similarly, the Health Impact Pyramid suggests five areas of focus for public health interventions organized in a vertical pyramid from top to bottom: personal education (e.g., nutrition education), clinical interventions (e.g., blood pressure medications), long-lasting protective interventions (e.g., immunizations), changing environments to make default decisions health-promoting (e.g., building walkable cities), and socioeconomic factors (e.g., educational attainment) (Frieden, 2010). While all five areas are important, the Health Impact Pyramid emphasizes that modifying environmental and socioeconomic factors (i.e., the base of the pyramid) is especially critical because interventions closest to the base have the potential to impact the greatest number of people simultaneously (Frieden, 2010).

Despite the recognized importance of the **social determinants of health**, a central challenge for public health practitioners is how to intervene effectively. Ventures into Public Health 3.0 are important (DeSalvo et al., 2017). But they may also seem daunting. Changing the social determinants, particularly ones that involve social and economic structures, "might require fundamental social transformation" (Frieden, 2010). And many major social determinants of health, such as poverty, are complex with many uncoordinated players both contributing to and attempting to ameliorate the problem (Kania & Kramer, 2011). In addition, practical barriers to changing the social determinants of health include knowledge gaps in what works and resolve gaps manifested in limited commitment to change.

The **HiAP** approach presents a promising vehicle to modify the social determinants. HiAP is a big, systems-change idea. HiAP, at its core, aims to integrate health concerns systematically across decisions made by sectors that typically do not consider health (IOM, 2011). These sectors include agriculture, education, housing, transportation, planning, and employment (IOM, 2011). Incorporating health considerations into decisions made by these sectors may help emphasize their collateral health consequences—even if a decision, on its face, appears not to be about health (IOM, 2011). HiAP often relies on wide-ranging approaches and intersectoral partnerships outside of public health to achieve this aim (IOM, 2011; Office of Disease Prevention and Health Promotion [ODPHP], U.S. Department of Health and Human Services [DHHS], 2019). HiAP is by nature interdisciplinary and cross-sectoral because the policies and practices that create the social determinants are interdisciplinary and cross-sectoral.

The HiAP idea may seem relatively straightforward. But what does HiAP look like on the ground? Adoption and implementation of the HiAP concept is malleable and differs widely across jurisdictions and communities. HiAP can be pursued through various formal and informal mechanisms and processes (IOM, 2011). It can be adopted and implemented in the forms that are most contextually appropriate. This flexibility is helpful because different social determinants may involve various stakeholders, policies, and practices and vary by community. However, flexibility also means that communities and jurisdictions must tailor their HiAP initiatives. Nevertheless, a thorough review by Rudolph and colleagues articulate five elements of successful HiAP implementation: (1) a focus on health and equity, (2) cross-sectoral partnerships, (3) mutually beneficial collaborations, (4) stakeholder engagement, and (5) modification of existing processes (Rudolph et al., 2013).

## HiAP in Public Health Practice

HiAP complements the work of health departments and public health systems. The U.S. public health system is by nature a complex, interdisciplinary, and cross-sectoral web of multiple governmental agencies, nonprofit organizations, business entities, and civil society organizations and the policies and practices they adopt and implement (IOM, 1988). HiAP involves engaging stakeholders that are part of this system.

HiAP initiatives are critical for health departments. For example, two of the 10 Essential Public Health Services are to "create, champion and implement policies, plans, and laws" and to "utilize legal and regulatory actions" (CDC, 2020). HiAP initiatives can involve supporting policies in other sectors, such as working with the educational sector to enhance educational attainment, or supporting legal actions that originate in other sectors, such as working with housing agencies to enforce housing codes (CDC, n.d.). Health department accreditation standards also call for health departments both to inform decision-makers and the public about health impacts of policies, including policies from outside the health sector, and to help develop data-driven, health-promoting policies (Public Health Accreditation Board [PHAB], 2013).

HiAP efforts can also be rooted in more traditional public health work. The cross sector collaboration aspects of implementing school-based immunization laws, for example, can be the foundation for or further HiAP efforts. And many of the skills needed for HiAP implementation are the same skills needed for implementing school-based vaccination laws: collaborating, monitoring and using data, tracking and changing policies and practices, engaging with stakeholders, and connecting science to policy and practice.

In addition, HiAP strategies can be structured around specific health targets centered on the social determinants of health. *Healthy People 2030*, for instance, contains objectives related to poverty, employment and income, food insecurity, educational attainment, criminal justice, and housing (ODPHP, n.d.). Achieving these objectives necessitates collaborating with sectors outside of health.

## SELECTED CONCEPTS AND FEDERAL AND STATE LEGAL FRAMEWORKS

### HiAP Efforts That Do Not Rely on Legal Mechanisms

The central aim of HiAP is to integrate health concerns into decisions made by sectors that affect health but usually do not consider health (IOM, 2011). Private sector organizations (e.g., retailers, farmers, financial institutions, landlords) frequently make business decisions with health consequences (e.g., pricing of more and less nutritious foods, antibiotics use in animal populations, economic investment in vulnerable communities, investment in housing stock), often with the backdrop of regulation. The private sector can be a crucial HiAP partner in part because of the magnitude, reach, and frequency of its decision-making.

However, government is a key player in HiAP initiatives because of its responsibility and accountability to the community. Governmental HiAP initiatives can be implemented in different ways, some of which do not involve modification of laws. For example, with federal funding assistance, Prince George's County, Maryland worked with partners from various sectors to operationalize HiAP through: (a) access to healthy foods for SNAP participants at farmers' markets, (b) trainings on preventing crime through environmental design, and (c) gap identification in existing school wellness policies (Institute for Public Health Innovation [IPHI], n.d.). Although initiatives like these may not involve changes to law, they are nevertheless subject to existing laws and policies, including ones that come with federal grants.

Governmental agencies can also formalize HiAP efforts through policies that do not rise to the level of law, such as strategic plans, state health improvement plans and community health improvement plans, internal agency policies, and land-use plans (Rudolph et al., 2013). For example, the 2018 to 2020 Strategic Plan for the health department in Licking County, Ohio contains an objective to assist other entities in adopting HiAP (Licking County Health Department [LCHD], 2018). Similarly, the Metropolitan Planning Organization (MPO) in Florida's Hillsborough County adopted a resolution that recognizes the connections between transportation and health, invokes HiAP, articulates a continued commitment to working with the health department to consider health in MPO decisions, and commits to "consider and report" impacts on health based on preselected "transportation and health indicators" (Hillsborough County Metropolitan Planning Organization, Florida [HCMPO], 2019). Such policies may help catalyze or implement HiAP.

## The Role of Law in Supporting HiAP

Legal mechanisms can create and enshrine HiAP efforts at every level of government. Law can be used "for institutionalizing an infrastructure for HiAP and for requiring agencies to ensure that the policies they pursue serve … health" (IOM, 2011). Legal mechanisms can also help create conditions that support HiAP implementation. Laws can allow leaders to create a collective agenda around a health issue, require or authorize collaboration across agencies, establish institutions for collaboration and assign responsibilities, and even provide funding (Gakh, 2015). And, like in other areas of public health, legal mechanisms can impede HiAP efforts.

Various legal tools may be used to pursue HiAP. They include statutes, ordinances, and resolutions adopted by legislative bodies; rules or regulations established by administrative entities like health departments or boards of health and orders issued by executive officials like governors and mayors; memoranda of understanding among governmental agencies or between governmental agencies and nongovernmental organizations; contracts and grants in which a governmental entity is a party; and litigation efforts.

Legal mechanisms can support HiAP through two complementary paths: (a) encouraging *private* entities to think about health impacts and (b) modifying *public* structures and processes— that is, how governmental entities function and interact with each other in order to consider health broadly. Both paths are forms of "public law," which focus on relationships among governmental entities or between governments and private parties (Garner, 2001, p. 571).

## Laws That Support HiAP by Regulating Private Parties

Through legal mechanisms, governments can encourage private entities to think about health, often without mentioning "HiAP" or "health equity." Guam law creates a process to abate "business privilege taxes" for "gross receipts derived from the construction of affordable housing," which is available to developers, contractors, or others who create at least 25 units of affordable housing (12 Guam Code Ann. § 58127.6 [West 2020]). Thus, a developer may be more likely to produce affordable housing units because the abatement has made their construction less expensive. In this instance, the government is using tax law as it applies to private parties to encourage the development of affordable housing—a health determinant tied to equity.

Similarly, over half of U.S. states and territories have used legal mechanisms to adopt Renewable Portfolio Standards, which require certain electricity suppliers to obtain a percentage of electricity from renewable energy sources (National Conference of State Legislatures [NCSL], 2020) such as wind and solar. Although market dynamics are also important in the use of renewable energy (NCSL, 2020), this type of standard encourages production and consumption of electricity generated from renewable sources, potentially reducing the carbon emissions that contribute to climate change.

## Laws That Support HiAP by Focusing on Government

Many law-based HiAP efforts target how governmental entities interact and make decisions. An example from Vermont demonstrates how law can create a stand-alone governmental entity focused on HiAP, align governmental agencies representing different sectors around health, and integrate health across governmental decisions. A gubernatorial executive order creates the Vermont HiAP Task Force comprising representatives from state agencies that make health-related governmental decisions, including education, agriculture, transportation, and natural resources (Vt. Exec. Order No. 07-15 [Oct. 6, 2015]). The order requires the Task Force to "identify strategies to more fully integrate health considerations into all state programs and policies" and requires its members to report "progress in embedding health impacts into their rulemaking, policies, and programs" (Vt. Exec. Order No. 07-15 [Oct. 6, 2015]). The state health department must lead the Task Force and create "guidance, criteria and analytic tools [ … to help] all branches of government in assessing potential positive or negative health impacts when proposing new agency rules, budgetary changes or major programmatic shifts" (Vt. Exec. Order No. 07-15 [Oct. 6, 2015]).

Legal mechanisms can also be used to integrate health into decision-making in more targeted ways, often by establishing partnerships. For example, at the federal level, the Patient Protection and Affordable Care Act (ACA) created the National Prevention, Health Promotion and Public Health Council (42 U.S.C. §300u-10). The requirement assembles a group of high-level federal leaders from sectors like transportation, education, agriculture, and labor to establish a National Prevention Strategy with specific objectives, tactics, and timelines for what the federal government and others can do to advance prevention nationwide (42 U.S.C § 300u-10). One practical "result" has been healthier food options and places to engage in physical activity around federal governmental buildings (IOM, 2015). Similarly, a Washington State statute requires the state board of health to conduct "health impact reviews" of proposed legislative and budgetary decisions at the request of the governor or state legislators, but permits limiting reviews based on feasibility concerns (Wash. Rev. Code Ann. § 43.20.285 [West, 2020]). Likewise, the Massachusetts "Healthy Transportation Compact," enshrined in state statute, sets out "a healthy transportation policy" centered on cooperation among several state departments, including health and transportation, in order to adopt "best practices" that focus on land-use policies that support walking and biking and the use of transportation-focused **health impact assessments** (Mass. Gen. Laws Ann. ch. 6C, § 33 [West, 2020]).

In each of these examples, the legal mechanisms *prioritize* and *require* at least thinking about health consequences but with flexibility about when and how. This means that they require considering collateral health impacts *some* of the time. Such flexibility may aid implementation. At the same time, it may not ensure that health is considered comprehensively across all decisions or that even when health is considered, health-maximizing decisions are ultimately made.

In addition to law-based efforts to connect sectors and integrate health into governmental decisions, laws can support HiAP by leaving room for HiAP activities. For instance, a Hartford, Connecticut municipal ordinance requires the health department to promote health equity using "best practices, effective collaboration with other partners and community members, [and] the promotion of a healthier living environment" (Hartford, Connecticut, Code of Ordinances § 2-92). Although this ordinance does not require or support decision-makers outside the health sector to consider health, its language arguably *authorizes* the health department to pursue HiAP. Likewise, by directing the state health department to establish an Office of American Indian Health to (a) reduce health disparities affecting American Indians, (b) coordinate related intra- and interdepartmental efforts, and (3) consult with Tribal governmental and Tribal health leaders and stakeholders, a Montana gubernatorial executive order (Mont. Exec. Order No. 06-2015 [Jun. 16, 2015]) may be implemented in a manner that supports HiAP.

Box 18.3 contains additional examples to illustrate how U.S. state and local governments have used legal mechanisms to formalize or advance government-focused HiAP efforts.

## Challenges to Law-Based HiAP Efforts

As in other areas of public health law, law (and policy) can impede HiAP. For instance, legal mechanisms formalize the same silos that HiAP efforts aim to dismantle. For good reasons, including effective management and administration, laws create and empower governmental agencies with sector-focused missions (e.g., departments of health, education, and transportation) with particular responsibilities, processes, and measures of success. It is difficult to imagine a public administration system that does not rely on subject-matter expertise and distribute governmental powers and duties among different agencies, particularly in larger jurisdictions. But a potential consequence is establishing silos that inhibit cross-cutting initiatives like HiAP.

## BOX 18.3  EXAMPLES OF STATE AND LOCAL LEGAL MECHANISMS THAT FORMALIZE OR SUPPORT HiAP INITIATIVES

**Jurisdiction:** State of Oregon

**Citation:** Oregon Health Authority & Oregon Department of Transportation. (2013). *Memorandum of Understanding Between the Oregon Health Authority, Public Health Division and the Oregon Department of Transportation.* https://www.oregon.gov/oha/ph/ProviderPartnerResources/HealthInAllPolicies/Documents/mou-oha-odot.pdf

**Legal Mechanism:** Memorandum of Understanding (MOU)

**Description:** Oregon law authorizes state governmental departments to enter into agreements with each other or with local governmental entities. An agreement between the state departments of health and transportation aims to connect these two departments and encourage them to collaborate. The primary focus of the initiative is to reduce injuries for users of all modes of transportation and to encourage walking, biking, and the use of public transportation. The MOU stipulates that the two departments agree to improve communication, hold regular meetings, coordinate efforts, update their respective boards, and jointly engage stakeholders. The departments also agree to share data and to collaborate on research.

**Advancing HiAP:** This MOU memorializes an agreement for cross-sector collaboration between the public health agency and another governmental agency that shapes a social determinant of health—the built environment. Through its aims of collaborative initiatives and data sharing, it plans to integrate health concerns into the work of the transportation sector.

**Jurisdiction:** State of Illinois

**Citation:** H.B. 2146, 101st Gen. Assembly (Ill. 2019). http://www.ilga.gov/legislation/fulltext.asp?DocName=&SessionId=108&GA=101&DocTypeId=HB&DocNum=2146&GAID=15&LegID=117830&SpecSess=&Session=

**Legal Mechanism:** State Statute

**Description:** This statute establishes a cross-sector working group to review legislation and make policy recommendations regarding promoting the social determinants of health "using a health in all policies framework." The working group must recommend how to integrate health into decision-making across sectors, promote collaboration across government, as well as "develop laws and policies to promote health and reduce health inequities" and recommend ways to implement them. The state health department must support the working group and other departments. The working group must meet at least twice a year and provide annual reports of findings and recommendations to the legislature. Its reports and recommendations must be considered when developing the state's health improvement plans.

**Advancing HiAP:** This statute requires various sectors and agencies to collaborate on establishing law and policy recommendations that integrate health concerns into decision-making through a HiAP lens.

**Jurisdiction:** Appleton, Wisconsin

**Citation:** Appleton, Wisconsin, Municipal Code §§ 7-200 - 7-202. https://www.appleton.org/home/showdocument?id=482

**Legal Mechanism:** Local Ordinance

*(continued)*

BOX 18.3 (*continued*)

**Description:** This ordinance recognizes the role of social factors in shaping health, the presence of health disparities, the impacts of chronic disease, and the HiAP approach. It defines HiAP as integrating health across decision-making in a collaborative manner and with stakeholder input. The ordinance also creates an Interdepartmental HiAP Team. Its members must select health equity indicators to track, work within their respective departments to improve selected indicators, and report on progress and challenges. The City must also integrate health equity practices into City plans, budgets, and performance systems; utilize a HiAP Strategy Document for implementation; periodically report on HiAP progress; and develop and operationalize a community engagement plan to integrate stakeholder perspectives into the HiAP initiative.

**Advancing HiAP:** This ordinance defines and prioritizes HiAP. It encourages integrating health across municipal decisions by creating a HiAP-focused cross-sector governmental entity; requiring integration of health equity concerns across municipal policies, plans, and programs; requiring periodic reporting on progress; and engaging with the community around health equity.

**Jurisdiction:** Richmond, Virginia

**Citation:** Richmond, Virginia, Resolution No. 2014-R262-2015-7. http://www.richmondgov.com/CampaignHealthyRichmond/documents/Attachment-01_Richmond-VA-Resolution.pdf

**Legal Mechanism:** City Council Resolution

**Description:** This municipal resolution adopts the "Policy for HiAP Framework." This framework aims to establish HiAP and "fair and just" concepts into the work of municipal government, including city plans, performance systems, and budgets in order to promote health equity. It defines HiAP, health, health equity, and determinants of health equity. It also focuses on addressing the needs of *all* residents through municipal decisions and actions to eliminate disparities. The resolution calls on the City's Chief Administrative Officer to apply HiAP and "fair and just" principles in all of its work; establish a cross-departmental team to coordinate efforts through metrics, strategic plans, work plans, guidelines, and analytical tools; and annually report on progress.

**Advancing HiAP:** This resolution prioritizes health and equity by requiring the municipal government to integrate them into its decisions primarily through cross-sector coordination and the alignment of metrics and plans.

**Jurisdiction:** State of New York

**Citation:** N.Y. Exec. Order No. 190 (Nov. 14, 2018). https://www.governor.ny.gov/news/no-190-incorporating-health-across-all-policies-state-agency-activities

**Legal Mechanism:** Gubernatorial Executive Order (Regulatory)

**Description:** This order recognizes the role of the social determinants of health, explains the "Health Across All Policies" approach, and recognizes the success of the state in some areas that constitute the social determinants. The order, which applies to state agencies in the governor's administration and other governmental entities, requires incorporating the livability domains and the state's prevention agenda into plans, policies, procedures, grants, contract solicitations, guidance "where practical and feasible," and appointing a liaison to the state's *ad hoc* committee.

BOX 18.3 (*continued*)

**Advancing HiAP:** This order requires, "where practical and feasible," agencies to integrate health and livability concerns into their work and to collaborate across sectors through a committee.

**Jurisdiction:** Tacoma-Pierce County Board of Health, Washington

**Citation:** Tacoma-Pierce County Board of Health, Washington, Resolution No. 2016-4495. https://www.tpchd.org/home/showdocument?id=532

**Legal Mechanism:** Board of Health Resolution

**Description:** This resolution broadly defines health, defines HiAP, and recognizes the importance of interagency collaboration to improve health outcomes. The resolution requires the Tacoma-Pierce County Health Department to "apply a Health in All Policies approach to its own work, including policy development and implementation, budgeting, and delivery of services"; incorporate the perspectives of stakeholders and communities through engagement; collaborate to ensure policies consider health impacts; and advocate for health equity and to improve the social determinants. It also encourages other decision-makers at all levels of government to consider the impacts of their decisions on health and health equity.

**Advancing HiAP:** This resolution requires the local health department to engage in HiAP work and to prioritize HiAP and health equity.

**Jurisdiction:** State of Colorado

**Citation:** Settlement Agreement, *Sierra Club et al. v. Chao, et al.* (D. Colo. No. 17-1679), (Dec. 20, 2018). https://www.codot.gov/projects/i70east/assets/reports-and-historic-documents/settlement-agreement

**Legal Mechanism:** Litigation (Settlement Agreement)

**Description:** This settlement agreement resulted from a lawsuit brought by the Sierra Club, Colorado Chapter, and others, against the federal and Colorado departments of transportation challenging the adequacy of the governments' assessments, as required by federal law, related to expansion of Interstate-70 through a Denver neighborhood. This document, which memorializes the settlement with the Colorado Department of Transportation, requires the Department to complete a comprehensive health assessment of causes of health disparities in the affected community. The assessment must be overseen by experts, including from the state department of health. The agreement also calls for enhanced air pollution monitoring in this area, notification and response when air pollution levels exceed a certain level, and reduction of pollution through planting of additional trees.

**Advancing HiAP:** This lawsuit is based on an alleged failure to comply with a federal requirement to analyze potential health and environmental effects of certain transportation projects. The settlement agreement that resulted from the litigation creates binding obligations meant to enhance the health of an impacted community experiencing health disparities both by understanding them and requiring the government to abate them.

The structure of governmental decision-making can also impede HiAP. On its face, the legislative and rulemaking processes in particular can seem open to community and stakeholder input. For example, state agencies in Alabama that make rules are often required to create those rules through open processes and to consider stakeholder feedback (Ala. Code § 41-22-5 [West, 2020]).

However, such requirements may be implemented in ways that discourage feedback. What kinds of stakeholders, for instance, are more likely to understand proposed agency rules and how they interact with current law, decipher how to submit comments, or be available to attend hearings during business hours?

The law-based HiAP initiatives discussed in this chapter highlight the *potential* of legal mechanisms to promote or support HiAP. But they also raise important questions. How are law-based HiAP efforts actually implemented? As in other areas of public health law, there may be a gap between HiAP laws as adopted and as implemented such that even laws that appear to make great strides in integrating health across governmental decisions do not actually do so in practice. A key question to consider with law-based HiAP efforts, particularly ones that focus on governmental processes, is to what extent they are or can be *enforced*. In other words, can HiAP advocates ensure they are implemented? And if so, is this through legal processes in which governmental entities can be compelled to engage in HiAP or through political action?

Much is still unknown about the effectiveness of HiAP—whether or not a HiAP effort includes law-based components. The ultimate goal of HiAP is to improve health determinants and outcomes and to promote health equity. But whether implementing HiAP, which involves changes to *process*, actually improves health outcomes remains to be seen. The most critical question for any law-based HiAP effort is whether, as adopted and implemented, it actually promotes or achieves HiAP goals (Hall & Jacobson, 2018).

## CONCLUSION

HiAP aims to systematically integrate the health perspective into decisions that may not otherwise consider health in order to improve the social determinants of health and to advance health equity. HiAP efforts are highly contextual. They can be implemented with or without legal mechanisms and often rely on a combination of law-based and other strategies. A law-based HiAP approach can use the tools of public health law, including legislation, regulation, and litigation. Law-based HiAP efforts can target how government operates and what it prioritizes; they can also encourage private sector decisions that promote health. It remains critical to determine if and how HiAP efforts, whether or not they are law-based, improve the social determinants of health, health outcomes, and health equity.

## CHAPTER REVIEW

### Review Questions

1. Explain the logic of HiAP as a tool to address the social determinants of health and to improve health equity.
2. You work at a state or local health department with a focus on chronic disease and health equity. You have been tasked with proposing a HiAP strategy for your jurisdiction.
   a. Discuss the advantages and disadvantages of utilizing a legal mechanism as part of this strategy.
   b. You and your colleagues decide to include a legal mechanism as part of the agency's HiAP strategy. What legal mechanism do you select and why? What factors would be relevant to this decision?
3. Select two examples of state or local legal mechanisms that support HiAP provided in this chapter. Retrieve them online and fully read the language.
   a. Describe the HiAP approach pursued in each example in your own words.
   b. Which approach do you think is more consistent with the definition and goals of HiAP and why?

c. What barriers to adopting this legal mechanism would you expect with each approach?

d. What implementation challenges would you anticipate with each approach?

e. How would you evaluate whether each approach is "successful"?

## Essay Question

Consider the model HiAP ordinance created by ChangeLab Solutions: (https://www.changelabsolutions.org/sites/default/files/HIAP_ModelOrdinance_FINAL_20150728.pdf). You work for an advocacy organization focused on health equity. Tailor this model ordinance to your city or county, making edits as you deem appropriate, so you can advocate for its adoption. Explain why you made the choices you made.

## Internet Activities

1. Find searchable statutes for your state. (Hint: They are often available through the state legislature's website or through a university library database.) Can you find statutory language that can be used to support HiAP work in your state?

   a. What concepts did you search for to find this language? What key terms did you use? What do these key terms and concepts suggest about HiAP and its definition?

   b. Do these laws focus on the relationship between the government and private parties, among governmental entities, or both?

   c. How could a public health practitioner utilize this statutory language to advance HiAP work?

   d. How could these provisions be strengthened to promote HiAP?

## REFERENCES

12 Guam Code Ann. § 58127.6 (West 2020).

42 USC § 300u-10.

Artiga, S., & Hinton, E. (2018). *Beyond health care: The role of the social determinants in promoting health and health equity.* Kaiser Family Foundation. https://www.kff.org/racial-equity-and-health -policy/issue-brief/beyond-health-care-the-role-of-social-determinants-in-promoting-health -and-health-equity

Centers for Disease Control and Prevention. (2020). *10 essential public health services.* https://www .cdc.gov/publichealthgateway/publichealthservices/essentialhealthservices.html

Centers for Disease Control and Prevention. (n.d.). *Ten essential public health services and how they can include addressing the social determinants of health and health inequities.* https://www.cdc.gov/ publichealthgateway/publichealthservices/pdf/ten_essential_services_and_sdoh.pdf

County Health Rankings & Roadmaps, University of Wisconsin School of Medicine and Public Health, Wisconsin Population Health Institute. (n.d.). *County health rankings & roadmaps: Our approach.* http://www.countyhealthrankings.org/our-approach

DeSalvo, K. B., Wang, Y. C., Harris, A., Auerbach, J., Koo, D., & O'Carroll, P. (2017). Peer reviewed: Public Health 3.0: A call to action for public health to meet the challenges of the 21st century. *Preventing Chronic Disease, 14,* 170017. http://dx.doi.org/10.5888/pcd14.170017

DiClemente, R. J., Salazar, L. F., & Crosby, R. A. (2007). A review of STD/HIV preventive interventions for adolescents: Sustaining effects using an ecological approach. *Journal of Pediatric Psychology, 32*(8), 888–906. http://dx.doi.org/10.1093/jpepsy/jsm056

Frieden, T. R. (2010). A framework for public health action: The health impact pyramid. *American Journal of Public Health, 100*(4), 590–595. http://dx.doi.org/10.2105/AJPH.2009.185652

Gakh, M. (2015). Law, the health in all policies approach, and cross-sector collaboration. *Public Health Reports, 130*(1), 96–100. http://dx.doi.org/10.1177/003335491513000112

Garner, B. A. (Ed.). (2001). *Black's law dictionary* (2nd pocket ed.). West Group.

Gostin, L. O. (2008). *Public health law: Power, duty, restraint* (2nd ed.). University of California Press.

Hall, R. L., & Jacobson, P. D. (2018). Examining whether the health-in-all-policies approach promotes health equity. *Health Affairs, 37*(3), 364–370. https://doi.org/10.1377/hlthaff.2017.1292

Hartford, Connecticut, Code of Ordinances § 2-92.

Hillsborough County Metropolitan Planning Organization, Florida. (2019, January 8). *Resolution No. 2019-1.* http://www.planhillsborough.org/wp-content/uploads/2019/06/HIAP-Resolution-and-Report.pdf

Institute for Public Health Innovation. (n.d.). *Highlights from the Community Transformation Grant for Prince George's County, Maryland: October 2012–September 2014.* http://www.institutephi.org/wp-content/uploads/2014/03/CTG-Highlights-Brochure_LoRes_112414.pdf

Institute of Medicine. (2011). *For the public's health: Revitalizing law and policy to meet new challenges.* National Academies Press.

Institute of Medicine. (2015). *Cross-sector responses to obesity: Workshop summary.* National Academies Press. https://doi.org/10.17226/21706

Institute of Medicine Committee for the Study of the Future of Public Health. (1988). *The future of public health.* https://www.ncbi.nlm.nih.gov/books/NBK218218/pdf/Bookshelf_NBK218218.pdf

Kania, J., & Kramer, M. (2011). Collective impact. *Stanford Social Innovation Review.* https://ssir.org/images/articles/2011_WI_Feature_Kania.pdf

Licking County Health Department. (2018). *Licking County Health Department Strategic Plan, 2018–2021.* http://www.lickingcohealth.org/documents/Final%202018-2021%20LCHD%20Strategic%20Plan.pdf

Marmot, M., Friel, S., Bell, R., Houweling, T. A., Taylor, S., & Commission on Social Determinants of Health. (2008). Closing the gap in a generation: Health equity through action on the social determinants of health. *The Lancet, 372*(9650), 1661–1669. https://doi.org/10.1016/S0140-6736(08)61690-6

Massachusetts Geneneral Laws Ann. ch. 6C, § 33 (West, 2020).

Max, J. L., Sedivy, V., & Garrido, M. (2015). *Increasing our impact by using a social-ecological approach.* Administration on Children, Youth, Family and Youth Services Bureau. https://www.healthyteennetwork.org/wp-content/uploads/2015/06/TipSheet_IncreasingOurImpactUsingSocial-EcologicalApproach.pdf

Montana Executive Order No. 06-2015 (Jun. 16, 2015).

National Conference of State Legislatures. (2020). *State renewable portfolio standards and goals.* http://www.ncsl.org/research/energy/renewable-portfolio-standards.aspx

National Research Council. (2011). *Improving health in the United States: The role of health impact assessment.* National Academies Press.

Office of Disease Prevention and Health Promotion, U.S. Department of Health and Human Services. (2019). *Healthy People 2020: The social determinants of health.* https://www.healthypeople.gov/2020/topics-objectives/topic/social-determinants-of-health

Office of Disease Prevention and Health Promotion, U.S. Department of Health and Human Services. (n.d.). *Healthy People 2030 social determinants of health.* https://health.gov/healthypeople/objectives-and-data/social-determinants-health

Public Health Accreditation Board. (2013). *Standards and measures.* https://www.phaboard.org/wp-content/uploads/2019/01/PHABSM_WEB_LR1.pdf

Ransom, M. M. (2016). *Public health law competency model: Version 1.0.* CDC. https://www.cdc.gov/phlp/docs/phlcm-v1.pdf

Rudolph, L., Caplan, J., Ben-Moshe, K., & Dillon, L. (2013). *Health in all policies: A guide for state and local governments.* American Public Health Association and Public Health Institute. https://www.apha.org/-/media/files/pdf/factsheets/health_inall_policies_guide_169pages.ashx?la=en&hash=641B94AF624D7440F836238F0551A5FF0DE4872A

Vermont Executive Order No. 07-15 (Oct. 6, 2015).

Washington Revised Code Ann. § 43.20.285 (West, 2020).

## Additional Resources

- **APHA/PHI Report**: Rudolph, L., Caplan, J., Ben-Moshe, K., & Dillon, L. (2013). *Health in all policies: A guide for state and local governments.* American Public Health Association and Public Health Institute.
  https://www.apha.org/-/media/files/pdf/factsheets/health_inall_policies_guide_169pages.ashx?la=en&hash=641B94AF624D7440F836238F0551A5FF0DE4872A
- **CDC HiAP Resource Center**: Centers for Disease Control and Prevention. (2015). *Health in all policies resource center.*
  https://www.cdc.gov/policy/hiap/index.html & https://www.cdc.gov/policy/hiap/resources
- **CDC HiAP Resource Center Intro Video:** Centers for Disease Control and Prevention. (2015). *Health in all policies resource center introductory video.*
  https://youtu.be/6ZBnRVqmwDo
- **ChangeLab Solutions Collaborative Health Slideshow:** ChangeLab Solutions. (2016). *Collaborative health slideshow.*
  https://www.youtube.com/watch?v=thYj8AlB3ms
- **ChangeLab Solutions HiAP Resources:** ChangeLab Solutions. (2019). *Health in all policies.*
  https://www.changelabsolutions.org/health-all-policies
- **Commission on Social Determinants of Health Final Report:** Commission on Social Determinants of Health. (2008). *Closing the gap in a generation: Health equity through action on the social determinants of health. Final Report of the Commission on Social Determinants of Health.* World Health Organization.
  https://www.who.int/social_determinants/thecommission/finalreport/en
- **WHO HiAP Training Manual:** World Health Organization. (2015). *Health in all policies training manual.*
  https://apps.who.int/iris/bitstream/handle/10665/151788/9789241507981_eng.pdf;jsessionid=967359F17A8F1F98A7F278EDD033BBD3?sequence=1

# 19

# Introduction to Legal Epidemiology

Lindsay K. Cloud and Ross D. Silverman

## Learning Objectives

By the end of this chapter, the reader will be able to:

- Discuss the relationship between law and policy and public health goals and outcomes.
- Define legal epidemiology.
- Recognize the basic practice of policy surveillance.
- Articulate the benefits of conducting a legal epidemiology project.

## Key Terminology

**Legal epidemiology:** the scientific study and deployment of law as a factor in the cause, distribution, and prevention of disease and injury in a population (Ramanathan et al., 2017).

**Policy surveillance:** the systematic, scientific collection and analysis of laws of public health significance (Burris, Hitchcock, et al., 2016).

**Transdisciplinary model:** melds legal and scientific facets of public health law to help break down enduring cultural, disciplinary, and resource barriers that have prevented the full recognition and optimal role of law in public health (Burris, Ashe, Levin, et al., 2016).

## Public Health Law Competencies

The chapter addresses the following competencies from the Public Health Law Competency Model (PHLCM, Ransom, 2016) and the Legal Epidemiology Competency Model (LECM, 2019).

**PHLCM: 1.1** Define basic constitutional concepts and legal principles framing the practice of public health across relevant jurisdictions.

**PHLCM: 1.2** Identify and apply public health laws (e.g., statutes, regulations, ordinances, and court rulings) pertinent to practitioner's jurisdiction, agency, program, and profession.

**LECM 1.1:** Articulate the importance of legal epidemiology concepts to inform health, fiscal, administrative, legal, social, and political research and discourse.

**LECM 3.1:** Identify opportunities for a legal evaluation study to address existing legal, health, or other issues.

---

### Spark Question

Provide an example of one law you believe has influenced public health. How would you study whether the law has had positive, negative, incidental, or no significant impact on public health over time?

---

## INTRODUCTION

Here, there, and everywhere – laws – and how they are structured and implemented (Burris, 2011), greatly influence our daily lives by shaping the environments where we live, learn, work, and play (Office of Disease Prevention and Health Promotion, n.d.). Laws enacted long before you were born can affect your overall health throughout each stage of life, beginning with where and how you were born and raised (Rothstein, 2017; Scrimshaw & Backes, 2020). In childhood, laws dictated which vaccinations were necessary before attending school to guard against infectious diseases. They shaped the school environment itself—from the curriculum you were taught, to whether and how often you had gym class, to the availability of counseling services, and even the selection of foods in your school cafeteria and vending machines (Chriqui et al., 2020). As an adolescent, you encountered the multitude of laws governing your ability to drive a car, from reaching a certain age and passing a test before obtaining a driver's license, to rules of the road concerning speed limits, wearing seatbelts, driving while intoxicated, and distracted driving. In adulthood, laws and policies regulate your work environment (e.g., employment protections, workplace safety), your marriages (e.g., family law), your interactions with the healthcare system (e.g., healthcare and insurance regulations), and even your wishes after death (e.g., wills, trusts, and estates).

Law's ubiquity has become particularly glaring during the COVID-19 pandemic. Since the first case of COVID-19 was confirmed in the United States on January 21, 2020, federal, state, and local governments have taken varying degrees of legal action that affect your daily routine from whether you are able to live in college housing, attend in-person classes, play a team sport, and attend social gatherings with friends. This recent surge of legal activity will influence health, well-being, and equity in the United States for generations to come; however, the direct and indirect effects of these laws, as well as their magnitude, remain unknown. In fact, the effects of laws on health are rarely evaluated after they are enacted, let alone before they are passed.

While law has influenced health and health equity for centuries, the extent of the association between law and health outcomes is less well known. This is partly because law's role in health has been understudied (Ibrahim et al., 2017). Historically, law has not been developed, implemented, and evaluated strategically or systematically, nor has the evidence generated from the few studies on environmental or behavioral impacts of policies been translated across public health issues—but it could be (Ramanathan et al., 2017). Enter the field of legal epidemiology. This chapter defines and characterizes the field of legal epidemiology, describes its practice, and discusses its importance to the public health field at large.

## DEFINING LEGAL EPIDEMIOLOGY

**Legal epidemiology** is the scientific study and deployment of law as a factor in the cause, distribution, and prevention of disease and injury in a population (Ramanathan et al., 2017). Essentially, legal epidemiology is a systematic approach to studying laws and policies and

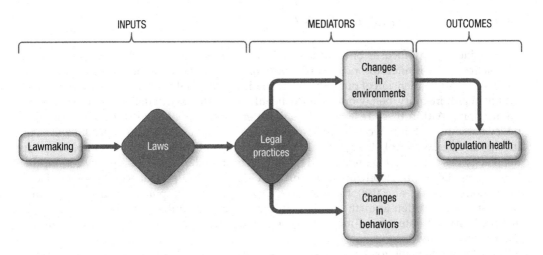

**FIGURE 19.1** Logic model of public health law research.

assessing their impact on population health (see Figure 19.1; Burris et al., 2010; Wagenaar & Burris, 2013). Its practice is centered on the notion that laws and legal practices can be studied in the same general manner, and with the same general scientific methods, as any other social phenomenon of importance to health. Legal epidemiology studies provide us with insights and empirical evidence about which laws and policies work to improve health, and sometimes more importantly, which ones do not.

## FROM CONCEPT TO PRACTICE

Legal epidemiology is one of several methods (e.g., systematic reviews, policy analysis, economic evaluations, content analysis, survey research, and community-based participatory research) investigators use in health policy research. However, it is the only method specifically developed to facilitate the quantitative measurement of the impact of laws and health equity. When you think of the practice of legal epidemiology, think: scientific, systematic, transparent, replicable, precise, and measurable.

### Who Are Legal Epidemiologists?

Although law is the central intervention in legal epidemiology studies, going to law school is not a prerequisite to engaging in its practice. Nonlawyers play a critical role in the practice and implementation of public health law (Burris, Ashe, Blanke, et al., 2016). Many public health practitioners are utilizing legal epidemiology methods, or its underlying concepts, without recognizing or labeling its practice as such. Further, with roots in both law and science, legal epidemiology emphasizes a transdisciplinary approach for the betterment of the public health law field at large. A transdisciplinary approach demands a true integration of expertise, theories, methods, and conceptual tools from various disciplines through long-term sharing and close collaboration (Burris, Ashe, Levin, et al., 2016; Stokols et al., 2008). Legal epidemiology teams can include lawyers, epidemiologists, public health practitioners, researchers, policy experts, statisticians, and social scientists, among other specialties.

## What Do Legal Epidemiologists Study?

Legal epidemiology focuses on laws and policies of importance to public health. Therefore, its practice is not limited to one area of research. Instead, these methods can be used to explore nearly any dimension of public health, including the social determinants of health, global health, health inequity, behavioral science, healthcare systems and delivery, and health communications. Within these research areas, legal epidemiologists focus on a wide variety of policy domains that influence population health, including mental health, reproductive health, infectious disease control, drug policy, housing, and income insecurity. For example, legal epidemiology has been used to understand the impact of state short-term emergency commitment laws on mental health stabilization (Hedman et al., 2016), the prevalence of abortion facility regulations (Jones et al., 2018), the effects of alcohol/pregnancy policies that vary by educational status in relation to birth outcomes and prenatal care utilization (Roberts et al., 2020), and the impact of state earned-income tax credit laws on birth outcomes by race and ethnicity (Komro et al., 2018).

In addition to being topically versatile, the unit of measurement for analysis includes any written legal text with the authority to regulate people, places, or things. Formal legal texts suitable for analysis exist at any level of governmental authority. Research may be conducted using international treaties and constitutions, national laws, executive orders, state statutes and regulations, case law, local ordinances, agency policies, and even institutional rules and standards (e.g., employment handbooks, hospital rules, and university policies). Oral speeches proclaiming legal action (e.g. a governor announcing a mandatory stay-at-home order) that are not memorialized in a formal document (e.g., an executive order) would not meet the inclusion criteria for a legal epidemiology study. Remember, written words can be objectively observed, and consequently measured.

## How Are Legal Epidemiology Methods Operationalized?

There are three foundational components of legal epidemiology used to measure the nature and distribution of law: legal prevention and control, legal etiology, and **policy surveillance** (Burris, Ashe, Levin, et al., 2016). Legal prevention and control is the study of laws and legal practices as *interventions* to prevent disease and injury, and as enablers of effective public health administration. Interventional law has been a common policy tool adapted to address issues in many health domains. For example, states have used interventional law to prevent injuries and deaths associated with driving motorized vehicles, attempting to keep pace with technological advances that have changed human behavior. As cell phones began to proliferate across America, lawmakers enacted laws that regulate cell-phone use while driving, which substantially vary by state based on the type of driver, the restricted behavior, and the penalties for infringement. To understand whether and how these varying restrictions work, researchers developed multistate studies investigating law as the primary intervention, with one study assessing the estimated decline in emergency department visits related to car crashes in states passing laws that banned texting-while-driving, compared to states lacking such laws (Ferdinand et al., 2019). In contrast, legal etiology is the study of laws and legal practices as likely *causes* of disease and injury. One study found a statistically significant increase in Florida's monthly total homicide and firearms homicide rates after passage of the state's stand-your-ground law, as compared to a sample of states without a stand-your-ground law (Humphreys et al., 2017). Policy surveillance is the ongoing, systematic collection, analysis, and dissemination of laws and policies across jurisdictions and over time that enables the creation of legal data that can be used for evaluation. For example, longitudinal policy surveillance data capturing over 30 years of changes to minimum wage laws for all 50 states was used to investigate the effects of state minimum wage laws on low birth weight and infant mortality in the United States (Komro et al., 2018). Policy surveillance methods can be used to create the underlying legal data for both legal prevention and control and legal etiology studies. In fact, policy surveillance datasets serve as the foundation of most legal epidemiology studies, thus its practice is explored in more detail in what follows.

## USING POLICY SURVEILLANCE TO ADVANCE LEGAL EPIDEMIOLOGY

*Policy surveillance*—the systematic, scientific collection and analysis of laws of public health significance—involves distinct but iterative phases (see Figure 19.2; Burris, Hitchcock, et al., 2016). These phases include: conceptualization and scoping; background research; creating a coding scheme and questions to analyze laws; collecting laws; building laws over time; applying the coding questions to laws to create data; quality control; publication and dissemination; as well as tracking and updating the law over time (Wagenaar & Burris, 2013). The policy surveillance process focuses on creating longitudinal legal data for evaluation and requires a team of three researchers due, in part, to its emphasis on redundancy in the research and coding phases.

Policy surveillance allows researchers to not only capture whether a law or policy exists within a jurisdiction, but also to capture the characteristics of key provisions of the law. Oftentimes, these details emerge as critical pieces of the puzzle in understanding the depth and breadth of laws and their influence on health.

To illustrate this concept, let us revisit laws related to school-based childhood immunization requirements. To understand the true impact of these laws, it would be important to capture which vaccination is required for school enrollment and entry. Through the policy surveillance research process, you would find that all state laws require the measles-mumps-rubella (MMR) vaccine, whereas only a few states require that students receive the human papillomavirus vaccine (HPV). To capture additional nuance, you would need to explore whether state laws offer nonmedical exemptions in lieu of obtaining a vaccine (e.g., exemptions based on religious or personal beliefs), and whether the state law applies to all schools (e.g., students attending

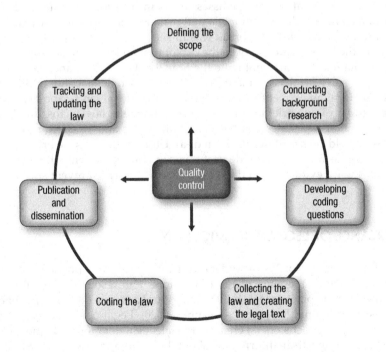

**FIGURE 19.2** The policy surveillance process.

private schools as well as public schools and day-care facilities). Creating legal data through policy surveillance capturing critical nuance and changes in the law over time facilitates health policy research and rigorous evaluation studies, such as examining the impact of school-based childhood immunization requirements on vaccination rates around the world (Vandelaer & Olaniran, 2015).

Legal epidemiology studies that assess laws across jurisdictions and over time using policy surveillance data can produce results with causal connections. Quasi-experimental studies using legal epidemiology data allow researchers to observe the effects of a law pre- and post-enactment; however, creating longitudinal legal data and deploying a legal evaluation can be time consuming and resource-intensive (Tremper et al., 2010). At this point, you may still be interested in law and policy as the primary target for health outcomes research, but do not have the time, experience, network, or resources to build longitudinal legal data just yet. Consider performing a legal assessment.

## THINK BIG, BUT START SMALL(ER) BY USING LEGAL ASSESSMENTS TO ADVANCE LEGAL EPIDEMIOLOGY

Legal assessment studies are the cross-sectional scientific collection and analysis of codified legal provisions of importance to health across jurisdictions (Centers for Disease Control and Prevention [CDC], n.d.-b). Legal assessment methods involve some, though not all, of the phases of the policy surveillance process (see Figure 19.2). Instead of collecting and building law over time, legal assessments capture a snapshot of the law across multiple jurisdictions at one particular point of time, generally requiring less time and resources than a policy surveillance project. While legal assessments lack (m)any repeated measures that strengthen causal claims for full-blown legal epidemiology studies, they can be quite valuable for understanding the general legal landscape of a particular area of law, providing the cross-sectional foundation for a future policy surveillance project, as well as facilitating advocacy efforts.

To envision the application of legal assessments in practice, imagine working at a state health department and a sudden salmonella outbreak occurs, affecting many children in your state. You learn the source of the outbreak was linked to an infected pet turtle at a local day care. One part of the investigation may be the exploration of laws concerning turtle sales, possession, and regulation. You may not have the time (or the need) to analyze turtle laws over time. Instead, you run a legal assessment to explore the current snapshot of these laws across a few states. The legal assessment provides you with the legal landscape necessary to expedite the writing of an issue brief on turtle-related salmonella laws across the United States, including the fact that two states ban the sale of all turtles and 16 states restrict or prohibit having turtles in child-care facilities (CDC, n.d.-a). Ultimately, the issue brief, using evidence from your legal assessment, can provide useful information to not only the public, but also to advocates lobbying for evidence-based lawmaking in an effort to prevent such an outbreak in the future.

## THE IMPORTANCE OF LEGAL EPIDEMIOLOGY

So why does this matter to you? As a student, you are the future of public health, and beyond this introductory chapter, there are plenty of free tools and resources to equip you with the information necessary to practice legal epidemiology and advance the field of public health law and practice (see Additional Resources; Benjamin, 2020). Legal epidemiology leads to better health faster, through its focus on: (a) creating reliable legal data for evaluation, (b) filling the need for accessible, nonpartisan information about the status and trends in the law, (c) tracking changes in law and policy over time to assess progress, (d) diffusing innovative policy ideas, and (e) building workforce capacity. Let us explore each in turn.

## Creating Reliable Legal Data for Evaluation

What gets measured can be improved and measuring the impact of law on health requires legal data (Chriqui et al., 2011). This is the real paradigm shift—these methods provide a rigorous and systematic approach for turning the text of law into data, and then using that data to evaluate the impact of laws and policies on health and health equity. Creating credible legal data that can be used in evaluation and social science publications can lead to more factual awareness about the law and increase evidence-based advocacy and policymaking. Between 2015 and 2020, more than 260 research papers have been published using policy surveillance data from two leading legal epidemiology resources that provide open-source legal data available for download at LawAtlas.org and PDAPS.org.

## Filling the Need for Accessible Nonpartisan Information About the Status and Trends in the Law

Creating and publishing transparent, nonpartisan information about the nuanced features of laws and policies across geographic regions and over time never felt more apt than during the COVID-19 pandemic where basic mitigation measures became highly politicized and therefore contested (e.g., face mask requirements). Legal epidemiology methods focus on observable features of the law—what the law says, not what we think the law is trying to say. States began passing a myriad of mitigation measures in March 2020. In addition to emergency declarations and stay-at-home orders, states issued other types of mandates including gathering bans, closing nonessential businesses (e.g., retail stores, movie theaters, and hair salons), mandating face mask use, implementing travel restrictions, and imposing restrictions on elective medical procedures. Polar charts (see Figure 19.3; Cloud et al., 2020) were created using underlying policy surveillance legal data (The Policy Surveillance Program, 2020), and provided the public with accessible, nonpartisan information on the status and trends of U.S. state laws that aimed to prevent the spread of COVID-19 and mitigate its impact on health.

## Tracking Changes in Law and Policy Over Time to Measure Progress

Tracking change over time to measure progress can be especially important in assessing and responding to an ongoing public health crisis. Although states were issuing new orders at an unprecedented pace, legal epidemiology methods facilitated the collection and analysis of nuanced features of these mitigation measures over time, now providing us with the legal data that tells a story (see Figure 19.3; Cloud et al., 2020). By March 15, 2020, 14 jurisdictions had taken some type of action, mostly imposing gathering bans. Less than 6 weeks later, by April 23, 2020 to be exact, almost every U.S. state had issued some type of mitigation measure, including nonessential business closures. By June 23, 2020, you already begin to see the easing of restrictions across states, with many businesses being allowed to partially reopen and many states lifting mandatory stay-at-home order restrictions. Being able to identify the intricacies and nuance within laws, and the ways laws vary when addressing similar issues in different jurisdictions, can be invaluable—not just for researchers studying the law, but also for the public, policy makers, advocates, public health practitioners, and others who use the law in their work.

## Diffusing Innovative Policy Ideas

Tracking and disseminating law and policy across jurisdictions allow policy makers to compare their jurisdiction with others in the hunt for new and innovative policy ideas. The City-Health Initiative is a great example of the creation of evidence-based policy-making and

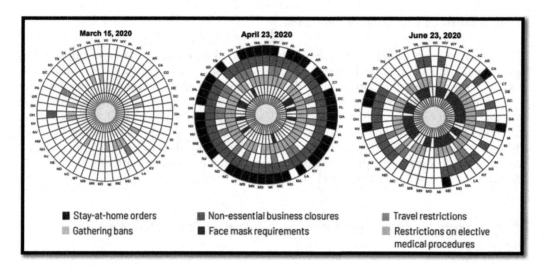

**FIGURE 19.3** State COVID-19 mitigation measures, March 15, 2020–June 23, 2020.

*Source:* Cloud, L K., and Moran-McCabe, Katie and Platt, Elizabeth and Prood, Nadya, A Chronological Overview of the Federal, State, and Local Response to COVID-19 (July 2020). Burris, S., de Guia, S., Gable, L., Levin, D.E., Parmet, W.E., Terry, N.P. (Eds.) (2020). Assessing Legal Responses to COVID-19. Boston: Public Health Law Watch, Available at SSRN: https://ssrn.com/abstract=3675780

advocacy using underlying legal data (CityHealth, n.d.). Policy surveillance data were created and analyzed using an algorithm based on expert-driven scoring criteria to rank the 40 largest U.S. cities and award medals (gold, silver, bronze, or none) based on the strength of their policies across nine public health topics (e.g., earned sick leave, affordable housing). This work led to tangible policy changes, as legislators were easily able to pinpoint what was needed to advance a particular policy area by comparing their jurisdiction to others and identifying which features of the law were working in other cities. Despite the innumerable challenges plaguing cities in 2020, 90% of the 40 largest cities earned an overall medal in at least one of the nine key policy topics, up from just 48% in 2017 during the first year of the CityHealth Initiative (CityHealth, 2020).

## Building Workforce Capacity

Legal epidemiology focuses on publishing (and supporting) open-source legal data that can be freely used, replicated, or updated through the transparency of its methods. Frameworks like the Ten Essential Public Health Law Services (see Table 19.1; de Beaumont, n.d.), and the Five Essential Public Health Law Services (Burris, Ashe, Blanke, et al., 2016) provide lawyers and nonlawyers with the tools to build workforce capacity. Legal epidemiology methods can support these services and ultimately strengthen how public health law functions.

## CONCLUSION

To evaluate the impact of law on health outcomes, it is necessary to have legal data suitable for research. Legal epidemiology—the scientific study and deployment of law as a factor in the cause, distribution, and prevention of disease and injury in a population—facilitates the quantitative measurement of the impact of law on health and health equity. The adoption of legal epidemiology methods can lead to greater research efficiency through its commitment to using

**TABLE 19.1  Selected Services From the 10 Essential Public Health Services (Revised Model, 2020)**

| ESSENTIAL PUBLIC HEALTH SERVICES | ROLE OF LEGAL EPIDEMIOLOGY |
|---|---|
| Service 5. Create, champion, and implement policies, plans, and laws that impact health | Service 5 requires evidence-based policymaking, which first requires data on what is working and what is not working. Legal epidemiology studies can provide the necessary evidence as to whether a particular law is having a positive, negative, incidental, or no effect on population health, ultimately improving policy-making recommendations and thereby improving overall health. |
| Service 8. Build and support a diverse and skilled public health workforce | Evaluating the effect of law in public health using legal epidemiology requires many different skills, including a close understanding of public health, legal research experience, and the ability to design and conduct quantitative and qualitative evaluation research. Rarely will one person encompass all of these capacities. Therefore, a transdisciplinary approach to public health law, in which professional boundaries break down and participants draw directly on each other's skills, can support a diverse and skilled public health workforce. |
| Service 9. Improve and innovate public health functions through ongoing evaluation, research, and continuous quality improvement | Legal epidemiology is an innovative method that supports the ongoing evaluation and research of laws and policies. Law and policy are not one-size-fits-all; a policy win in one region can often fail in another, and what worked in the 1980s may not work in 2021. Like all industries, public health law needs to keep up with people, places, and time, and tracking changes in the law over time is one key way to measure its influence. |

transparent, reproducible, and credible research methods to turn the text of law into quantitative data, reducing costs and increasing productivity through adopting technology for use in its research processes (e.g., MonQcle, n.d.), and producing data with multiple uses.

Over the past decade, the field of legal epidemiology has blossomed through the creation, refinement, and dissemination of its foundational theory, methods, texts, and tools (Wagenaar & Burris, 2013). As courses and certificates in its practice are being developed and incorporated into educational programs across the United States and abroad, students and new public health professionals are critical to the future development and growth of this evolving field.

## CHAPTER REVIEW

### Review Questions

1. Define legal epidemiology.
2. List and describe the three basic foundational components of legal epidemiology.
3. Using the multitude of examples in this chapter, explain how law is being used to advance public health today.
4. Legal epidemiologists can measure any observable, written text including constitutions, statutes, regulations, ordinances, case law, agency policies, and institutional rules. True/False
5. Legal epidemiology addresses three important goals, *EXCEPT*:
   a. to make law understandable to a wide variety of audiences
   b. to preempt other levels of government from passing laws
   c. to identify and quantify attributes and trends in law and policy
   d. to compare legal data to identify associations between law and health

## Essay Question

Healthcare-associated infections (HAIs) occur during the course of healthcare delivery, affecting one in 20 patients in U.S. hospitals. Widespread recognition that HAIs are preventable has led states to exercise legal authority in the last decade to stop HAIs from occurring. These "state HAI laws" create prevention programs, incentivize public and private engagement in prevention activities, and allow public health entities to collect and analyze HAI data from healthcare facilities. You are a public heath analyst and your state is considering implementing such a law. Your supervisor wants to know how other states are using the law to address HAIs, and whether they are working to reduce HAI rates.

You decide a legal epidemiology study is needed, so you prepare an outline for your supervisor. Consider the following in your outline.

1. Create a resource list of up to five organizations, secondary sources, and/or people who will help you get started researching this topic.
2. List two states that you would include in your analysis and why.
3. How will collecting and analyzing the laws of other jurisdictions help inform the work in your state?
4. Consider the features of the law that are important to measuring impact.
5. What health outcomes would you consider in your study?

## Internet Activities

1. You work at a research institution that studies the impact of laws on health. You are looking for new project opportunities to support your work in legal epidemiology. Do an internet search on a public health law topic of your choice and answer the following questions:
   a. What public health law topic did you choose and why?
   b. Is there an existing dataset already published on your topic? If so, cite and describe the resource (e.g., Is the resource up to date? Does it have all of the information that you need? In your opinion, is it reputable?).
   c. In roughly five to eight sentences, make the case to your boss as to why a legal epidemiology project will or will not work for your chosen topic.
2. You are a policy analyst in a local public health department. You have been asked to provide options in policy and law to address your community's shortage of available housing. There has been a dramatic decline in housing sales, and an increase in demand for rental units. Your community has a low socioeconomic status. After conducting some background research, you learn about a concept called "inclusionary zoning," and you are interested in learning how legal epidemiology might support your efforts. After watching the webinar entitled Legal Epidemiology in Practice: Exploring Local Inclusionary Zoning Laws, answer the following questions.
   a. What is "inclusionary zoning"?
   b. What steps did the Cook County, Illinois Department of Health take in their legal epidemiology study addressing inclusionary zoning?
   c. Which jurisdictions did they include? Why?
   d. What barriers did they face in doing this work?
   e. How do the researchers plan to use their findings?

## REFERENCES

Benjamin, G. C. (2020). Perspectives from the field: Using legal epidemiology to advance public health practice. *Journal of Public Health Management and Practice, 26,* S93–S95. http://dx.doi.org/10.1097/PHH.0000000000001108

Burris, S. (2011). Law in a social determinants strategy: A public health law research perspective. *Public Health Reports (Washington, D.C.: 1974), 126*, (Suppl. 3), 22–27. https://doi .org/10.1177/00333549111260S305

Burris, S., Ashe, M., Blanke, D., Ibrahim, J., Levin, D. E., Matthews, G., Penn, M., & Katz, M. (2016). Better health faster: The 5 essential public health law services. *Public Health Reports, 131*(6), 747–753. https://doi.org/10.1177/0033354916667496

Burris, S., Ashe, M., Levin, D., Penn, M., & Larkin, M. (2016). A transdisciplinary approach to public health law: The emerging practice of legal epidemiology. *Annual Review of Public Health, 37*, 135–148. https://www.ncbi.nlm.nih.gov/pmc/articles/PMC5703193

Burris, S., de Guia, S., Gable, L., Levin, D. E., Parmet, W. E., & Terry, N. P. (Eds.). (2020). *Assessing legal responses to COVID-19.* Public Health Law. https://static1.squarespace.com/static/5956e16e6b8f5b8c45f1c216/t/5f4d68a37ff9343b77604f16/1598908819812/Chp1_COVID PolicyPlaybook-Aug2020.pdf

Burris, S., Hitchcock, L., Ibrahim, J., Penn, M., & Ramanathan, T. (2016). Policy surveillance: A vital public health practice comes of age. *Journal of Health Politics, Policy and Law, 41*(6), 1151–1173. https://read .dukeupress.edu/jhppl/article/41/6/1151/40084/Policy-Surveillance-A-Vital-Public-Health-Practice

Burris, S., Wagenaar, A. C., Swanson, J., Ibrahim, J. K., Wood, J., & Mello, M. M. (2010). Making the case for laws that improve health: A framework for public health law research. *The Milbank Quarterly, 88*(2), 169–210. https://doi.org/10.1111/j.1468-0009.2010.00595.x

Centers for Disease Control and Prevention. (n.d.-a). Menu of state hospital influenza vaccination laws. *Public Health Law.* https://www.cdc.gov/phlp/docs/menu-shfluvacclaws.pdf

Centers for Disease Control and Prevention. (n.d.-b). *The legal epidemiology competency model version 1.0.* https://www.cdc.gov/phlp/docs/menu-legalepimodel.pdf

Chriqui, J. F., Leider, J., Temkin, D., Piekarz-Porter, E., Schermbeck, R. M., & Stuart-Cassel, V. (2020). State laws matter when it comes to district policymaking relative to the whole school, whole community, whole child framework. *The Journal of School Health, 90*(12), 907–917. https://doi .org/10.1111/josh.12959

Chriqui, J. F., O'Connor, J. C., & Chaloupka, F. J. (2011). What gets measured, gets changed: Evaluating law and policy for maximum impact. *The Journal of Law, Medicine and Ethics, 39*(Suppl. 1), 21–26. https://doi.org/10.1111/j.1748-720X.2011.00559.x

CityHealth. (2020). *2020 policy assessment.* https://static1.squarespace.com/static/5ad9018bf93fd4ad7295 ba8f/t/5fcedf6c10aae77571615f68/1607393203369/2020+CityHealth+Annual+Report.pdf

CityHealth. (n.d.). *Homepage.* https://www.cityhealth.org

Cloud, L K., Moran-McCabe, K., Platt, E., & Prood, N. (2020). A chronological overview of the federal, state, and local response to COVID-19. In S. Burris, S. de Guia, L. Gable, D. E. Levin, W. E. Parmet, & N. P. Terry, (Eds.). *Assessing legal responses to COVID-19.* Boston: Public Health Law Watch, Available at SSRN: https://ssrn.com/abstract=3675780

de Beaumont. (n.d.). *10 essential public health services.* https://debeaumont.org/10-essential-services

Ferdinand, A. O., Aftab, A., & Akinlotan, M. A. (2019). Texting-while-driving bans and motor vehicle crash–related emergency department visits in 16 US States: 2007–2014. *American Journal of Public Health, 109*, 748–754. https://doi.org/10.2105/AJPH.2019.304999

Hedman, L. C., Petrila, J., Fisher, W. H., Swanson, J. W., Dingman, D. A., & Burris, S. (2016). State laws on emergency holds for mental health stabilization. *Psychiatric Services, 67*(5), 529–535. https:// doi.org/10.1176/appi.ps.201500205

Humphreys, D. K., Gasparrini, A., & Wiebe, D. J. (2017). Evaluating the impact of Florida's "stand your ground" self-defense law on homicide and suicide by firearm: An interrupted time series study. *JAMA Internal Medicine, 177*(1), 44–50. https://doi.org/10.1001/jamainternmed.2016.6811

Ibrahim, J. K., Sorensen, A. A., Grunwald, H., & Burris, S. (2017). Supporting a culture of evidence-based policy: Federal funding for public health law evaluation research, 1985–2014. *Journal of Public Health Management and Practice, 23*(6), 658–666. https://doi.org/10.1097/PHH.0000000000000598

Jones, B. S., Daniel, S., & Cloud, L. K. (2018). State law approaches to facility regulation of abortion and other office interventions. *American Journal of Public Health, 108*(4), 486–492. https://doi .org/10.2105/AJPH.2017.304278

Komro, K. A., Markowitz, S., Livingston, M. D., & Wagenaar, A. C. (2018). Effects of state-level earned income tax credit laws on birth outcomes by race and ethnicity. *Health Equity, 3*(1), 61–67. https:// doi.org/10.1089/heq.2018.0061

MonQcle. (n.d.). *Homepage.* https://monqcle.com

Office of Disease Prevention and Health Promotion. (n.d.). *Social determinants of health.* https://www .healthypeople.gov/2020/topics-objectives/topic/social-determinants-of-health

The Policy Surveillance Program. (2020). *COVID-19: State emergency declarations & mitigation policies.* https://lawatlas.org/datasets/covid-19-emergency-declarations

Ramanathan, T., Hulkower, R., Holbrook, J., & Penn, M. (2017). Legal epidemiology: The science of law. *The Journal of Law, Medicine and Ethics, 45*(1 Suppl.), 69–72. https://www.ncbi.nlm.nih.gov/ pmc/articles/PMC5690565/#R1

Ransom, M. M. (Ed.). (2016). *Public health law competency model: Version 1.0.* https://www.cdc.gov/ phlp/docs/phlcm-v1.pdf

Ransom, M. M., Ramanathan, T., & Yassine, B. (Eds.). (2018). *The legal epidemiology competency model: Version 1.0.* https://www.cdc.gov/phlp/publications/topic/resources/legalepimodel/index.html

Roberts, S. C., Mericle, A. A., Subbaraman, M. S., Thomas, S., Kerr, W., & Berglas, N. (2020). Variations by education status in relationships between alcohol/pregnancy policies and birth outcomes and prenatal care utilization: A legal epidemiology study. *Journal of Public Health Management and Practice, 26,* S71–S83. https://doi.org/10.1097/PHH.0000000000001069

Rothstein, R. (2017). *The color of law: A forgotten history of how our government segregated America.* Liveright.

Scrimshaw, S. C., & Backes, E. P. (2020). *Birth settings in America: Outcomes, quality, access, and choice* National Academies Press.

Stokols, D., Hall, K. L., Taylor, B. K., & Moser, R. P. (2008). The science of team science: Overview of the field and introduction to the supplement. *American Journal of Preventive Medicine, 35,* S77– S89. https://doi.org/10.1016/j.amepre.2008.05.002

Tremper, C., Thomas, S., & Wagenaar, A. C. (2010). Measuring law for evaluation research. *Evaluation Review, 34*(3), 242–266. https://doi.org/10.1177/0193841X10370018

Vandelaer, J., & Olaniran, M. (2015). Using a school-based approach to deliver immunization— Global update. *Vaccine, 33*(5), 719–725. https://doi.org/10.1016/j.vaccine.2014.11.037

Wagenaar, A. C., & Burris, S. (Eds.). (2013). *Public health law research: Theory and methods.* Jossey-Bass.

## Additional Resources

- **LawAtlas.org** has more than 125 open-source legal datasets that use scientific legal mapping to capture the characteristics of laws and policies of public health significance.
- **PDAPS.org** is home to 20+ scientific legal maps on drug abuse–related topics, and is widely used as a source of rigorous legal data for researchers, policymakers, and the public.
- **CityHealth.org** is an initiative of the de Beaumont Foundation and Kaiser Permanente that is powered by policy surveillance data collected by the Center for Public Health Law Research team at Temple University. It uses a rating tool powered by MonQcle to award medals to the 40 largest U.S. cities on their policies across nine domains, such as earned sick leave and affordable housing policies.
- **National Environmental Health Association Webinar Series: An Introduction to Legal Epidemiology**
  https://www.neha.org/node/59017
- **"Advancing Legal Epidemiology,"** *Journal of Public Health Management and Practice*
  https://journals.lww.com/jphmp/toc/2020/03001
- **The Legal Epidemiology Competency Model Version 1.0**
  https://www.cdc.gov/phlp/publications/topic/resources/legalepimodel/index.html
- **Legal Epidemiology Series; Public Health Law Academy Training**
  https://www.changelabsolutions.org/good-governance/phla/legal-epidemiology
- **Center for Public Health Law Research Theory & Methods Library**
  http://publichealthlawresearch.org/theory-methods
- **Policy Surveillance Training Resources**
  http://publichealthlawresearch.org/resource/policy-surveillance-training-resources

# 20

# Public Health Law and Ethics

Kelly K. Dineen, Molly Berkery, Montrece McNeill Ransom,
Emely Sanchez, and Gabrielle Metoyer

## Learning Objectives

By the end of this chapter, the reader will be able to:

- Distinguish between public health law and public health ethics.
- Characterize moral norms and the varying way they can be expressed.
- Recognize ethical issues in public health practice.
- Apply the "stakeholders, facts, norms, options" (SFNO) framework to public health ethical dilemmas.

## Key Terminology

**Clinical healthcare ethics:** A systematic framework to evaluate the conduct and integrity of healthcare professionals providing clinical healthcare.

**Ethics:** A systematic examination and application of moral principles held by a society (Beauchamp & Childress, 2001; Ortmann et al., 2016).

**Legal ethics:** A systematic framework to evaluate the conduct of attorneys in representing clients, primarily using a state's legal "Rules of Professional Conduct."

**Morals:** Standards of behavior or beliefs about what is right and what is wrong.

**Norms:** Rules or expectations that are socially enforced.

**Prima facie:** A Latin term meaning "at first sight"; In the context of law and ethics, however, it refers to evidence or information that on its face or first review appears to sufficiently provide a complete argument. Such prima facie evidence would be taken as fact, but subject to rebuttal or counter argument (Legal Information Institute, n.d.).

**Professional code of ethics:** A written expression of the moral *norms* (including principles, virtues, and values) that guide and ground behavior by members of a profession in carrying out their professional roles.

**Public health ethics:** A systematic framework to evaluate the conduct and integrity of public health practitioners and researchers in implementing, evaluating, complying with, and enforcing public health laws, policies, and programs.

## Public Health Law Competencies

This chapter addresses the following competencies from the Public Health Law Competency Model (PHLCM; Ransom, 2016).

**1.1** Define basic constitutional concepts and legal principles framing the practice of public health laws across relevant jurisdictions.

**1.3** Describe the protocol for contacting and best practices for engaging with legal and/or ethical advisors, and other key public health law resources.

**2.3** Recognize the legal authority and limits of critical system partners and others who influence health outcomes.

---

### Spark Question
In your opinion, what is the difference between ethics and morals?

---

## INTRODUCTION

Despite its explicit focus on justice and population level change, the field of **public health ethics** is relatively new. At its core, public health ethics is about practical decision-making, often when the law is unclear. Other scholars note that "decisions fall into the realm of ethics when they pertain to things within our control that will either show respect or not show respect to human beings" (Dubois, 2008, p. 47). Having a grounding in public health ethics is important because the day-to-day decisions made by public health practitioners impact the "health and well-being of diverse groups of individuals, groups, and communities" (American Public Health Association [APHA], 2019). Public health ethics include the systematic evaluation of the **morals** of those decisions, both before and after the decision is made and action is taken. According to Dawson and Upshur, "public health ethics is concerned with everything related to the values that capture the aims, methods, practice, and policy related to public health" (Dawson & Upshur, 2013, p. 103).

While public health ethics borrow from principles of clinical, biomedical, and research ethics, the direct application of those individual fields to an **ethics** of public health is not sufficient to address the myriad issues central to the practice of public health. Public health is focused primarily on the everyday decision-making needed to carry out its legal authority to protect and promote the health of the public (Goldberg, 2013; Jennings, 2007). Ethical considerations underlie numerous aspects of public health practice ranging from health department resources to human subjects research to clinical care to the distribution of vaccines during pandemics to media strategies related to high-risk patients/populations. The very nature of the practice of public health underscores a central ethical dilemma: to balance individual freedoms and liberties with the government's ethical and legal responsibility to protect the health of citizens and provide some protection from harm.

Public health law and public health ethics are complementary and in certain instances include clinical, biomedical, and research ethics, but can also be distinguished in a variety of ways (see Table 20.1). Public health often depends upon the law to set minimum standards and empower public health practitioners to advance strategies to educate, promote health, and prevent the spread of disease. Law underlies governmental police power to protect the health of citizens as well as the ability to collect and allocate public monies (Childress et al., 2002). Public health law provides the authority for and outlines the limitations on governmental action. Public health law encourages and discourages certain behaviors.

Public health ethics include ongoing analysis, deliberation, and justification for public health action and public health policy, often when law is unwritten, vague, or does not apply. The law can provide a floor for decision-making when confronted with an ethical dilemma and

TABLE 20.1 *Law v. Ethics*

| PUBLIC HEALTH LAW | PUBLIC HEALTH ETHICS |
|---|---|
| ■ Provides authority and limitations on federal and state governmental power<br>■ Incentives and disincentives for behavior | ■ Provides ongoing analysis, deliberation, and justification for public health action and policy<br>■ Often applicable when law is indeterminate |
| Formal Institution<br>■ Statutes<br>■ Regulations<br>■ Case Law | Less formal<br>■ Moral norms, values<br>■ Professional codes<br>■ Based on previous experience and incidents |
| Public proceedings with a "reasonable person" standard | Publicly justifiable positions based on ethical reasoning |

may prohibit or compel certain actions. However, the law does not answer questions about ethical approaches and public health decision-making benefits from explicit values considerations from the outset and from a framework to resolve dilemmas as they arise.

This chapter addresses basic concepts of public health ethics, reviews and explains the predominant moral norms that underlie public health ethics, and provides a framework for analyzing and resolving ethical problems for the public health practitioner.

## MORAL NORMS

The application of public health ethics necessarily involves an understanding of moral norms that guide a public health practitioner's decision-making when facing ethical dilemmas. As described in the following, these norms can be expressed in ethical principles, public health values, and professional codes of ethics. Legal norms, also discussed in this section, are also relevant to the resolution of ethical dilemmas, as decision-makers must appreciate the ways in which relevant laws may limit the number of ethically acceptable options for actions.

## Four Core Ethical Principles

The words "moral" and "ethical," while frequently used interchangeably, have distinct meanings. **Morals** are traditions of belief about right or wrong; the rules that emerge from those traditions of belief are moral **norms**. Moral norms are the foundation for what a culture considers moral conduct. "Ethics," on the other hand, is the systematic examination and application of morality (Beauchamp & Childress, 2001; Ortmann et al., 2016). Moral norms can be in the form of values, virtues, or principles (Ortmann et al., 2016). As described by Beauchamp and Childress, the four **prima facie** principles are (a) autonomy, (b) justice, (c) beneficence, and (d) nonmaleficence (Beauchamp & Childress, 2001, pp. 10–12). These four principles have been consistently relied upon in clinical ethics and have contributed to public health ethics work and are described as follows.

### Autonomy

The principle of respect for persons requires respect for an individual's inherent dignity and capacity for rational choice; this includes the obligation to honor autonomy, which is the right of persons to determine what is done to or for them without coercion or undue interference from others. It means respecting the liberty of individuals to make choices and act (Childress et al., 2002). Public health ethics is also concerned with relational autonomy, which emphasizes the interdependence of individual actors and their impact on others (Jennings, 2016; providing a review of the evolving literature in relational autonomy and liberty). Respect for persons extends beyond just those who have capacity and also supports dignity "within transactions, exchanges, and relationships" (APHA, 2019, p. 8).

Ethical issues arise because what may best promote the health of populations may require individual sacrifices or even harms, and as such, a limitation on an individual's *autonomy*. One example of this is the legal requirement of all 50 states mandating children be vaccinated in order to attend school. According to Dawson and Verweij, "Personal autonomy, cherished in modern individual health care, might not be given priority in public health care, where other values, such as the protection of the health of individuals and groups, the prevention of harm to others, and the promotion of health equity are central" (2007, p. 2).

## Justice

Justice is "a group of norms for fairly distributing benefits, risks and costs" (Beauchamp & Childress, 2001, pp. 12–13; for a comprehensive review of the evolution of theories justice in public health, see Goldberg, 2013). One example of this is health equity and the prioritization of vaccines to communities with high numbers of Black, Latinx, and Indigenous residents during a pandemic because of the disproportionate rates of hospitalizations and deaths from COVID-19 in those communities. It includes both distributive justice (equitable distribution of benefits and burdens) and procedural justice (fair deliberative procedure that includes public participation, especially of affected parties; Childress et al., 2002; Ortmann et al., 2016). According to Ortmann et al., "justice has always functioned dually, applying to individuals but more importantly serving as an overarching principle for adjudicating competing claims in relation to the group or to other members of society" (2016, p. 22). Jennings asserts that justice "requires a deliberative and inclusive decision-making process in order to ensure that authority and power in public health is [sic] exercised in fair and productive ways" (Jennings, 2020, p. 190).

## Beneficence

Beneficence is a group of norms pertaining to relieving, lessening or preventing harm, and providing benefits and balancing benefits against risks and costs (Jennings, 2020, pp. 12, 13). The principle of beneficence presupposes compassion and requires the promotion of others' well-being through positive action and the desire to do good. A public health example of beneficence would be laws that require seatbelts in all automobiles. Installation of seatbelts might place a burden on the automobile manufacturers, but this burden is outweighed by the reduction of motor vehicle deaths and injuries caused by lack of appropriate safety restraints.

## Nonmaleficence

Nonmaleficence means to do no harm. It is distinct from beneficence in the sense that choosing not to harm first is qualitatively different than minimizing harms relative to benefits (Ortmann et al., 2016). Within the public health sphere, nonmaleficence might take the form of a public health department and local government reviewing building planning proposals to ensure communities do not lose access to parks, public transit, or healthy food options as new areas of the city are developed.

## Public Health Moral Considerations and Values

Childress and colleagues identified several moral considerations in public health ethics that reflect and incorporate these four core principles. These include (a) producing benefits; (b) avoiding, preventing, and removing harms; and (c) producing the maximal balance of benefits over

**TABLE 20.2  Health Equity and Public Health Ethics**

| PUBLIC HEALTH LAW | PUBLIC HEALTH ETHICS |
|---|---|
| 1. Institutional Review Board (IRB) or Independent Ethics Committee (IEC) by Title 45 Code of Federal Regulations Part 46 | 1. Including core ethical principles in human-subject public health research |
| 2. Executive Order on Ensuring an Equitable Pandemic Response and Recovery | 2. Including ethical principles in the distribution and allocation of resources, including vaccines, to populations disproportionally impacted by the pandemic |
| 3. Health Insurance Portability and Accountability Act (HIPAA) | 3. Including core ethical principles in the collection, use, and distribution of personally identifiable health data— including public health data for disease surveillance |
| 4. Executive Order on Federal Actions to Address Environmental Justice in Minority Populations and Low-Income Populations | 4. Including ethical principles in the distribution and allocation of environmental hazards and waste, especially in low-income and minority communities |

*Sources:* Biden, J. (2021, January 21). *Executive order on ensuring an equitable pandemic response and recovery.* https://www.whitehouse.gov/briefing
-room/presidential-actions/2021/01/21/executive-order-ensuring-an-equitable-pandemic-response-and-recovery; Centers for Disease Control and Prevention.
(2003). *HIPAA privacy rule and public health: Guidance from CDC and the U.S. Department of Health and Human Services.* Morbidity and Mortality
*Weekly Report, 52* (Early Release), 1–24. http://www.cdc.gov/privacyrule/Guidance/PRmmwrguidance.pdf; Food and Drug Administration. (n.d.).
*IRB-frequently asked questions.* Retrieved February 17, 2021, from https://www.fda.gov/regulatory-information/search-fda-guidance-documents/institutional-
review-boards-frequently-asked-questions; Institutional Review Board, 45 C.F.R. §46. https://www.ecfr.gov/cgi-bin/retrieveECFR?gp=&SID=83cd09e1c0f
5c6937cd9d7513160fc3f&pitd=20180719&n=pt45.1.46&r=PART&ty=HTML; U.S. Environmental Protection Agency. (n.d.). *Summary of executive order
12898—Federal actions to address environmental justice in minority populations and low-income populations (59 FR 7629; February 16, 1994).* Retrieved
July 23, 2020 from https://www.epa.gov/laws-regulations/summary-executive-order-12898-federal-actions-address-environmental-justice

harms and costs (i.e. utility). These three considerations, according to the authors, "provide prima facie warrant for many activities in pursuit of the goal of public health" (Childress et al., 2002, p. 172). The 2019 Public Health Code of Ethics also identifies the principles of beneficence and nonmaleficence under the core value of health and safety (APHA, 2019).

## Community, Solidarity, and Care

Public health also places emphasis on the community as an entity formed by interactive and interdependent members. It is not merely a sum of its parts but a special ecosystem of relationships, interests, and values. According to Ortmann and colleagues,

> Public health values community in two obvious senses. First, it recognizes that the success of most health interventions depends on a community's acceptance, cooperation, or participation. Second, it recognizes that to be successful, public health must respect the community's values and gain the trust of its members. Yet there is a third, deeper sense in which community represents a value. A community is, to emphasize again, neither a statistical abstraction nor a mere aggregate of individuals but rather a network of relationships and emotional bonds between people sharing a life in common organized through a political and moral order. (Ortmann et al., 2016, pp. 7–8)

Solidarity is a concept grounded in the community, honoring the dignity of and showing respect for community members, regardless of their productivity, abilities, or social standing (Jennings, 2019). It means all members of the community have moral worth and are deserving of consideration and care. Three progressing levels of demonstrating solidarity are (a) standing up for, (b) standing up with, and (c) standing up as. Jennings describes care as a "social relational practice based on the recognition that others are due moral consideration or attentiveness, which should be accommodated in ways appropriate to their particular needs, vulnerability, and circumstances" (Jennings, 2018, p. S20). The byproducts of solidarity and care are the "affirmation of and attention to others" (Jennings, 2018, p. S23). One example of solidarity in action is wearing masks and abiding by public health recommendations on social distancing during the COVID-19 pandemic. These acts acknowledge that our behavior may impact others and the community and that some personal inconvenience is necessary to positively impact the health of the community, including members who may be at higher risk of serious illness.

## Professional Codes of Ethics

Public health, like many other professions, has a **professional code of ethics**. A code of ethics expresses the virtues expected of professionals, the norms and values of the profession, and the profession's relationships with and among members of the profession and society (Jennings, 2018). The Public Health Code of Ethics was updated in 2019 and includes six core values with corresponding obligations, explained in Table 20.2.

Professional codes of ethics often include virtues the members of the profession should cultivate. Unlike honoring a moral principle, such as maximizing benefits to others, virtues focus on the professional's way of being a moral person. Virtues are often described as habits of character that predispose individuals to behave ethically (Beauchamp & Childress, 2001). Commonly expected professional virtues include veracity, compassion, knowledge development, courage, and professional competence (Pellegrino & Thomas, 1993). Veracity is the "comprehensive accurate and objective transmission of information" as well as the way the professional fosters understanding (Beauchamp & Childress, 2001, p. 289). Another critical virtue for health professionals is humility (Dubois et al., 2013). The virtue of humility encompasses several other practices, including self-knowledge, reflection and perspective taking, and intellectual honesty (admitting what you do not know and seeking help; Dineen, 2016). Cultivating these virtues can better prepare public health practitioners for recognizing and resolving ethical problems.

## TABLE 20.3  2019 Public Health Code of Ethics, Core Values

| CORE VALUE | PROFESSIONAL OBLIGATIONS, MORAL NORMS, AND VIRTUES |
|---|---|
| Professionalism and Trust | ■ Use of scientific evidence to guide decisions<br>■ Honesty and transparency (including examination of and disclosure of conflicting interests and influences)<br>■ Professional competence and accuracy |
| Health and Safety | ■ Beneficence (promotion of public safety, health, and well-being)<br>■ Nonmaleficence (prevention, minimization, and mitigation of health harms) |
| Health Justice and Equity | ■ Promotion of the equitable distribution of burdens, benefits, and opportunities for health (distributive justice)<br>■ Remediation of structural and institutional inequities (justice) |
| Interdependence and Solidarity | ■ Promotion of positive (and mitigating negative) relationships among individuals, societies, and environments to protect and promote flourishing<br>■ Attending to intergenerational resource conflicts |
| (Respect for) Human Rights and Civil Liberties | ■ Respect for persons (respect for personal autonomy and self-determination)<br>■ Privacy (maintain individual privacy)<br>■ Attend to power disparities (advocate for absence or avoidance of institutional and interpersonal domination) |
| Inclusivity and Engagement | ■ Engagement of diverse stakeholders (individual, community, and public) in decision-making (procedural justice) |

*Source:* Adapted from American Public Health Association. (2019). *Public health code of ethics,* 5–6. https://www.apha.org/-/media/files/pdf/membergroups/ethics/code_of_ethics.ashx

## Legal Norms

It is especially important to also consider legal norms in evaluating whether proposed actions are ethically appropriate. According to Daniel Goldberg, "the mission of public health is morally charged, and public health law at its most robust can help illuminate what laws and policies should exist and are of highest ethical priority" (2013, p. 392). Legal norms include state, tribal, local, and federal legislation, regulation, and case law. As mentioned earlier, law puts boundaries on public health action. Law often outlines what a practitioner *must* do, authorizes what they *can* do, and in some instances describes what they *cannot* do. This can be explicitly authorized or inferred from statutes and case law. An example of a public health norm prescribed by law would be restaurant inspection (see Table 20.3).

When reading public health laws, or any laws, it is important to pay close attention to what is permissible and what might be mandatory. A law that reads "the public health officer or his or her agent *shall* inspect restaurants annually…" is very different from "the public health officer or his or her agent *may* inspect restaurants annually." The first phrasing, using "shall," creates a burden on the health department to perform annual restaurant inspections, while the latter, using "may," creates an option for the health department to inspect annually; it is not mandatory.

In other instances, the law may conflict with what *ought* to be done, prohibiting public health practitioners from taking the most ethically appropriate action. For example, public health practitioners utilizing a harm reduction model confront laws that criminalize the possession of syringes. Such laws severely limit the ability to operate syringe services programs, making it difficult to address the high rates of infectious disease among people who inject drugs in many communities (Centers for Disease Control and Prevention [CDC], 2016).

Legal advice from an attorney may also provide a framework for decision-making, but it is not often definitive when it comes to ethical decision-making. Legal advice or legal counsel is the "guidance given by lawyers to their clients" during the course of representation (Advice of Counsel, 2019). Practically, providing legal advice or counsel means the attorney has researched the legal question and applicable law, identified problems and solutions, and then provided the client with options and guidance about what might be the best strategy for the client's case. In the context of a health department, the legal advice an attorney might give could be about any number of subjects. A public health department attorney might provide legal counsel related to restaurant inspection enforcement; quarantine and isolation, management and compliance with rules for grants and other funding streams, involuntary commitment proceedings, nuisance proceedings related to public health threats, health department employment disputes, and more. Keep in mind with each of these examples, the attorney is acting on behalf of the health department, not the individuals employed by the health department.

A lawyer may not, however, be able to provide advice about what a public health practitioner *ought* to do in an ethical dilemma. This is particularly true in three specific situations: (a) when several, legally viable options are available, (b) where the law does not require or prohibit a specific action, and (c) where there is no legal precedent to guide the decision-making. This is where having a framework for resolving ethical issues becomes critical for thinking through options, and delineating justification for or against taking a specific action.

### TABLE 20.4  Public Health Norm Prescribed by Law

California Health and Safety Code § 113725.2 states

"Local enforcement agencies, and the department when adequate funding is made available to the department, **shall** conduct routine training on food facility inspection standardization to promote the uniform application of inspection procedures." (emphasis added)

*The use of the word "shall" creates a mandatory action on behalf of the health department; the department has to conduct routine training about food facility inspection.*

## FRAMEWORK FOR RESOLVING ETHICAL PROBLEMS

Both ethical and legal decision making require a deliberate consideration of the facts, questions, and conflict at hand, a clear understanding of the options available, the capacity to decide, and reasoning or justification for making that decision. And, in both ethical and legal decision making, in the end reasonable, ethical minds might still disagree on the final decision.

An ethical framework is a "tool or approach for practically addressing ethical challenges that often includes a stepwise procedure" (Ortmann et al., 2016, p. 14). Ethical frameworks generally take a pragmatic approach that procedurally allows for using a variety of substantive moral norms and values to resolve ethical problems. There are a variety of frameworks available, any of which could be used effectively. This chapter will offer the SFNO model, first described by James M. Dubois, with incorporation of the public health ethics literature.

### TABLE 20.5  SFNO Approach to Analyzing Ethical Problems

"So Far No Objections"
**Stakeholders:**
- Who has a *stake* in the decision being made? Why?
- Who will be significantly affected by the decision made? Why? Please be specific.

**Facts:**
- What additional *facts* are necessary to inform your decision-making process?
- What factual issues might generate disagreement?
- What facts are relevant to a solution?

**Norms:**
- What ethical principles, *norms,* or values are at stake?
- **Which do you think are relevant, and which might appear to conflict or generate disagreement?**

**Options:**
- Consider a *wide variety* of alternatives. Resist the urge to quickly reach a recommendation.
  - ☐ What actions or policies deserve serious consideration?
  - ☐ Explore the values behind the alternatives (cognitive dissonance and perspective taking foster ethical and professional development).
- Narrow the options to arrive at a few ethically acceptable options.
  - ☐ If the ethical ideal is not possible, which compromise solutions are most attractive?
- *Justification* criteria may be helpful in explaining your reasons for selecting one or two options as superior.
  - ☐ *Permissibility:* Would the action being considered be ethically wrong even if it were to have a good outcome?
  - ☐ *Necessity:* Is it necessary to infringe on the values or **norms** under consideration in order to achieve the intended goal?
  - ☐ *Effectiveness:* Will the action be effective in achieving the desired goal (based on evidence and experience)?
  - ☐ *Proportionality:* Is the desired goal important enough to justify overriding another principle or value?
  - ☐ *Least infringement and Reciprocity:* Is the policy or action designed to minimize the infringement of the principle or value that conflicts with it? Have we done what is reasonable to offset the potential harms and losses that the proposed action imposes on individuals and communities?
  - ☐ *Proper process/Public justification:* Has the decision been made using proper processes? Have all potentially affected stakeholders had a meaningful opportunity to participate?

*Source:* Adapted from Dubois, J. M. (2008b). *Solving ethical problems: Analyzing ethics cases and justifying decision: Ethics in mental health research.* Oxford University Press; Volpe, R. L., Bakanas, E., Dineen, K. K., Dubois, J. (Eds.). (2016). *Guidance for facilitators & facilitation guide in exploring integrity in medicine: The Bander Center for Medical Business Ethics Casebook* (2nd ed.). Saint Louis University.
Justification criteria synthesized from Dubois, J. M. (2008b). *Solving ethical problems: Analyzing ethics cases and justifying decision: Ethics in mental health research.* Oxford University Press; Childress, J. R., Faden, R. R., Garre, R. D., Gostin, L. O., Kahn, J., Bonnie, R. J., Kass, N. E., Mastroianni, A. C., Moreno, J. D., & Nieburg, P. (2002). Public health ethics: Mapping the terrain. *Journal of Law, Medicine and Ethics, 30*(2), 170–178. https://doi.org/10.1111/j.1748-720X.2002.tb00384.x; American Public Health Association. (2019). *Public health code of ethics,* 1–30.

## The SFNO Framework

SFNO is an easily memorized acronym that stands for (a) Stakeholders, (b) Facts, (c) Norms, and (d) Options (Dubois, 2008a) (See Table 20.5). The phrase "so far no objections" is a helpful way to memorize the acronym. The SFNO model is simply an organizing device that allows those involved in a public health decision to identify and reflect on important considerations for and implications of their proposed actions. The model is helpful in working through both cognitive and social ethical dilemmas. Table 20.4 contains the key steps of the SFNO model. Two case studies, analyzing and applying the SFNO model, follow.

---

### HYPOTHETICAL CASE STUDY #1: NEEDLE EXCHANGE

Louis is the director of the Public Health Department of Baron County. Louis recently proposed a community outreach syringe services program (SSP) with a local community drug and alcohol rehabilitation nonprofit, New Beginnings, for drug use reduction in a neighborhood with a high population of people who inject drugs (PWID). One goal of the SSP is to prevent the occurrence and spread of the hepatitis C virus (HCV). The HCV is commonly spread by sharing needles or other equipment used to prepare and inject drugs. The HCV can be treated, but without treatment can lead to cirrhosis of the liver and death. There is currently no vaccine for the HCV (CDC, n.d.-b).

The SSP would offer free, sterile hypodermic syringes and needles (injection supplies) while safely disposing of used equipment using one of two models. Under the first model, individuals would be able to exchange used injection supplies for sterile injection supplies only if they submit to regular HCV screening. Under the second model, HCV testing would be offered, but not mandatory for supply exchange.

Several residents of Baron County are opposed to the proposed SSP and fear it would only promote drug use in the neighborhood. There are currently no state, county, or local laws prohibiting or expressly allowing SSPs. However, there is a state law that prohibits the use of medical paraphernalia for nonmedical reasons.

1. Who are the stakeholders?
2. What are the relevant facts?
3. What norms are relevant?
4. What are the available options?

---

## Stakeholders

In hypothetical case study #1, Louis must consider all of the stakeholders, or in other words, the individuals who will be directly or indirectly impacted by his proposed SSP. In this case study, the stakeholders are the PWID in the neighborhood, the residents of the neighborhood and Baron County, the healthcare providers implementing the SSP, as well as those who treat infections and HCV in PWID, New Beginnings, and law enforcement and first responders. Additional stakeholders may include volunteers and local businesses.

## Facts

In this case, factual disagreements will be over whether the state law that prohibits the use of medical paraphernalia (syringes) for nonmedical reasons could prevent the needle exchange program. It will be important to build support with local law enforcement to ensure the SSP, if implemented, is not targeted by law enforcement for arrest of the PWID participating in the services. Ensuring the operation of the SSP will not place New Beginnings in legal jeopardy is also critical.

Several residents are opposed to the program and fear potential promotion of drug use. It will be important to explore the source of and basis for their fears because they are not supported by facts. Research has demonstrated that SSPs do not increase drug use but do reduce harms to PWID and law enforcement and first responders (by reducing needlestick injuries from discarded used needles in the community). SSPs also help PWID into treatment (SSP clients are five times as likely to enter addiction treatment), reduce overdose deaths, and overall infection rates (CDC, n.d.-c). Baron County and the surrounding area have a high population of PWID already. With this comes greater risk of exposure and a higher prevalence of the HCV which is most commonly spread by sharing needles. Untreated HCV can be fatal. SSPs are an effective tool for community-based prevention and intervention of infection and disease (www.cdc.gov/ssp/syringe-services-programs-factsheet.html.) The program would offer free, sterile injection supplies and involve HCV testing at some level. Disease screening is also critical as a tool to prevent disease burden and death.

Another important consideration is whether PWID would feel comfortable identifying themselves by participating in the program. Existing social stigma and discrimination against PWID is pervasive and PWID reasonably fear becoming a target of more harm. This could impact the success of the program. It will be important to address this as well as the widespread misperceptions within the community about PWID and SSPs.

## Norms

The most immediately relevant moral norms are beneficence (promoting health and safety), reducing harm, showing respect to persons, justice and equity, and norms based in solidarity and community. Providing these services would express solidarity with and respect for the dignity and worth of PWID, who face stigma and discrimination every day. It would also address equity by serving a drastically underserved population. Providing these services, of course, reduces harm by reducing the chance of infection, enhancing early detection, and facilitating treatment. Mandating the HCV testing may reduce harm by catching more infections, but it may also enhance harm by compromising the autonomy (or free choice) of PWID and by reducing service use as a result. Coercive programs can be especially harmful to PWID who are likely to have been in the criminal legal system and avoid coercion as a result. It may be more ethical to consider voluntary only or infrequent (*e.g.* once every 6 months) mandatory testing. Inclusivity and engagement are norms that would be honored by involving SSP clients in decision-making about mandatory testing. Inclusivity and engagement are norms that also ground working with community members and law enforcement, which will also enhance effectiveness.

Services may also benefit PWID by helping them access addiction treatment. This also reduces harm to the community by decreasing the rates of infections in the community and the rate of needlestick injuries with contaminated discarded needles.

Another important norm is justice and equity. The existing inequities for PWID mean most of their health needs are not being met and the SSP is an important opportunity to take a small step to ameliorate this. Doing this will require significant educational and outreach campaigns to the community to address opposition.

The legal norms of current state law will also need to be addressed. It is currently illegal for PWID to use drugs. However, the goal and purpose of SSPs is not law enforcement but promoting health and harm reduction. Consulting an attorney to determine the legal risks in this context will be a critical step toward making the SSP possible as will working with the local law enforcement community to prevent unintended harms of arrest and incarceration of PWID in the community.

## Options

The options in Case Study #1 include: (a) a decision to not offer the SSP because of the opposition and legal risks; (b) offer the SSP and require HCV screening in exchange for supplying sterile syringes and needles; (c) offer the SSP and make HCV screening optional, or (d) consider a hybrid approach in which the SSP begins by making HCV optional and tracks uptake and infection rates. Option (d) has the benefit of not compromising the autonomy of PWID while also keeping a close eye on levels of harm from infection. The risk is that some harms to the PWID may go undetected but that may be justified in this case because the need to build trust with PWID may outweigh catching every single case of HCV. Effectiveness is a critical justification because if PWID feel coerced, they may not use the SSP at all. Option (d) is also proportionate because it is likely that, as trust builds, many clients will agree to screening and will have the benefit of sterile injection supplies. Option (d) also fulfils the justification criteria of least infringement because while it may compromise the ability to treat all HCV infections early, it does still allow the PWID to build a relationship and may lead them to addiction treatment, have voluntary testing, and access sterile injection supplies—therefore reducing the risks of future infections.

---

### HYPOTHETICAL CASE STUDY #2: VACCINE EXEMPTIONS

Karliyah is an epidemiologist who specializes in infectious disease prevention and vaccine development. She also serves on the state's Vaccination Policy Committee. Karliyah is concerned because her state is facing a mumps outbreak. While the laws in her state require all Pre-K and school-aged children to be vaccinated for mumps in order to attend school, there are exemptions to the vaccination requirement for religious or personal belief reasons. Karliyah is concerned because mumps is a highly contagious virus, easily spread through contact with saliva or respiratory droplets from the mouth, nose, or throat (CDC, n.d.-d). Mumps can cause inflammation of the testicles, ovaries, pancreas, brain, and spinal cord. It can also cause lifelong complications, including sterility and deafness (CDC, n.d.-a). Karliyah's office has started to get calls from several vaccine-hesitant families in the area where the mumps outbreak has the highest case numbers. The governor is considering an emergency order that would remove the religious and personal belief exemptions to vaccines for the current mumps outbreak. Karliyah has not yet heard whether the governor would be willing to sign such a law.

1. Who are the stakeholders?
2. What are the relevant facts?
3. What norms are relevant?
4. What are the available options?

---

## Stakeholders

In hypothetical case study #2, the stakeholders are Karliyah (as a resident and stakeholder in the Vaccination Policy Committee), the residents of her state, including parents and school children in her district, and vaccine-hesitant families, the governor, lawmakers, and other authoritative actors such as the state Department of Education and Department of Health.

## Facts

In this case, factual disagreements will be about the potential removal of religious and personal belief legal exemptions to address a public health outbreak and potential public health emergency. State law requires children to be vaccinated from certain communicable diseases. Removing the exceptions may lead some people to violate the law; and understanding there are penalties such as fines for noncompliance is an important fact. Also, the constitution does not require an exception for religious reasons in the case of children in schools, but federal antidiscrimination laws do require exceptions be made for children with an underlying condition (disability) that makes vaccination dangerous for them. Facts about the harms of mumps are also important. Mumps is a highly contagious virus, easily spread through contact with saliva or respiratory droplets from the mouth, nose, or throat. Pre-K and school-aged children are considered high-risk for the spread of mumps because of their health behaviors. Targeting mumps and its spread early in childhood development can prevent negative health consequences. Mumps can cause inflammation of the testicles, ovaries, pancreas, brain, and spinal cord. It can also cause lifelong complications, including sterility and deafness. Vaccine-hesitant families are vocal about potential enforcement and are living in areas with the highest case numbers. Vaccine hesitancy can contribute to increased spread of the disease and delay control of the potential public health emergency.

## Norms

The most immediately relevant legal norms are the state laws on vaccine mandates, religious freedom, disability discrimination law, and the rights of parents to make decisions for their children. The moral norms are based in community and solidarity, promoting health and well-being, reducing harms, and respecting the autonomy of parents to make decisions for their children. Parental autonomy is a long-honored principle, but it can be outweighed by the best interest of the child and the state's interests in community well-being by preventing disease outbreaks. Potential harms reach beyond the individual to include increased risk of a larger epidemic, and the benefits of mandating the vaccine by removing exemptions. The cultural expression and protection of individual freedoms and the community's relationship with the law are also relevant norms to consider. In this case study, we see a tension arise between an individual right and the public good among members of the community who are vaccine hesitant. Group identity influences social and moral norms and is a major force of conformation which then sets behavioral standards for different people.

## Options

The options in Case Study #2 include: (a) mandating the vaccine for school entry by removing the religious and philosophical exemptions and promote outbreak mitigation strategies; (b) removing one exemption, commonly the philosophical exemption, and promote outbreak mitigation strategies; or, (c) making no changes regarding vaccine exemptions and requirements for school entry, while continuing to promote other outbreak mitigation strategies. Option (a) means that some will get the vaccine who would not have previously, but under coercion while infringing on parental autonomy and possibly religious beliefs. This may be justified by necessity, effectiveness, and proportionality (provided the scope of the potential outbreak warrants the intrusion). Option (b) protects individual religious freedoms while removing the philosophical objection. This is less intrusive but may mean more people will fall ill from mumps, and may ultimately not be effective. Option (c) honors the parents' rights but at the cost of the community's health and is the least desirable option from a public health perspective.

## CONCLUSION

Ethics underlies all public health action, and ethical problems are an unavoidable feature of dynamic public health. Finding ethical solutions requires compassionate consideration of community values and morals, understanding of applicable laws and rules, as well as the ability to think flexibly and creatively to create inclusive solutions. Public health practitioners can further improve their capacity for ethical engagement by working with public health legal counsel to better understand the role of law in "Can I?", "Must I?" or "May I?" situations and by building cooperative relationships with community stakeholders. Working through SFNO provides a framework to work through some of the tangles that naturally occur around ethical issues (Dubois, 2008a).

## CHAPTER REVIEW

### Review Questions

1.  An ethical decision is one that is both morally acceptable to the community and _____.
2.  What does SFNO stand for?
3.  Compare and contrast public health law and public health ethics.

### Essay Question

You are a local public health inspector, and you have received a complaint about a person with a serious hoarding disorder. When you arrive at the property, you find that the resident is 84 years old, estranged from his family, and is living on a fixed income. The community is rural, suburban, and primarily African American. You notice a newly developed subdivision across the street, and it occurs to you that you have received an increasing number of complaints about this home and others in the vicinity. Upon inspection, you also notice vector control and other concerns. There is a local ordinance that recognizes hoarding as a danger to human health, and as such, this home *can* legally be declared a nuisance. Using the SFNO framework, how might you address this issue? How might you justify your decision?

### Internet Activities

1.  Download CDC's Good Decision Making in Real Time: Public Health Ethics Training for Local Health Departments Student Manual at the following: www.cdc.gov/os/integrity/phethics/docs/Student_Manual_Revision_June_3_2019_508_compliant_Final_with_cover.pdf
    ■  Complete Section B, Module 1 Case Study on Smoke-Free Policies in Outdoor Public Spaces and summarize your findings.
2.  Take the World Health Organization's online quiz, The Ethics of Public Health Surveillance: www.who.int/ethics/quiz-surveillance-ethics/en
3.  Write a summary of your results including a description of the ethical issue and the applicable WHO Guideline on the Ethics of Public Health Surveillance.

## REFERENCES

Advice of Counsel. (2019). *Black's law dictionary* (11th ed.).

American Public Health Association. (2019). *Public health code of ethics*. https://www.apha.org/-/media/files/pdf/membergroups/ethics/code_of_ethics.ashx

Beauchamp, T. L., & Childress, J. F. (2001). *Principles of biomedical ethics* (6th ed.). Oxford University Press.

Centers for Disease Control and Prevention. (2016, February). *Syringe Services Programs (SSPs) developing, implementing, and monitoring programs.* https://www.cdc.gov/hiv/pdf/risk/cdc-hiv-developing-ssp.pdf

Centers for Disease Control and Prevention. (n.d.-a). *Complications of mumps.* Retrieved March 20, 2021, from https://www.cdc.gov/mumps/about/complications.html

Centers for Disease Control and Prevention. (n.d.-b). *Hepatitis C information.* Retrieved March 20, 2021, from https://www.cdc.gov/hepatitis/hcv/index.htm

Centers for Disease Control and Prevention. (n.d.-c, May 23). *Syringe service programs: Summary of information on the safety and effectiveness of syringe services programs (SSPs).* Retrieved March 20, 2021, from https://www.cdc.gov/ssp/syringe-services-programs-summary.html

Centers for Disease Control and Prevention. (n.d.-d). *Transmission of mumps.* Retrieved March 20, 2021, from https://www.cdc.gov/mumps/about/transmission.html

Childress, J. R., Faden, R. R., Garre, R. D., Gostin, L. O., Kahn, J., Bonnie, R. J., Kass, N. E., Mastroianni, A. C., Moreno, J. D., & Nieburg, P. (2002). Public health ethics: Mapping the terrain. *Journal of Law, Medicine and Ethics, 30*(2), 170–178. https://doi.org/10.1111/j.1748-720X.2002.tb00384.x

Dawson, A., & Upshur, R. (2013). A model curriculum for public health ethics. In D. Stretch, G. Marckmann, & I. Hirschberg (Eds.), *Ethics in public health and health policy* (pp. 103–118). Springer.

Dawson, A., & Verweij, M. (2007). Introduction. In A. Dawson & M. Verweij (Eds.), *Ethics, prevention, and public health* (pp. 1–12). Oxford University Press.

Dineen, Kelly K., Addressing Prescription Opioid Abuse Concerns in Context: Synchronizing Policy Solutions to Multiple Public Health Problems (2015). Law & Psychology Review, 2016, Saint Louis University School of Law Legal Studies Research Paper Series No. 2016-13, Available at SSRN: https://ssrn.com/abstract=2819463

Dineen, K. K. (2016). Addressing prescription opioid abuse concerns in context: Synchronizing policy solutions to multiple complex public health problems. *Law and Psychology, 30*(Rev. 1).

Dubois, J. M. (2008a). *A framework for analyzing ethics cases.* https://www.researchgate.net/publication/242419386_A_FRAMEWORK_FOR_ANALYZING_ETHICS_CASES

Dubois, J. M. (2008b). *Solving ethical problems: Analyzing ethics cases and justifying decision: Ethics in mental health research.* Oxford University Press.

Dubois, J. M., Kraus, E., Mikulic, A., Cruz-Flores, S., & Bakanas, E. (2013). A humble task: Restoring virtue in an age of conflicted interests. *Academic Medicine, 88*(7), 924–928. https://doi.org/10.1097/ACM.0b013e318294fd5b

Goldberg, D. (2013). Ethics and public health law: On the need to ask the right questions. *Journal of Public Health Management and Practice, 19*(5), 391–392. https://www.nursingcenter.com/journalarticle?Article_ID=1576622&Journal_ID=420959&Issue_ID=1576621

Goldberg, D. (2017). Justice, compound disadvantage, and health inequities. In D. Goldberg (Ed.), *Public health ethics and the social determinants of health* (pp. 17–32). Springer.

Jennings, B. (2007). Public health and civic republicanism: Toward an alternative framework for public health ethics. In A. Dawson & M. Verweij (Eds.), *Ethics, prevention, and public health.* Oxford University Press.

Jennings, B. (2016). Reconceptualizing autonomy: A relational turn in bioethics. *Hastings Center Report, 46*(3), 11–16. https://doi.org/10.1002/hast.544

Jennings, B. (2018). Solidarity and care coming of age: New reasons in the politics of social welfare policy. *Hastings Center Report, 48*(S3), S19–S24. https://doi.org/10.1002/hast.908

Jennings, B. (2019). Relational ethics for public health: Interpreting solidarity and care. *Health Care Analysis, 27,* 4–12. https://doi.org/10.1007/s10728-018-0363-0

Jennings, B. (2020). Ethics codes and reflective practice in public health. *Journal of Public Health, 42*(1), 188–193. https://doi.org/10.1093/pubmed/fdy140

Jonsen, A. R., Siegler, M., & Winslade, W. J. (2006). *Clinical ethics: A practical approach to ethical decisions in clinical medicine* (6th ed.). McGraw-Hill.

Legal Information Institute. (n.d.). *Prima facie.* Cornell Law School Legal Information Institute. https://www.law.cornell.edu/wex/prima_facie

Ortmann, L. W., Barrett, D. H., Saenz, C., Bernheim, R. G., Dawson, A., Valentine, J. A., & Reis, A. (2016). Public health ethics: Global cases, practice, and context. In D. H. Barrett, L. H. Ortmann, A. Dawson, C. Saenz, A. Reis, & Bolan, G. (Eds.), *Public health ethics: Cases scanning the globe* (pp. 3–36). Springer.

Pellegrino, E. D., & Thomas, D. C. (1993). *The virtues in medical practice.* Oxford University Press.

Ransom, M. M. (Ed.). (2016). *Public health law competency model: Version 1.0.* https://www.cdc.gov/phlp/docs/phlcm-v1.pdf

## Additional Resources

- **Visit CDC's Office of Scientific Integrity website to learn more about public health ethics**
  https://www.cdc.gov/od/science/integrity/phethics/index.htm
- **Watch the webinar, entitled, Ethical Issues in Public Health Data Use**
  http://www.nwcphp.org/training/ethical-issues-public-health-data-use

# 21

# Public Health Executive Decision-Making and the Law:

## Responsibilities, Strategies, and Consequences

Denise Chrysler, Lance Gable, Donna E. Levin, and Peter D. Jacobson

## Learning Objectives

By the end of this chapter, the reader will be able to

- Apply the analysis "Can I?"; "Must I?"; and "Should I?" when assessing a public health official's authority to act against a public health threat.
- Analyze the difference between exercise of discretion and abuse of discretion.
- Explain the framework of duty for health officers.
- Compare tools to assist public health decision-making.
- Examine various approaches for holding public officials accountable.

## Key Terminology

**Civil law:** The area of law that allows for actions brought to enforce, redress, or protect private rights (Black's Law Dictionary, 6th ed.).

**Criminal law:** The area of law that pertains to or relates to the law of crimes, or the administration of penal justice, or that relates to or has the character of crime. (Black's Law Dictionary, 6th ed.)

**Discretionary Authority:** The power or authority to take or not take action.

**Duty to Warn:** The legal obligation to warn people of a danger.

**Gross Negligence:** A severe degree of negligence taken as reckless disregard. Blatant indifference to one's legal duty, others' safety, or their rights.

**Negligence:** A failure to behave with the level of care that someone of ordinary prudence would have exercised under the same or similar circumstances. The behavior usually consists of actions, but can also consist of omissions when there is a duty to act (https://www.law.cornell.edu/wex/negligence).

**Qualified immunity:** Protects public officials from being sued for damages unless they violated "clearly established" law of which a reasonable official in their position would have known (https://definitions.uslegal.com/q/qualified-immunity).

**Wanton and Willful Misconduct:** Reckless disregard for others' safety and rights and knowing harm or injury may result.

## Public Health Law Competencies

This chapter addresses the following competencies from the Public Health Law Competency Model (PHLCM; Ransom, 2016).

1.2  Identify and apply public health laws (e.g., statutes, regulations, ordinances, and court rulings) pertinent to practitioner's jurisdiction, agency, program, and profession.

2.3  Recognize the legal authority and limits of critical system partners and others who influence health outcomes.

---

### Spark Question

Should a health officer be immune from liability for failing to warn the public of a potential disease outbreak in a timely manner? Why or why not?

---

## INTRODUCTION

Public health executive decision-making has never been easy. The uncertain epidemiological trajectory of infectious disease exposure, the economic and political consequences of making the wrong decisions, and the general distrust of public officials have always made decision-making difficult.

The Flint water crisis (Jacobson et al., 2018; see Boxes 21.1 and 21.2) and resulting unresolved civil and criminal litigation against governmental officials have brought greater attention to the legal challenges and risk-management responsibilities health officers face on a daily basis. While it is tempting to assume that the criminal charges filed in Flint constitute an extreme outlier, complacency among public health practitioners would be risky. For example, the Illinois attorney general opened a criminal investigation of the state's governor and health commissioner following Legionella deaths, and state officials in Florida have been accused of delaying notice of well water contaminated with perfluoro octane sulfonate (PFOS) and perfluorooctanoic acid (PFOA) because of an impending election. Thus, it is timely to examine the liability implications of public health executive decision-making.

---

### BOX 21.1 THE FLINT WATER CRISIS: WERE RACE AND POVERTY A FACTOR?

*The facts of the Flint water crisis lead us to the inescapable conclusion that this is a case of environmental injustice. Flint residents, who are majority Black or African American and among the most impoverished of any metropolitan area in the United States, did not enjoy the same degree of protection from environmental and health hazards as that provided to other communities.*

Flint Water Advisory Task Force, Final Report, March 2016, p. 54.

In April 2014, reportedly as a cost-saving measure, public officials in Flint changed the source of drinking water from Lake Huron of the Great Lakes to the Flint River "without necessary corrosion control treatment to prevent lead release from pipes and plumbing." As a result, an estimated 140,000 Flint residents, mostly Black and poor, were exposed to lead and other contaminants in drinking water for at least 18 months despite complaints from community members about the water being brown.

After the involvement of concerned residents and independent researchers, Flint was re-connected to the Detroit water system on October 16, 2015. A federal emergency was declared in January 2016. Since then, multiple criminal charges and civil lawsuits have

BOX 21.1   *(continued)*

been brought against governmental officials and private employees at the center of the crisis. The most serious criminal charges, involuntary manslaughter, were made against Michigan's state health official and four others (Ruckart et al., 2019).

There are many who argue that race and poverty factored into the governmental decision-making in Flint, and that the residents were victims of environmental racism. Then presidential candidate Hillary Clinton put it this way in the January 17, 2016 Democratic presidential debate:

> We've had a city in the United States of America where the population, which is poor in many ways and majority African American, has been bathing and drinking in lead-contaminated water. And the governor of that state acted as though he didn't really care. He had requests for help that he basically stonewalled. I'll tell you what: If the kids in a rich suburb of Detroit had been drinking contaminated water and being bathed in it, there would've been action.

Hillary Clinton, January 17, 2016
https://www.chicagotribune.com/politics/ct-flint-water-race-20160122-story.html

The full impact of the crisis may not be clear for many years, but according to the Centers for Disease Control and Prevention (CDC), lead exposure can damage children's brains and nervous systems, lead to slow growth and development, and result in learning, behavioral, hearing, and speech problems (https://www.cdc.gov/features/leadpoisoning/index.html). As noted by Dr. Mona Hanna-Attisha, Flint's whistleblower, "If you were going to put something in a population to keep them down for generations to come, it would be lead." (https://www.nytimes.com/2016/01/30/us/flint-weighs-scope-of-harm-to-children-caused-by-lead-in-water.html)

BOX 21.2   THE 2014–2105 LEGIONNAIRES' DISEASE OUTBREAK

In addition to the lead exposure discussed in Box 21.1, the Flint community suffered Legionnaires' disease outbreaks at McLaren Flint Hospital in both 2014 and 2015. Although there is some dispute about the source of the Legionella, the switch to the Flint River was the likely factor (Jacobson et al., 2020). This Legionnaires' outbreak was one of the largest in U.S. history, and while the issue of whether Legionella caused or contributed to these deaths remains highly contested, studies show that 12 out of 91 (13%) of those affected by the disease died.

Legionnaires' disease is a severe form of pneumonia that can be fatal if not properly diagnosed and treated. This means public education and awareness are critical to protecting public health.

Although state and local health departments were conducting surveillance and recorded many Legionnaires' cases at McLaren Flint Hospital during the 2014 to 2015 outbreak, they did not notify the public until after the spike had subsided in 2016. And there is some evidence that the only notification to the medical community came halfway through the outbreak, in an email sent to 15 infection-control personnel at three local hospitals.

The Michigan Health Department's delay in alerting the public about the hospital's Legionnaires' disease outbreaks and the hospital's perceived failure to protect patients from the Legionella bacteria has resulted in numerous lawsuits against the state governor and McLaren Flint Hospital, including one for $100 million. While unresolved at the time of publishing, the circumstances leading to these lawsuits provide a solid example for exploring the liability implications of public health decision-making.

In this chapter, we first examine the civil liability aspects of failure to notify the public of a disease outbreak, using the Legionella outbreak in Flint (see Box 21.2) as the model case. Under a state's Public Health Code, what constitutes the duty to promote and protect the public's health? A related question is, what guidance does the Code provide as to when a state or local health officer should notify the public about a disease outbreak? Then, we address more generally the public health executive decision-making process in exercising discretionary power to protect the public's health. Finally, we consider alternative mechanisms for holding public health officials accountable for their decisions.

Our guiding approach is that the attorney's role is to provide legal advice about the health officer's authority and limits. After that, responsibility rests with the health officer to determine the nature and extent of the public health threat and the appropriate response based on their best professional judgment. As such, it is critically important that current and emerging public health practitioners are deliberate and thoughtful in their decision-making in a public health emergency or crisis and consider potential legal and health consequences of those decisions.

## THE FRAMEWORK FOR DEFINING DUTY

Public health statutes and codes provide a broad grant of authority to protect and promote the public's health. To exercise the scope of authority, state codes establish a general duty "… to prevent disease, prolong life, and promote the public health" (Michigan Compiled Laws [MCL] 333.221[1]). The Michigan Public Health Code is reasonably representative of how state laws outline the health officer's responsibilities:

> (2) The department shall: (a) Have general supervision of the interests of the health and life of the people of this state; (b) Implement and enforce laws for which responsibility is vested in the department; (c) Collect and utilize vital and health statistics; (d) Make investigations … as to (i) The causes of diseases and especially epidemics … .[1]

As this language suggests, the statutes and codes do not define a health officer's duty with specificity or provide decision-making guidance. Instead, the duty is broadly stated "… to safeguard properly the public health; to prevent the spread of diseases and the existence of sources of contamination; and to implement and carry out the powers and duties vested by law in the department" (MCL 333.2226[d]). Lacking adequate specificity, it seems fair to conclude that the general duty language in state public health codes is aspirational.

Aside from equally general statements of the duty to protect the public's health, no public health organization offers a more precise definition. Likewise, neither states nor public health organizations, including CDC, have issued protocols or criteria to guide decision-making regarding notice to the public.[2] The one exception, described in the following, is not necessarily recognized as the industry standard, though it provides a useful way of thinking about disclosure.

Given the lack of specificity in state codes (and the absence of provisions regarding notice to the public), how should duty and breach of duty be defined?[3] That is, how can health officers implement the general duty language in determining whether and how to notify the public? As a point of departure, a general **negligence** framework (duty, breach of duty, causation, and damages) would define duty broadly as taking appropriate actions to implement the

---

[1] MCL 333.2221. This section is based on an analysis of nine state public health codes that one of the authors (Jacobson) conducted.
[2] Based on an online search of national public health organizations' websites and Jacobson's conversations with individuals at these organizations.
[3] "Duty" is not defined in two of the leading texts—Wiley and Gostin, and Turnock. Turnock notes the following: "… public health practice is the development and application of preventive strategies and interventions to promote and protect the health of the public." Further he observes that in exercising the police powers to protect the public's health, "… its use is a duty, rather than a matter of choice, although its form is left to the discretion of the user."

responsibilities established in state codes to protect and promote the public's health. To determine the nature and extent of the duty, it would be appropriate to ask what a reasonable health officer would have done under the circumstances to keep the public informed, prevent further exposure, and enable the public to ensure its own health.

This would essentially establish a general negligence standard of exercising the best professional judgment under the circumstances based on industry custom.[4] If so, the plaintiff would need to identify professional guidelines and protocols for notifying the public or demonstrate how other health officers have handled similar situations in the past.

A final consideration is the **duty to warn** analogy from general tort law. Even if there is no clear notice provision, a court could impose a duty to warn of obvious disease exposures. The case law seems split on this issue. Police are generally given great deference, but several cases have upheld liability against 911 dispatchers.[5] One distinction from those cases is the health officer's specific statutory duty to protect the public's health.

## Immunity

Regardless of how duty is defined and even if the failure to issue public notice of an outbreak constitutes an abuse of discretion, that alone might not be enough to impose liability. Most states offer **qualified immunity** from liability to governmental employees and to the state government itself, thereby establishing a more demanding liability standard and in effect requiring **gross negligence** or **wanton and willful misconduct** to be liable. In Michigan, for example, the government is immune from liability absent gross negligence, defined as "conduct so reckless as to demonstrate a substantial lack of concern for whether an injury results."[6]

### TABLE 21.1  Distinguishing Criminal and Civil Law

|  | CIVIL LAW | CRIMINAL LAW |
|---|---|---|
| Definition | Legal resolution of disputes arising from alleged violations of private rights (e.g., injuries) | Legal resolution of alleged violations of criminal offenses |
| Burden of Proof | "Preponderance of evidence": The burden of proof falls on the plaintiff. One must produce evidence beyond the balance of probabilities. | "Beyond a reasonable doubt": The burden of proof is always on the state/government. |
| Penalty/Punishment | Usually involves some type of compensation for injuries or damages as well as disposition of property and other disputes. | A guilty defendant is punished by incarceration and/or fines, or in exceptional cases, the death penalty. Crimes are divided into two broad classes: Felonies and Misdemeanors. |
| Who files the lawsuit? | Private party | Government/State |

---

[4] As a general rule, governmental officials have considerable flexibility for discretionary duties, though they may be liable for not adhering to mandatory (usually ministerial) duties. To be sure, there are other possibilities, including a fiduciary duty to the public, a stewardship model, an abuse of discretion approach, or a standard of substantial departure from the norm (used to determine a constitutional violation in *Youngberg v. Romeo*, 1982).

[5] See, e.g., *De Long v. County of Erie*, 60 N.Y.2d 296 (1983); *Hutcherson v. City of Phoenix*, 192 Ariz. 51 (1998); *Munich v. Skagit Emergency Communication Center*, 175 Wash.2d 871 (2012).

[6] MCL 691.1407 states that "… each officer and employee of a governmental agency … is immune from tort liability … while in the course of employment or service or caused by the volunteer while acting on behalf of a governmental agency if all of the following are met: (a) The officer, employee, member, or volunteer is acting or reasonably believes he or she is acting within the scope of his or her authority. (b) The governmental agency is engaged in the exercise or discharge of a governmental function. (c) The officer's, employee's, member's, or volunteer's conduct does not amount to gross negligence that is the proximate cause of the injury or damage."

More specifically, Michigan offers qualified immunity for state and local public health employees except for Wanton and willful misconduct (MCL 333.2228[2]). Although the Code does not define "willful and wanton misconduct," Michigan case law holds that it may be found "… if the conduct alleged shows an intent to harm, or, if not that, such indifference to whether harm will result as to be the equivalent of a willingness that it does" (*Jennings v. Southwood*, 1994).

Either of these standards creates a high bar for civil liability, let alone for proving the intent required to sustain a criminal conviction. At best, as in Flint, the failure to notify might be mistaken. As such, it is unlikely that failure to notify the public will result in either civil or criminal liability.

## Industry Standards

At this point, there is no industry standard or CDC recommendation to guide notice. No national public health organization has issued protocols or criteria to guide decision-making on when to notify the public. Only the Association of Health Care Journalists, in collaboration with the Association of State and Territorial Health Officials (ASTHO) and the National Association of City and County Health Officials (NACCHO), has issued any guidance, but it is not recognized as an industry standard.[7] The 2010 guidance proposes public notification when (a) the information will be helpful for individual protection from harm; (b) a major public health event or natural disaster is anticipated or has occurred; (c) public attention has been attracted, and risks need to factually and effectively be communicated; and (d) the event provides a "teachable moment."

Nonetheless, while it seems likely the general duty just discussed would incorporate a duty to notify the public of a disease outbreak, the absence of guiding protocols provides the health officer with wide discretion. As stated in *Youngberg v. Romeo (1982)*, "[I]t is conceded by petitioners that a duty to provide certain services and care does exist, although even then a State necessarily has considerable discretion in determining the nature and scope of its responsibilities …. Nor must a State choose between attacking every aspect of a problem or not attacking the problem at all."[8]

With regard to notice, it seems prudent to anticipate that most public health professionals would err on the side of disclosure. For example, "In public health practice, the primary ethic is to warn the public at risk when the warning can help avoid the risk of harm or allow patients to seek treatment. If in doubt, notify the public of the concern and steps to take, and let the public handle the risk."[9] Still, the decision is complicated and not always obvious. Much depends on whether the parameters of the exposure are defined clearly enough to justify public notice.

The health officer must weigh the benefits and costs of either notifying the public or choosing to wait. As with many similar decisions, health officers must make their best professional judgment under conditions of uncertainty, without the luxury of complete information.

Determining whether and when to notify the public of a disease outbreak is therefore within the health officer's professional judgment. Absent specific guidance, a health officer must use their experience and discretion in making the decision. Each situation must be examined under the specific circumstances that arise. To sustain a negligence lawsuit, the plaintiff would need to surmount the immunity provisions and show either gross negligence or wanton and willful misconduct. Those are both high barriers. Even if the plaintiff could meet the higher standard, they would then need to show that the failure to notify the public caused the injury or

---

[7] These principles are: public health officials have discretion to decide amount and manner for releasing information; openness is paramount; withhold information *only* when clearly justified reason to keep confidential (Association of Health Care Journalists, 2010).

[8] In *Youngberg*, the Court adopted the following from Judge Seitz's concurring opinion from the Third Circuit's decision: "I would hold that the jury should be instructed that the defendants are liable if their conduct was such a substantial departure from accepted professional judgment, practice, or standards in the care and treatment of this plaintiff as to demonstrate that the defendants did not base their conduct on a professional judgment" (*Youngberg v. Romeo*, 1982).

[9] Personal communication to Jacobson from a national public health organization executive.

death. This, too, would be difficult to show in most cases because causation for morbidity and mortality is complex and often based on multiple factors. For example, individuals exposed to Legionella are usually already suffering from conditions that pose serious medical risks.

Likewise, to sustain either a manslaughter or criminal misconduct-in-office charge, the prosecutor would need to prove beyond a reasonable doubt that the health officer's failure to give notice constituted Wanton and willful misconduct. To do so, the prosecution must show either intentionality (i.e., that the health officer willfully and intentionally ignored evidence of the outbreak, withheld evidence, or obstructed contrary investigations) or gross negligence.

## EXECUTIVE DECISION-MAKING FOR PUBLIC HEALTH OFFICIALS

Decision-making is at the core of a public health director's responsibility. As the health officer for the state, Tribal, county, or local health department, the executive is responsible for making decisions to address situations that pose a threat to the community's health. The executive is called upon to use their professional judgment, informed by evidence and facts, to take the best course of action within the confines of the agency's legal authority. Starting with the legal landscape in which the decision must be made, the executive must ask three key questions: Can I? Must I? Should I?

**Can I?** focuses on whether the agency has the legal authority to act, and if so, in what way? The public health agency's authority is based on the police power, which reserves for the states the power to protect the welfare, safety, and health of the public (*Jacobson v. Massachusetts*, 1905). An agency's authority will also be specified in many respects by the jurisdiction's statutory and regulatory provisions, and judicial interpretations of these provisions. The parameters of authority may include both specific grants of and limitations on authority, for example, preemption of an official's ability to act by a higher level of government and constitutional safeguards for individual rights such as liberty and due process.

**Must I?** asks whether there are legal requirements that mandate action, and if so, is there direction on how the agency must act specifically? Sometimes action is directed by a funding source, and sometimes, even though a legal directive exists, the agency has a great deal of discretion in determining how to fulfill its obligation. If you must act, the action does not have to address every aspect of the problem—initial or selective action is permissible but cannot be biased or otherwise impermissibly motivated (*Youngberg v. Romeo*, 1982).

**Should I?** is a policy question that requires the executive to determine whether and how **discretionary authority** should be exercised. *Discretionary authority* must be used reasonably and impartially, never in an arbitrary and capricious manner. With leeway to decide what is wise and what is best, use of discretionary authority is tough terrain. The expectation is that the executive will make the "right" decision even when all relevant facts may not be ascertainable and evidence may be inconclusive. This is easier said than done, and to be sure, there will be no scarcity of those in the public, at higher levels of government and in the media, who will question the judgments of health officials with the benefit of hindsight.

Recognizing the need for simple, step-by-step guidance to aid public health officials faced with these difficult decisions, one of the authors[10] created the Public Health Executive Decision-Making Tool, which provides a straightforward path to support executive decision-making when circumstances pose a public health threat or danger. The tool outlines a clear approach for analyzing a public health threat as it unfolds and for documenting the decision-making process. It posits the key questions to evaluate the risk of taking action based on information that is currently known or understood, versus waiting for more information before acting.

The tool suggests that a public health official should establish a "situation room," which should include the members of that official's agency and other experts who can be called upon to advise on policy, law, disease information, other types of health threats, and risk

---

[10] Denise Chrysler.

communication. This team should be prepared to meet as often as necessary, sometimes several times a day.

The tool includes decision-making prompts to help officials document what is known and when about the situation, the daily changes in that knowledge, and the resultant impact on decisions. This documentation can be used to provide updates to other executive branch officials or to develop a transparent record justifying the decisions at a later date. In addition, with legal guidance, it may be possible to preserve the option to claim attorney–client privilege for some or all of these records. For accuracy and transparency, it would be appropriate to assign a staff member the responsibility for ongoing note-taking.

## Using the Executive Decision-Making Tool

**Assess the Situation:** With your team in place, describe the facts as known and understood at the time. Focus on asking the right questions and not assuming the answers. Anticipate a quick evolution of facts and circumstances. Start at the beginning every time the situation is reassessed to validate the information you have. Based on the facts, determine what the potential danger or threat is, and list each of them (e.g., potential disease[s] or conditions).

**Consider the Consequences:** Determine the likelihood of the occurrence of each danger or threat based on current evidence. If the danger or threat occurs or continues, what are the potential consequences, for example, the "list of horribles"? As such, it is important during this step to consider the impact of these outcomes on different populations, especially the most vulnerable. This is where health equity considerations may fit in. According to the Association for State and Territorial Health Officials, "Effective leaders for health equity are well-informed decision-makers with a shared understanding of the principles and practices of advancing health equity and have the skills and ability to inspire and motivate individuals and organizations to take action to improve health outcomes." (2018, p. 20).

**Discuss Mitigation:** Consider the options and how the threat and/or danger can be addressed. What measures or mitigation might be used? What have others done in similar situations to mitigate impact or likelihood of reoccurrence? Consider the range of actions and their pros and cons, being mindful of the disparate effect on different populations.

**Assess the Level of Certainty:** Weigh the potential harm of implementing measures or mitigation prematurely against delaying these actions. Before taking action, consider whether there are any other options; what resources are needed to execute and maintain the chosen course of action; how you know when you are "done"; and how you measure success. Not acting is also a decision, not a default. If action is not taken now, will you be held accountable for not acting? What do you not know today that you should know? Is that information knowable, and if so, what is the timeframe for knowing? List the pros and cons of acting versus waiting. Staff input is key—encourage free discussion and respectful challenge.

**Communicate:** If not from the very beginning of your decision-making process, then soon after, you will be confronted with how much notice and information should be provided to the public. This requires careful deliberation and balance. Key considerations include whether notice will make a difference for those notified; what, if any, reasons there are for lack of transparency; and what is in the best interest of the public's health. The public health mission must be your north star—paramount over any political pressure or expediency.

**Try to "Shapeshift":** What and when would *you* want to know about the threat or danger? Put yourself in the position of others, e.g., facility resident, patient, parent, consumer, or member of the general public. Avoid paternalism—deciding you know best—even if others would clearly or most likely want the information you are not sharing.

**Rely on Others:** Finally, remember that risk communication is an area of expertise and rely on those with the expertise to reach out to the affected and/or general public and the media. Bring in others who should be part of the communication, perhaps other agencies or other stakeholders. Plan for ongoing communication; tell those you are informing when to expect further communication; and let the public know how to communicate with you.

## ACCOUNTABILITY FOR PUBLIC HEALTH OFFICIALS

One of the most challenging aspects of public health executive decision-making arises after decisions have been made and actions taken that have led to unanticipated or undesirable negative health consequences. Ideally, the structural and political mechanisms of our democracy place constraints and parameters on the actions of governmental officials that incentivize these officials to make decisions that will avoid causing harm to the public and hold these officials appropriately accountable when they intentionally or inadvertently cause harm (or are perceived to have done so). As described previously, the specific parameters that outline the duties of public health officials are ambiguous, leaving much room for discretion. Nevertheless, in general, public health officials are subject to the same expectations that face all governmental officials. Members of the public expect governmental officials to perform their roles responsibly and competently. Further, in a democratic society, governmental officials operate with the knowledge that their decisions have real consequences and if these consequences cause harm, accountability for those decisions may follow.

In reality, the effectiveness and consistency of holding officials accountable when they cause harm varies considerably. The aftermath of the Flint water crisis provides a cautionary example for those who presume that governmental officials whose decisions cause harm will be held personally accountable. Accountability for public health officials can be achieved through an assortment of nonexclusive mechanisms we classify as: *internal* (invoking formal or informal powers of oversight and review within established governmental processes); *external* (methods relying on public or political pressure, transparency, and advocacy); and *legal* (using **civil** or **criminal law** to seek redress or punishment).

### Internal Accountability

Internal accountability measures for governmental accountability arise from processes available within the government itself. Ideally, these mechanisms should help avoid harm to the public. While the specific mechanisms differ between jurisdictions, most state and local governments have formal and informal processes for ensuring oversight of and accountability for officials. Some common approaches include internal oversight conducted by an official designated for this role (e.g., an inspector general or ombudsperson), post hoc reviews of decisions by a more senior official within the same executive agency, or the development of an after-action report by agency officials to evaluate the appropriateness of prior decisions. Additionally, standing or ad hoc oversight committees can investigate the circumstances surrounding problematic decisions. These approaches may allow others within the government to correct and reverse bad decisions and/or sanction, admonish, or remove decision-makers who made decisions that caused harm. Furthermore, these efforts may provide an opportunity to formulate recommendations for systemic change that go beyond the actions of specific individuals.

Unfortunately, these internal accountability mechanisms did not work effectively to prevent the Flint crisis or hold officials responsible in the aftermath. Two independent panels were convened to assess the causes of the crisis, but neither of these groups had direct authority to implement their recommendations (Davis et al., 2016). Likewise, both the U.S. Congress and the Michigan Legislature held oversight hearings (Stamas et al., 2016), but neither of these efforts resulted in accountability for the officials responsible for the decisions linked to harm. These oversight mechanisms have the most potential to achieve lasting systemic change, but often falter as political and economic considerations overtake the impetus to act.

## External Accountability

Accountability may also emerge from outside of the government, initiated by community members, advocates, researchers, or journalists who can identify potential or ongoing risks of harm and alert the decision-makers or the public about these risks. External accountability is an informal and multifaceted endeavor and can be pursued through direct contact with governmental officials as well as via traditional and social media. These strategies can be implemented rapidly, highlight health risks that might otherwise be ignored and may be still ongoing, and produce significant public and political pressure for governmental officials to respond. Thus, external, informal methods of accountability are those most likely to be utilized while there is an ongoing risk to health to alert public health officials to relevant information that may prompt them to act.

In Flint, however, external accountability mechanisms did not produce quick results. Despite a nearly immediate public reaction to the switch in Flint's water supply by community members, journalists, and scientists, it was not until Dr. Mona Hanna Attisha's study on elevated blood lead levels in Flint children was released 18 months later that the state acknowledged the lead in the water supply and began to take some steps to remediate the harm (Hanna-Attisha et al., 2016). It was even longer before the public was informed of the Legionella outbreak (Zahran et al., 2018). These examples highlight a major limitation of external, informal accountability methods: if the communities affected lack sufficient political clout, the information being presented may be ignored and the attempts to call attention to an emerging risk may be unsuccessful or tragically delayed. Residents of Flint were disempowered by longstanding structural racism and community disinvestment (Hammer, 2017), and were deprived of democratic representation through a state-appointed emergency manager who was installed to make all decisions about city finances (Jacobson et al., 2018). While community voices eventually spurred state officials to act, this action came too late to avoid serious harm to the public's health.

To be sure, external advocacy and transparency can achieve some (albeit minimal) measure of retrospective accountability. In 2019, former Michigan Governor Rick Snyder was denied an opportunity to participate as a visiting fellow at Harvard when a public outcry arose over the perception that Harvard was rewarding a state official who had failed to stop the Flint water crisis.

## Legal Accountability

Yet another type of accountability can be sought through judicial processes. Civil lawsuits can allow for individuals who have alleged harm based on the decisions of governmental officials to seek damages for those harms. Numerous civil suits have been filed related to the Flint water crisis, claiming that officials engaged in gross negligence, Wanton and willful misconduct, recklessness, and civil rights violations for decisions that caused or exacerbated harms from switching the city's water supply to the Flint River or for failing to warn the public about the risk of a Legionnaires' outbreak (*Burgess v. United States*, 2019; *Mays v. City of Flint*, 2017). These claims present powerful arguments that attempt to link officials' decision to the eventual harm suffered by residents and to obtain compensation from the state for those actions.

But as described in this chapter, civil claims filed against governmental officials face a number of powerful obstacles. In circumstances where the allegation is that public health officials failed to warn about an outbreak, plaintiffs will struggle to establish that a duty of care has been violated, and more serious allegations of gross negligence, Wanton and willful misconduct, and recklessness will be even harder to prove. Likewise, establishing causation between the decisions of governmental officials and the harms suffered by members of the public will be challenging since many factors may contribute to the sequence of events that leads to harm. Significantly, the broad protection afforded by qualified immunity will insulate public health officials from most tort claims based on their decisions in office, particularly decisions that are just calls about when to notify the public of an outbreak. At least one of the cases related to the Flint crisis survived the qualified immunity hurdle, with a court finding that officials from the Michigan Department of Environmental Quality committed "an egregious violation of the right to bodily integrity" and allowing claims of civil rights violations to proceed against these officials (*Guertin et al. v. State of Michigan et al.*, 2019). Qualified immunity provisions, however, limit the usefulness of civil litigation as a method of accountability for governmental officials.

Criminal prosecution is infrequently used as a method of accountability for governmental officials since most conduct does not give rise to violations of criminal law. When criminal charges are brought against governmental officials, it is most often to prosecute corruption rather than seek accountability for decisions that harmed members of the public. As a result, criminal prosecution provides perhaps the most visible mechanism to impose responsibility for those found to have violated the law through imprisonment or criminal fines. In the Flint case, prosecutors in Michigan brought a range of serious criminal charges against 15 governmental officials, including involuntary manslaughter charges against two public health officials.[11]

Nonetheless, there are serious potential downsides to using criminal prosecution to impose accountability on public health officials. If officials perceive that criminal penalties will follow if they fail to act and prevent harm, there may be an incentive to overreact to small risks, which can undermine support for and compliance with public health initiatives in the future. Such prosecutions, especially if they are perceived as arbitrary or politically motivated, may also deter people from seeking these important positions (Gable & Buehler, 2017).

Numerous state and local officials were involved in the decisions that resulted in both the Flint water supply's lead contamination and created conditions conducive to the flourishing of Legionella bacteria. Other officials who could have investigated more rigorously or intervened sooner instead waited and downplayed the risks of harm. Even so, Flint residents complain that there has been little accountability for the consequences. The existing accountability measures failed to protect the public's health and prevent harm. Neither the subsequent civil and criminal litigation nor the considerable political pressure provided meaningful retrospective accountability for those involved in the decision-making who were allegedly responsible for the harm.

## CONCLUSION

We conclude that the duty language in state public health codes is aspirational in nature and is not defined with greater specificity. Even when a code lists a particular duty to disseminate information (e.g., Florida), which not all codes do, it lacks specificity as to when/how much information should be shared with the public. Whether health officers should adopt public notification as the default option, with appropriate caveats about the strength of the evidence, is for professional organizations to decide.

But there are potentially serious adverse consequences if the law imposes liability and encourages routine notice for ubiquitous agents such as Legionella. Among other concerns, the public may be unduly scared and hence postpone needed care, or the public may become inured to the constant notices and simply ignore them altogether. Notice should be provided when it is clear that people can use the information to protect themselves from harm. Otherwise, reliance on the health officer's professional judgment remains the optimal legal approach.

---

[11] Most of the high-profile criminal charges have either been dropped or are being reconsidered. Despite *nolo contendere* pleas from lower officials, the difficulty of sustaining criminal indictments against top officials suggests the inadequacy of criminal law to provide redress in these types of situations.

## CHAPTER REVIEW

### Review Questions

1. The responsibility rests with legal counsel to determine the nature and extent of the public health threat and the appropriate response based on their best professional judgment. True/False
2. To sustain either a manslaughter or criminal misconduct-in-office charge, the prosecutor would need to prove beyond doubt_____ that the health officer's failure to give notice constituted willful and wanton misconduct.
3. Criminal prosecution is often used as a method of accountability for governmental officials. True/False
4. List and define the three types of accountability that health officials face.

### Essay Question

What measures would you impose to hold public health officials accountable? Would you focus on legal or nonlegal sanctions? What trade-offs are involved in your approach?

### Internet Activities

1. Review the *CDC's Crisis and Emergency Risk Communication: Media and the Law* publication (https://emergency.cdc.gov/cerc/ppt/CERC_Media%20and%20Public%20Health%20 Law.pdf) and address the following:
   ■ In addition to laws related to discretionary authority and liability, what other laws or legal issues might impact when or how a public health official shares information in a public health emergency or crisis?
   ■ In your own words, what does it mean for public health information to be "of public concern"? Why does this matter in claims against a health department related to sharing information about a public health emergency or crisis?
2. Listen to the following podcasts:
   ■ **WDET's 'Created Equal' Podcast Debuts Second Season, Examining Flint Water Crisis** https://wdet.org/posts/2019/10/21/88756-wdets-created-equal-podcast-debuts -second-season-examining-flint-water-crisis
   ■ **How to Save the World Podcast, Episode 15: The Flint Water Crisis and Environmental Racism** https://soundcloud.com/howtosavetheworldpodcast/episode-15-the-flint -water-crisis-environmental-racism.
   Address the following:
   ■ In what ways do you think environmental racism influenced governmental decision-making during the Flint water crisis?
   ■ What evidence is offered by the podcast hosts to support your opinion?
   ■ How might you integrate health equity and environmental racism considerations as you move through the elements of the Public Health Decision-Making Tool in times of emergency or crisis? https://www.networkforphl.org/resources/public -health-decision-making-tool

## REFERENCES

Association for State and Territorial Health Officials. (2018). Foundational practices for health equity. https://www.astho.org/Health-Equity/Documents/Foundational-Practices-for-Health-Equity

Association of Health Care Journalists. (2010, October). *Guidance on the release of information concerning deaths, epidemics or emerging diseases.* https://healthjournalism.org/releaseguidance

*Burgess v. United States*, 375 F. Supp. 3d 796 (E.D. Mich. 2019).

Davis, M. M., Kolb, C., Reynolds, L., Rothstein, E., Sikkema, K. (2016, March). *Flint Water Advisory Task Force Final Report: Office of the Attorney General, State of Michigan.* Interim Report of the Flint Water Crisis Investigation. https://www.michigan.gov/documents/snyder/FWATF_FINAL _REPORT_21March2016_517805_7.pdf

Gable, L., & Buehler, J. W. (2017). Criticized, fired, sued, or prosecuted: Hindsight and public health accountability. *Public Health Reports, 132*(6), 676–768. https://doi.org/10.1177/0033354917730820

*Guertin et al. v. State of Michigan et al.*, No. 5:16-cv-12412 (6th Cir., Jan. 4, 2019).

Hammer, P. J. (2017). The flint water crisis, the Karegnondi water authority and strategic-structural racism. *Critical Sociology, 45*(1), 103–119. https://doi.org/10.1177/0896920517729193

Hanna-Attisha, M., LaChance, J., Sadler, R. C., & Schnepp, A. C. (2016). Elevated blood lead levels in children associated with the Flint drinking water crisis: A spatial analysis of risk and public health response. *American Journal of Public Health, 106*(2), 283–290. https://doi.org/10.2105/ AJPH.2015.303003

*Jacobson v. Massachusetts*, 197 U.S. 11 (1905).

Jacobson, P. D., Boufides, C. H., Bernstein, J., Chrysler, D., Citrin, T. (2018, January). *Learning from the flint water crisis: Protecting the public's health during a financial crisis.* http://www.debeaumont .org/wordpress/wp-content/uploads/FlintReport.pdf

Jacobson, P. D., Boufides, C. H., Chrysler, D., Bernstein, J., Citrin, T. (2020). The role of the legal system in the flint water crisis. *The Milbank Quarterly, 98*(2), 554–580.

*Jennings v. Southwood*, 521 N.W.2d 230 (Mich. 1994).

*Mays v. City of Flint*, 871 F.3d 437 (6th Cir. 2017).

Michigan Compiled Laws 333.2221.

Michigan Compiled Laws 333.2228(2).

Michigan Compiled Laws 691.1407.

Ruckart, P. Z., Ettinger, A. S., Hanna-Attisha, M., Jones, N., Davis, S. I., & Breysse, P. N. (2019). The Flint water crisis: A coordinated public health emergency response and recovery initiative. *Journal of Public Health Management and Practice, 25*(Suppl. 1, Lead Poisoning Prevention), S84–S90. https://doi.org/10.1097/PHH.0000000000000871

Stamas, S. J., Ananich, J., McBroom, E. et al. (2016, October). *Report of the Joint Select Committee on the Flint water emergency.* http://flintwaterstudy.org/wp-content/uploads/2016/10/FINAL-Report-of-the-Joint-Select-Committee.pdf

*Youngberg v. Romeo*, 457 U.S. 307, 317 (1982).

*Youngberg v. Romeo* 457 U.S. 307 (1982).

Zahran, S., McElmurry, S. P., Kilgore, P. E., Mushinski, D., Press, J., Love, N. G., Sadler, R. C., & Swanson, M. S. (2018). Assessment of the Legionnaires' disease outbreak in Flint, Michigan. *Proceedings of the National Academy of Sciences, 115*(8), E1730–E1739. https://doi.org/10.1073/ pnas.1718679115

## Additional Resources

- **Executive Decision-Making and Liability for Public Health Officials (Webinar Recording), Network for Public Health Law**
  https://www.youtube.com/watch?v=0j8dJishxpY
- **Public Health Decision-Making Tool**
  https://www.networkforphl.org/resources/public-health-decision-making-tool
- **TEDMED, Flint's Fight for America's Children, Mona Hanna-Attisha**
  https://www.tedmed.com/talks/show?id=627338

# AFTERWORD

## The Future of Public Health and the Law: Reducing the Racial Equity Gap

*We do know that health inequities at their very core are due to racism .... There's no doubt about that. As a Black man, my status, my suit and tie don't protect me.*

DR. GEORGES BENJAMIN, executive director of the
American Public Health Association (Vestal, 2020)

At the heart of this text is a focus on health equity and the role of law in protecting and promoting public health. Our goal was to present a text that not only provides a comprehensive, user-friendly overview of foundational and interventional public health law, but also highlights ways in which public health practices, policies, and laws impact health equity and health disparities.

As this book goes to press, this goal seems even more relevant and urgent than ever before. On January 30, 2020, the World Health Organization (WHO) declared the relentless coronavirus disease, COVID-19, a Public Health Emergency of International Concern (Gostin et al., 2020). Several months later, on May 25, 2020, the world watched in horror for 8 minutes and 46 seconds as George Floyd was killed by law enforcement officers on camera. In the middle of the COVID-19 pandemic, Americans organized protests, marches, demonstrations, and petitions advocating for systemic changes to protect and uplift the livelihood of America's most vulnerable populations.

While some have only one pandemic to grapple with, Black Americans are facing a double burden: the disproportionate impact of COVID-19 and systemic, structural racism. While this double burden is not new to the minority experience, it is perhaps the first time since the civil rights protests of the 1960s that Black American voices are getting a place on the international stage (Anderson, 2003). It is becoming clearer to people that although the law may have changed since the 1960s, so much of how laws are implemented and enforced has not.

Events like the killing of George Floyd—of Breonna Taylor, Manuel Ellis, James Spurlock, Ahmaud Arbery, Rashard Brooks, and on and on—have triggered in many in the Black American community a feeling of exhaustion, helplessness, anger, and hopelessness. Much of the media and political response to these events have not been trauma-informed. Trauma-informed messaging recognizes that traumatic experiences and their mental and emotional impacts tie closely into behavioral health problems. Much of what we saw on our social media feeds and on the news retraumatized us and others with histories of racism and discrimination-related traumas. According to one study, within a week of George Floyd's death, anxiety and depression among Black Americans were higher than any other racial or ethnic group (Fowers & Wan, 2020).

These mental health statistics, coupled with the disproportionate burden of illness and death among Black Americans from COVID-19 (Millett et al., 2020), provide evidence of what many Black Americans in public health have been saying and what research has shown—*structural racism is a public health issue*. Racism structures opportunity and assigns value based on skin color, resulting in conditions that unfairly advantage some and unfairly disadvantage others. "Racism hurts the health of our nation by preventing some people the opportunity to attain their highest level of health" (Burak, 2020). We cannot reach our goals of health equity without addressing racism.

Studies show that the racism and discrimination that Black Americans experience in our daily lives create stress that affects our internal organs and overall physical health (Smedley, 2012). This results in a higher prevalence of chronic diseases such as high blood pressure, asthma, and diabetes, as well as a shorter life span. Considering maternal and child health, according to a 2019 study by the U.S. Department of Health and Human Services (DHHS) Office of Minority Health, we also know that in the Black population:

- Infant mortality is 2.3 times higher than in non-Hispanic Whites;
- Infants are 3.8 times as likely to die from complications related to low birth weight as compared to non-Hispanic White infants;
- The sudden infant death syndrome (SIDS) mortality rate is over twice that of non-Hispanic Whites; and
- Mothers are 2.3 times more likely than non-Hispanic White mothers to receive late or no prenatal care.

Healthcare is just one area where racism and discrimination impact health outcomes. The reality, as seen throughout this text, is that healthcare, access, and delivery determines only about 25% of our health. The remaining 75% of what determines our health, as a population, is our total environment or ecology—this includes the social environment in which we live, work, learn, play, worship, and age (Hood et al., 2016). These social determinants of health result in upstream challenges related to, for example, limited income opportunities, lack of quality childcare, inferior schools, less safe neighborhoods, unstable housing, limited legal and social support, limited access to healthy food, poor access to transportation, and fewer community recreational facilities. The downstream effects include disproportionate rates of heart disease, stroke, cancer, diabetes, respiratory conditions, obesity, arthritis, pedestrian fatalities, and more (Merck, 2018).

This means that racial health disparities are not just the result of disparate access and treatment in the realm of healthcare. As Will Jawando, a Montgomery County (Maryland) council member, said, "whether it is police-involved killings or disparate health outcomes where [Black-American] patients can't get treatment because they are not seen as being sick, or financial redlining in certain ZIP codes, food deserts, or people of color getting hit by cars more often because their communities aren't walkable—it's all ultimately due to racism" (Vestal, 2020). Impacting infectious disease, this systemic racism has led to rapidly expanding inequity amidst the COVID-19 pandemic, impacting both risk of infection and chances of survival (Mosley & Hagan, 2020).

As we hope this book has effectively highlighted, when you consider most public health issues and conditions, you will find striking disparities and health inequities based on determinants of health that are driven by race. Racial disparities are not the result of individual behaviors or lack of adherence to medical and healthcare guidance (Associated Press, 2020). They are the result of deeply embedded structural racism that exists across all segments of our society—from our courthouses to our hospitals, from our schools to our workplaces.

My interest in racial health disparities is personal and professional. My first professional publication, almost 20 years ago, was a section in a book chapter where I wrote about lead poisoning, health disparities, and the law. That work opened my eyes up to how law can be used to limit exposure to a toxic substance and how implementing public health laws can positively impact health outcomes. Yet, I also learned that while these laws helped reduce the number of lead-poisoned children, this reduction served to highlight significant, continued, racial disparities in lead exposure. Even though fewer children are poisoned by lead, there are still more non-White kids with lead poisoning. The question for me was—and still is—why?

I have learned that the answer to that question is complex and involves the myriad upstream and downstream factors mentioned earlier. But resolving the problem of racial health inequities through public health law necessarily involves acknowledging that race is a critical social determinant of health. Perhaps it is even *the* most significant determinant of health.

There is an old African proverb that says that the child who is not embraced by the warmth of the village will burn it down to feel its warmth. The protests that followed George Floyd's death have been a visual depiction of this proverb in real-time. The seemingly continuous killing of unarmed Black people—right in the middle of a pandemic that has had a dramatically disparate impact on Black and Brown communities—continues to serve as a painful reminder that, for many Black Americans, belonging in this country is conditional. These events reminded many of us that far too often we do not feel the warmth of the laws and legal protections outlined in our country's founding documents, including those protections contemplated in foundational public health laws. These events also signaled to the nation that our health, our lives, our existence depend on foundational, sustainable change at the individual, community, and systemic level. If we want to see a change in the racial health equity gap, the status quo will not work. Public health law can play a role to reverse hundreds of years of racism that is built into the core of our country.

More than 200 U.S. jurisdictions (cities, counties, and states) have heard this call and declared racism a public health issue (Singh, 2020). These declarations are meant to catalyze change across all sectors of government and engender impact across all social determinants of health—criminal justice, education, healthcare, housing, transportation, budgets, taxes, economic development, and social services—all toward the goal of shrinking the health gap between Black Americans and the rest of the population.

This policy approach underscores the fact that the law itself is also a critical social determinant of health. Laws and regulations, how they are enforced, against whom they are enforced, and the structural frameworks they create have a profound effect on public health. The racism built into our system of laws, structures, and institutions has resulted in a system that significantly limits the access that Black Americans have to the services and conditions required to be healthy.

Even as states, cities, and counties declare racism as a public health issue, it will take more than a declaration or words on paper to see real change. We already have a lot of really good words on paper that say that discrimination is illegal. You have read about many of them in the pages of this textbook. So, naming the problem is a good first start. As Gary LeRoy, president of the American Academy of Family Physicians, stated, "the elimination of health disparities will not be achieved without first acknowledging racism's contribution to health and social inequalities" (LeRoy, 2020). But, it is *just a start*. The reality is that without financial resources, mandates, or a prescription for action written into law, it will be difficult to get to the meaningful, comprehensive, systemic change that is needed.

It cannot just be talk or words on paper. It is time for action. It is time for public health practitioners to identify and work to overcome conscious and unconscious bias in our research, our practices, and our policies. It is time to balance public health leadership across race and gender. The next generation of public health, social services, and healthcare practitioners—the readers of this book—is being called upon to lead this charge.

Leading this charge involves accepting that creating policies and programs that address the social determinants of health, health equity, or health disparities will do little to address the racial health equity gap without addressing structural, systemic racism. Looking at the social determinants, health equity, and health disparities through a lens that does not consider racism and discrimination, and that does not adequately name, define, or consider the effects of racism and discrimination—as has been our practice in the field—does very little to mitigate racial health disparities and has the potential to worsen existing health disparities. By focusing on structural racism in public health, you are not privileging Black people nor other people of color over other vulnerable groups. To the contrary, by understanding how racism works in our society, you can better understand the legal, structural, and economic gaps that harm all kinds of vulnerable populations. This understanding is critically important to reducing the health equity gap.

As the future of public health and public health law, it is your responsibility to use all of the tools in the public health toolbox, including foundational and interventional public health laws, to address the injustices caused by racism so that we can close the health equity gap. It is your responsibility to learn about and use tools like legal epidemiology to study the impact of our laws on public health and, more specifically, the impact of these laws and legal structures on the health of Black Americans and other people of color. This means that you will have to do more than just evaluate and understand how laws create the conditions that have a negative impact on health. You will need to be prepared to step into the muddy waters of public health advocacy around issues that fall outside of the traditional domain of public health. Policymakers do not allocate resources or implement regulations to address inequities because of their reliance on sound data (legal epidemiological or otherwise). They respond to social movements, to economic implications, to pressure. As the next generation of public health leaders, you are being asked to reimagine the discipline of public health and what it asks of us, in a post-COVID world.

The field, and the health of the public, needs this of you if we are to realize the hope that is at the core of the mission of public health: "fulfilling society's interest in assuring conditions in which people can be healthy" (Institute of Medicine (U.S.) Committee for the Study of the Future of Public Health, 1988). Not just some people, but all people.

Our hope is that the information shared in this text supports you toward that end.

MONTRECE MCNEILL RANSOM, JD, MPH

## REFERENCES

Anderson, C. (2003). *Eyes off the prize: The United Nations and the African American struggle for human rights, 1944–1955.* Cambridge University Press.

Associated Press. (2020, June 11). *Ohio lawmaker, an ER doctor, asks if hygiene is why 'colored' people get COVID-19.* https://www.latimes.com/world-nation/story/2020-06-11/senator-asks-if-hygiene -is-reason-colored-people-get-virus

Burak, E. W. (2020, June 2). We need to name it: Racism is a public health crisis. *Georgetown University Health Policy Institute Center for Children and Families.* https://ccf.georgetown.edu/2020/06/02/ we-need-to-name-it-racism-is-a-public-health-crisis

Fowers, A., & Wan, W. (2020, June 12). Depression and anxiety spiked among Black Americans after George Floyd's death. *Washington Post.* https://www.washingtonpost.com/health/2020/06/12/ mental-health-george-floyd-census

Gostin, L. O., Habibi, R., & Meier, B. M. (2020, May 10). Has global health law risen to meet the COVID-19 challenge? Revisiting the international health regulations to prepare for future threats. *Journal of Law, Medicine and Ethics, 48,* 376–381. http://doi.org/10.2139/ssrn.3598165

Hood, C. M., Gennuso, K. P., Swain, G. R., & Catlin, B. B. (2016). County health rankings: Relationships between determinant factors and health outcomes. *American Journal of Preventive Medicine, 50*(2), 129–135. https://doi.org/10.1016/j.amepre.2015.08.024

Institute of Medicine (U.S.) Committee for the Study of the Future of Public Health. (1988). *The future of public health: Summary and recommendations.* National Academies Press (U.S.). https://www .ncbi.nlm.nih.gov/books/NBK218215

LeRoy, G. (2020, May 31). *AAFP condemns all forms of racism.* https://www.aafp.org/media-center/releases-statements/all/2020/aafp-condemns-all-forms-of-racism.html

Merck, A. (2018, October 8). *The upstream-downstream parable for health equity.* https://salud-america.org/the-upstream-downstream-parable-for-health-equity

Millett, G. A., Jones, A. T., Benkeser, D., Baral, S., Mercer, L., Beyrer, C., Honermann, B., Lankiewicz, E., Mena, L., Crowley, J. S., Sherwood, J., & Sullivan, P. (2020). Assessing differential impacts of COVID-19 on Black communities. *Annals of Epidemiology, 47,* 37–44. https://doi.org/10.1016/j.annepidem.2020.05.003

Mosley, T., & Hagan, A. (2020, June 22). *California surgeon general: Systemic racism is linked to COVID-19 pandemic.* WBUR. https://www.wbur.org/hereandnow/2020/06/22/california-surgeon-general-covid-19-racism

Singh, M. (2020, June 12). 'Long overdue': Lawmakers declare racism a public health emergency. *The Guardian.* https://www.apha.org/topics-and-issues/health-equity/racism-and-health/racism-declarations

Smedley, B. D. (2012). The lived experience of race and its health consequences. *American Journal of Public Health, 102*(5), 933–935. https://doi.org/10.2105/AJPH.2011.300643

Vestal, C. (2020, June 15). *Racism is a public health crisis, say cities and counties.* Pew Trusts. https://pew.org/2AsZVRC

# GLOSSARY

**Administrative agency:** "An organization within the executive branch government, with the authority to implement and administer legislation" (Change Lab, 2020). (Chapter 4)

**AFAB:** Assigned female at birth. (Chapter 15)

**AMAB:** Assigned male at birth. (Chapter 15)

**Americans With Disability Act (ADA):** A federal law, passed in 1990, that prohibits discrimination against people with certain disabilities. (Chapter 10)

**ASAB:** Assigned sex at birth; the sex assigned to a child when born, which is based on primary sex characteristics and chromosomes. (Chapter 15)

**Bleach poisoning:** The chlorine in bleach can poison individuals if overexposed. Bleach poisoning can occur from injection, inhalation through the nose or mouth, or ingestion if the chlorine is in liquid form. (Chapter 5)

**Built environment:** Those environments that are man-made or -modified, including homes, schools, workplaces, highways, urban sprawl, and various mobile and stationary sources of air pollution. (Chapter 13)

**Case Law:** Law made by the judiciary. Case law refers to collection of decisions made by courts that establish authority on a particular topic. (Chapter 1)

**Ceiling preemption:** When a higher level government prohibits lower level governments from requiring anything more than or different from what the higher level law requires. (Chapter 3)

**Chronic disease:** Conditions that last 1 year or more and require ongoing medical attention and/or limit activities of daily living. (Chapter 8)

**Cisgender:** A category for persons whose gender identity aligns with their sex assigned at birth. (Chapter 15)

**Cisnormativity:** Systemic prejudice that assumes most people are cisgender and works in favor of cisgender people. (Chapter 15)

**Civil Law:** The area of law that allows for actions brought to enforce, redress, or protect private rights. (Chapter 21)

**Climate change:** Climate change is defined by *National Geographic* as the long-term alteration of temperature and typical weather patterns in a place. The World Health Organization argues that climate change threatens good health, including clean air, safe drinking water, food supply, and safe shelter. (Chapter 13)

**Clinical healthcare ethics:** A systematic framework to evaluate the conduct and integrity of healthcare professionals providing clinical healthcare. (Chapter 20)

**Collaborative practice agreements:** Formal, written relationships between healthcare providers that allow for certain expanded services for patients and the healthcare team. (Chapter 8)

**Command and control regulation:** The direct regulation in an industry or activity that states what is permitted and what is illegal. (Chapter 13)

**Community health worker:** A trusted member of (and/or someone who has an unusually close understanding of) the community served, and who serves as a link between health and social services and the community to facilitate access to services and improve the quality and cultural competence of service delivery. (Chapter 8)

**Community-clinical linkages:** Connections between community and clinical sectors to improve population health. (Chapter 8)

**Consent:** When all partners freely choose, with clear understanding, to engage in a specific activity at the moment the activity will take place. (Chapter 9)

**Cooperative federalism:** A form of government in which federal, state, and local governments interact cooperatively and collectively to solve common problems. (Chapters 2 and 8); An assignment of responsibility from one level of government to another, sometimes with funding to meet the assigned responsibilities. (Chapter 1)

**Cordon sanitaire:** The restriction of movement of people into or out of a defined geographic area. (Chapter 7)

**Criminal Law:** The area of law that pertains to or relates to crimes, or the administration of penal justice, or which relates to or has the character of crime. (Chapters 2 and 8)

**Delegation:** Powers and authority granted from one governmental entity to another (Gostin & Wiley, 2016). (Chapter 4)

**Delegation of authority:** Division of authority and powers downward to the subordinate levels of government. (Chapter 2)

**Determinants of health:** The range of personal, social, economic, and environmental factors that influence health status. (Chapter 17)

**Dialysis:** A treatment for when a person's kidneys fail to perform certain natural functions. Dialysis treatment helps to remove waste, salt, and extra water from the body as well as regulate certain necessary chemicals in the person's blood such as potassium and sodium. (Chapter 5)

**Dillon's Rule:** Express grants of authority to local governments; grants of authority to local governments are specific and should be narrowly interpreted. (Chapter 1)

**Discretionary authority:** Power or authority to take or not take action. (Chapter 21)

**Disease reporting:** An ongoing and systematic collection of health data specifically related to incidence of infectious diseases; is accomplished by state, Tribal, local, and territorial public health agencies employing mandatory notification requirements when a disease case of public health concern is identified. (Chapter 7)

**Due process:** Fair treatment through the normal judicial system, especially as a citizen's entitlement. (Chapter 7)

**Duty to warn:** The legal obligation to warn people of a danger. (Chapter 21)

**Eliminated:** Absence of naturally occurring cases and continued transmission of an infectious disease in a certain geographical area for at least 12 months. (Chapter 6)

**Emergency declaration:** A legal designation vested in federal, state, Tribal, local, or territorial executive branch officials authorizing the use of optional and expedited public health powers relating to individuals, groups, or property during exigencies. (Chapter 11)

**Emergency liability protection:** A limitation on exposure to civil or criminal liability or penalties for actions taken during or in response to a public health emergency. (Chapter 11)

**EMR/EHR:** Electronic medical or health records; A digital or online version of patient health information. (Chapter 15)

**Enabling Act:** Legislation passed at the federal or state level granting specific authority to an administrative agency to act for a specific purpose (Gostin & Wiley, 2016). (Chapter 4)

**Enumerated powers:** Specific powers granted to Congress by the U.S. Constitution. (Chapter 2)

**Environmental Law:** Regulations, statutes, local, national, and international legislation, and treaties designed to protect the environment from damage and to explain the legal consequences of such damage toward governments or private entities or individuals. (Chapter 13)

**Environmental Public Health Law:** Environmental laws that affect health by limiting exposures to disease-causing agents, targeting unhealthy features of the environment, influencing the creation and maintenance of community spaces for physical activity, and regulating the use and disposal of harmful industrial materials like lead. (Chapter 13)

**Epidemic:** Disease occurrence in excess of the expected levels in a certain geographical area or specific population. (Chapter 6)

**Equal protection:** Refers to the idea that a governmental body may not deny people equal protection of its governing laws. The governing body must treat an individual in the same manner as others in similar conditions and circumstances. (Chapter 7); the government must treat an individual in the same manner as others in similar conditions and circumstances. (Chapter 2)

**Eradicated:** Complete, worldwide end of an infectious disease so that no additional transmission of the disease occurs. (Chapter 6)

**Erin's Law:** Requires that all public schools in each state where it is mandated implement child sexual abuse prevention programming. (Chapter 9)

**Ethical framework:** A tool or process for evaluating and resolving an ethical problem. (Chapter 20)

**Ethics:** A systematic examination and application of moral principles held by a society. (Chapter 20)

**Executive order:** Legally binding directives issued by a president, governor, or other leader of an executive branch. (Chapter 1)

**Executive Branch:** The branch of government that executes and enforces law. (Chapter 1)

**Express preemption:** When a law explicitly states that it preempts lower level lawmaking authority. (Chapter 3)

**Federal Indian Law:** The body of law governing the rights, relationships, and responsibilities of Tribes, states, and the federal government. (Fletcher, 2016, § 3). (Chapter 14)

**Federal Tort Claims Act:** A 1946 federal statute that permits private parties to sue the United States in federal court for most torts committed by persons acting on behalf of the United States. (Chapter 5)

**Federalism:** A system of governance where a jurisdiction is governed equally by two levels of government. (Chapters 1, 6, and 16); The legal structure which governs the distribution and allocation of powers between the federal and state governments in the United States (Gostin & Wiley, 2016; Hodge, 2016). (Chapter 4)

**Federalist system:** A system of government in which power is distributed between national and regional governmental bodies with differing responsibilities. In the United States, the federalist system encompasses the distribution of power between the federal government and state governments. (Chapter 11)

**Field preemption:** When a higher level government prohibits lower level governments from passing or enforcing any laws on an issue, reserving the entire area (the field) of regulation to itself. (Chapter 3)

**Floor preemption:** When a higher level government passes a law that establishes a minimum set of requirements and allows lower level governments to pass and enforce laws that impose more rigorous requirements. (Chapter 3)

**Gender expression:** The physical (e.g., clothing, hair style), behavioral (e.g., mannerisms, vocal intonation), and relational (e.g., pronouns, chosen name) ways in which someone expresses their gender and engages with others to have their gender seen. (Chapter 15)

**Gender identity:** An individual's internal sense of self, which may be a man or transgender man, woman or transgender woman, nonbinary (e.g., genderqueer, genderfluid, agender), or another gender. It is crucial to note the distinction of gender from sex, which is rooted in biological indicators (e.g., primary sex characteristics and chromosomes). (Chapter 15)

**Global health:** Addressing public health in a globalizing world, global health looks beyond the efforts of individual nations to encompass the larger set of determinants that affect the health of the entire world. (Chapter 12) Global health recognizes that all countries face interconnected public health threats, requiring collective global action to improve health and achieve equity in health for all people worldwide. (Chapter 12)

**Global Health Law:** Global health law describes legal frameworks that structure global public health. These frameworks encompass the legal institutions, processes, and instruments—both hard and soft law—that support global health and shape how a vast landscape of state and non-state actors engage in disease prevention and health promotion. This legal engagement is anchored in the fundamental premise that, in a globalizing world, threats to public health increasingly transcend national frontiers and require cross-border coordination. (Chapter 12)

**Gross negligence:** A severe degree of negligence taken as reckless disregard. Blatant indifference to one's legal duty, others' safety, or their rights. (Chapter 21)

**Health equity:** Refers to the attainment of the highest level of health for all people or means striving for the highest possible standard of health for all people and focusing on the needs of those at greatest risk for poor health, due to their social conditions. (Chapter 13); the idea that everyone should have an equal opportunity to reach their maximum potential in terms of health. Achieving health equity requires removing barriers to achieving good health, especially for underserved and marginalized communities. (Chapters 8 and 16); when all have a fair chance to reach their health potential and when health potential is not impeded by social factors or positions. (Chapter 18)

**Health Impact Assessment (HIA):** A systematic process that uses research, data, analysis, and stakeholder feedback to determine the possible health effects and their distribution of a policy, project, or plan and to recommend ways to maximize health. (Chapters 13 and 18)

**Health in All Policies (HiAP):** A systematic approach to incorporate health concerns across decisions that normally do not consider health but nevertheless have health consequences. (Chapter 18)

**Health inequities:** Differences in health that are socially produced, systemic, and unfair. (Chapter 17)

**Healthy housing/home:** Housing that is designed, constructed, maintained, and rehabilitated in a manner that is conducive to good occupant health. (Chapter 13)

**Herd immunity:** A form of indirect protection of a community from an infectious disease that occurs when a large enough percentage of a population has become immune to an infection, thus providing a measure of protection for individuals who are not immune. This may also be referred to as "community immunity." (Chapter 6)

**Heteronormativity:** Systemic prejudice that assumes most people are heterosexual and works in favor of heterosexual/straight people. (Chapter 15)

**Home Rule:** The degree of autonomy a local government can exercise. In home rule states local authority exists so long as it is not expressly restricted by the state. (Chapters 1 and 3)

**I/T/U:** The three-tiered healthcare delivery system that includes Indian Health Service facilities, Tribal health programs, and urban Indian health centers. (Chapter 14)

**Immunization:** The process by which a person is made immune to an infectious disease. Sometimes this term is used interchangeably with "vaccination." (Chapter 6)

**Immutable characteristic:** An immutable characteristic is a physical attribute that is perceived as being unchangeable, entrenched, and innate. (Chapter 2)

**Implied preemption:** When a law passed by a higher-level government contains no explicit preemption-related language but is nevertheless found to preempt the authority of a lower-level government. (Chapter 3)

**Inherent authority:** The innate authority of Tribes as sovereigns to govern their people and lands. (Chapter 14)

**Intermediate determinants of health:** The places where people live and work. (Chapter 17)

**International Health Law:** The traditional approach to the application and use of international law to address public health challenges that is driven solely by relationships among states. Historically, international health law structured multilateral cooperation (across multiple states) under international law to respond to public health threats. As compared to global health law, international health law does not include nonstate actors and does not necessarily focus on the promotion of social justice in public health. (Chapter 12)

**International Health Regulations (IHR):** The IHR are an international legal agreement that aims to prevent, detect, control and provide a public health response to the international spread of disease. Overseen by the World Health Organization (WHO) and last revised in 2005, this legal instrument enshrines a broad range of state obligations, including the requirement that states build core public health capacities, that they maintain public health responses that are commensurate with the risk to human health, and that they acknowledge and act cooperatively in accordance with WHO guidance (Chapter 12).

**International Human Rights Law:** Comprises the area of international law focused on legal standards to address basic needs and frame necessary entitlements to uphold a universal moral vision for the advancement of dignity and justice. As a basis for global justice, international human rights standards and obligations frame government responsibilities and facilitate legal accountability to realize the highest attainable standard of health for all. (Chapter 12)

**International Law:** Law that is developed between national governments (states) in written form, whether embodied in a single treaty or related instruments, and is legally binding on governments. When governments seek to cooperate with other countries to confront a common health threat, international law often becomes central to crafting a coordinated approach. (Chapter 12)

**Isolation:** Separates a person or group of persons known to be contagious with a communicable disease from others who are not sick to prevent disease transmission. (Chapter 7); The physical confinement and separation of an individual/groups who are reasonably believed or known to be infected with a contagious/possibly contagious disease from non-isolated individuals/groups, to limit transmission of the disease. (Chapter 11)

**Judicial Branch:** The branch of government that adjudicates disputes and interprets law. (Chapter 1)

**Judicial review:** Courts' review of an executive agency' actions when an aggrieved party files a lawsuit to challenge a newly promulgated regulation or issuance of a public health order. (Chapters 1 and 4)

**Jurisdiction:** The area over which a government, court, or other legal entity can exercise its power. (Chapter 1)

**Law:** Unless otherwise specified, law includes statutes, regulations, municipal ordinances, judicial opinions, at the federal, state, local, Tribal, and territorial levels. (Chapter 17)

**Legal epidemiology:** The scientific study and deployment of law as a factor in the cause, distribution, and prevention of disease and injury in a population. (Chapter 19)

**Legal ethics:** A systematic framework to evaluate the conduct of attorneys in representing clients, primarily using a state's legal "Rules of Professional Conduct." (Chapter 20)

**Legislative Branch:** The branch of government that creates law. (Chapter 1)

**Legislative Process:** The process by which legislation is proposed and potentially passed. (Chapter 1)

**LGBTQ:** The acronym for the community of lesbian, gay, bisexual, transgender, queer, and additional sexual and gender minorities. (Chapter 15)

**Life course approach:** The interaction of biological, behavioral, psychological, social, and environmental factors impacting health outcomes throughout the course of an individual's life. (Chapter 16)

**Life course vaccination:** The concept that vaccination provides protection and health benefits to people throughout their lives, at different stages and circumstances. (Chapter 6)

**Litigation:** Criminal or civil actions in a court of law; using legal processes in courts of law to resolve disputes. (Chapter 1)

**Mandated reporter:** A person who, because of their profession, is legally required to report any suspicion of child abuse or neglect to the relevant authorities. (Chapter 9)

**Medicaid:** A federal healthcare program jointly financed by state governments established in 1965 through an amendment to the Social Security Act of 1935 to provide health insurance coverage for low-income people. (Chapter 8)

**Medications for opioid use disorder:** Prescription medications that have been shown to reduce the negative impacts of opioid use disorder. There are currently three such medications approved by the Federal Drug Association: buprenorphine, methadone, and naltrexone. (Chapter 10)

**Model State Emergency Health Powers Act:** A model act drafted with national input by the Centers for Law and the Public's Health at Georgetown and Johns Hopkins Universities in 2001 that provides a menu of model emergency powers and authorities that adopting states or other governments can use to define, declare, and respond to public health emergencies. (Chapter 11)

**Morals:** Standards of behavior or beliefs about what is right and what is wrong. (Chapter 20)

**Mutual aid agreement:** A compact formed between two or more governmental entities (e.g., states, Tribes, localities, and territories) to share personnel and materials in the event of an emergency or disaster. (Chapter 11)

**Naloxone:** A medication that reverses the respiratory depression and other physical symptoms associated with opioid overdose. (Chapter 10)

**Negligence:** In the legal context, a failure to behave with reasonable care that someone of ordinary prudence would have exercised under the same or similar circumstances. (Chapter 5); A failure to behave with the level of care that someone of ordinary prudence would have exercised under the same or similar circumstances. The behavior usually consists of actions but can also consist of omissions when there is a duty to act. (Chapter 21)

**Nonbinary:** A collection of genders that are not exclusively a man/masculine or woman/ feminine, including genderqueer, gender fluid, and agender.

**Nonpharmaceutical interventions (NPIs)** are actions, apart from getting vaccinated and taking medicine, that people and communities can take to help slow. (Chapter 7)

**Norms:** Rules or expectations that are socially enforced.. (Chapter 20)

**Nuisance:** Condition, activity, or situation (e.g., a loud noise or foul odor) that interferes with the use or enjoyment of property; especially a nontransitory condition or persistent activity that either injures the physical condition of adjacent land or interferes with its use or with the enjoyment of easements on the land or of public highways (Black's Law Dictionary, 9th Ed.). (Chapter 13)

**Obesity:** Overweight and obesity are both labels for ranges of weight that are greater than what is generally considered healthy for a given height. (Chapter 5)

**Opioid:** A substance used to treat moderate to severe pain. (Chapters 5 and 10)

**Ordinance:** An example of a local law passed by a county or municipal government. (Chapter 1)

**Outbreak:** Appearance of a disease within a geographic area or among a specific population. (Chapter 6)

**Overdose Good Samaritan Laws:** Laws that shield someone from being arrested or prosecuted for certain charges if they summon emergency assistance for a suspected overdose. In many cases, these protections also apply to the person who overdosed. (Chapter 10)

**Pandemic:** An epidemic occurring worldwide, or over a very wide area, crossing international boundaries, and usually affecting a large number of people.

**Patient Protection and Affordable Care Act of 2010 (ACA):** A federal healthcare law enacted in 2010 to ensure affordable health insurance coverage, expand the Medicaid program, and support innovative healthcare delivery models. (Chapter 8)

**Police powers:** Inherent authority that allows states to promote general welfare within their boundaries (Chapter 1); The intrinsic authority to exercise reasonable control over persons and property to promote the health, safety, welfare, and morals of the public. (Chapter 2)

**Policy surveillance:** The systematic, scientific collection and analysis of laws of public health significance (Chapter 19)

**Preemption:** A legal doctrine that provides that a higher level government may limit, or even eliminate, the power of a lower level government to regulate a certain issue. (Chapter 3); legal theory in which a higher authority of law will displace the law of a lower authority of law when the two authorities conflict. (Chapter 6); the law of a "higher" level of government overrides the law of a lower jurisdiction. (Chapter 1); The legal notion that laws created at a higher level of government override the laws created at lower levels of government. Higher levels of government may also specifically reserve powers to legislate in a subject area even where they are silent in that area (Hodge, 2016). (Chapter 4)

**Prima facie:** This is a Latin term meaning "at first sight." In the context of law and ethics, however, it refers to evidence or information that on its face or at first review appear to sufficiently provide a complete argument. Such prima facie evidence would be taken as fact, but subject to rebuttal or counter argument. (Chapter 20)

**Procedural due process:** Procedural due process is the constitutional requirement that when the government acts in such a way that denies a person a life, liberty, or property interest, the person must be given notice, the opportunity to be heard, and a decision by a neutral decision-maker. (Chapter 2)

**Professional code of ethics:** A written expression of the moral norms (including principles, virtues, and values) that guide and ground behavior by members of a profession in carrying out their professional roles. (Chapter 20)

**Promulgate:** To publish; to announce officially; to make [a law whether statutory or administrative] public as important or obligatory. (Chapters 4 and 13); The process by which an agency puts forth and files an administrative rule. (Chapter 4)

**Public Health Emergency of International Concern (PHEIC):** An extraordinary event that is determined, as provided in the IHR: (1) to constitute a public health risk to other states through the international spread of disease and (2) to potentially require a coordinated international response. Where the WHO director-general has declared a PHEIC, this triggers greater international coordination through the WHO, facilitating the coordinated exchange of information for enhanced risk assessment and response across stakeholders. (Chapter 12)

**Public health ethics:** A systematic framework to evaluate the conduct and integrity of public health practitioners and researchers in implementing, evaluating, complying with, and enforcing public health laws, policies, and programs. (Chapter 20)

**Public health surveillance:** "The ongoing, systematic collection, analysis, and interpretation of health data, essential to the planning, implementation and evaluation of public health practice, closely integrated with the dissemination of these data to those who need to know and linked to prevention and control." (Thacker, 1992) (Chapter 7)

**Punitive preemption:** When a state government not only preempts local laws on a subject but also punishes local officials and local governments that attempt to enact or enforce preempted laws. (Chapter 3)

**Qualified immunity:** Protects public officials from being sued for damages unless they violated "clearly established" law of which a reasonable official in their position would have known. (Chapter 21)

**Quarantine:** Separates and restricts the movement of a person or group of persons who were exposed to a contagious disease to see if they become sick. (Chapters 7 and 11)

**Rape:** Penetration, no matter how slight, of the vagina or anus with any body part or object, or oral penetration by a sex organ of another person, without the consent of the victim. (Chapter 9)

**Regulation:** Legally binding instruments made by agencies (Chapter 1); A rule promulgated by an administrative agency with the binding effect of law (Koyuncu, 2008) (Chapter 4)

**Reproductive health:** A state of complete physical, mental, and social well-being, not merely the absence of disease or infirmity, in all matters relating to the reproductive system and to its functions and processes. It is focused on the availability and accessibility of healthcare services, facilities, and research that impact reproductive and sexual health. (Chapter 16)

**Reproductive justice:** Reproductive justice links reproductive rights with the social, political, and economic inequalities that affect a woman's ability to access reproductive healthcare services. It is focused on the ways in which persisting social inequalities mean that issues around access to reproductive healthcare have a greater impact on marginalized communities than privileged ones. (Chapter 16)

**Reproductive rights:** The idea that there are certain rights, recognized in and protected by law, founded in protections of privacy, bodily integrity, and personal autonomy. Focused on ensuring all people can exercise the right to make their own reproductive choices, including but not limited to, decisions around contraception and abortion. (Chapter 16)

**Rulemaking:** The process of interpreting legislative guidance found in a statute and promulgating new regulations. (Chapter 1)

**Scope of practice:** Roles and responsibilities that a healthcare provider is allowed to undertake within the scope of their professional license. (Chapter 8). The specific activities certain types of healthcare practitioners are authorized to perform, based on statutory, regulatory, licensure, or professional rules. (Chapters 6 and 11)

**SCOTUS:** Abbreviation for the Supreme Court of the United States. This is the highest federal court in the nation. (Chapter 16)

**Separation of powers:** A Separation of powers means vesting the legislative, executive, and judicial powers of government in separate bodies. (Chapter 2)

**Sexting:** Sending sexually explicit digital images, videos, text, and/or emails, usually sent through a mobile device. (Chapter 9)

**Sexual assault:** A nonconsensual sexual act proscribed by federal, Tribal, or state law, including when the victim lacks capacity to consent. (Chapter 9)

**Sexual battery:** An unwanted form of contact with an intimate part of the body that is made for purposes of sexual arousal, sexual gratification, or sexual abuse. (Chapter 9)

**Sexual violence:** Use of force or manipulation into unwanted sexual activity without consent. (Chapter 9)

**Social determinants of health:** The factors that affect the health of communities and populations (Chapter 17); Factors that impact a person's health. These may include biological, socioeconomic, psychosocial, environmental, behavioral, or social characteristics. (Chapter 16). Social factors, systems, and conditions created through choices that shape how resources and power are distributed and that affect health outcomes and can impede health equity. (Chapters 15 and 18)

**Social distancing measures:** Nonpharmaceutical interventions to prevent or slow the spread of communicable disease by restricting when, where, and how people gather together. (Chapter 7)

**Socioeconomic position:** Description of the access to resources and to power based on an individual's social position. (Chapter 17)

**Soft law:** A set of instruments that are not legally binding but that express or lead to commitments with legal implications – as seen in codes of conduct, voluntary resolutions, and global declarations. As compared with legally-binding hard law, soft law can be used, among other things, to reinforce legally-binding commitments, serve as the basis for the development of legally-binding instruments, and interpret norms set out by treaties. (Chapter 12)

**Sovereign immunity:** A government's protection from being sued in its own courts without its consent, including protection of governmental personnel from being held personally liable for acts related to their official duties. (Chapter 11)

**State:** Under international law, a state is an organized political community, a nation or territory under one government and capable of accepting binding obligations under international law. States are distinguished from non-state actors – non-governmental organizations, private businesses, and individual advocates that have power to effect change but are not bound by international law. A state that is bound by an international law is referred to as a "state party" to that law. (Chapter 12)

**Statute:** A law passed by a legislature and enacted through a constitutional process (Chapter 1)

**Statutory rape:** Sexual intercourse with a person under the age of lawful consent. (Chapter 9)

**Structural determinants of health:** The context, socioeconomic position of individuals, and the institutions and mechanisms that create and maintain stratifications that affect health. (Chapter 17)

**Substantive due process:** Substantive due process is the notion that due process not only protects certain legal procedures, but also protects certain fundamental human rights. (Chapter 2)

**Transdisciplinary model:** Melds legal and scientific facets of public health law to help break down enduring cultural, disciplinary, and resource barriers that have prevented the full recognition and optimal role of law in public health. (Burris S, Ashe M, Levin D, Penn M, &; Larkin M. A transdisciplinary approach to public health law: the emerging practice of legal epidemiology. Ann Rev Public Health. 2017;(37):135-148.) (Chapter 19)

**Transgender:** A category for persons whose gender identity does not align with their sex assigned at birth. This is an umbrella term to describe all gender-diverse individuals, although not all gender-diverse individuals may use this language. For example, some nonbinary individuals do not identify as transgender. (Chapter 15)

**Tribal consultation:** The requirement for federal agencies to consult with Tribes when taking actions that impact Tribes or American Indian and Alaska Native people. (Chapter 14)

**Tribal law:** The laws of each individual Tribe. (Chapter 14)

**Tribal set-aside:** Term used by federal agencies for funds allocated to American Indian/ Alaska Native (AI/AN) programs to differentiate from funding for programs available to all populations. (Chapter 14)

**Tribal sovereignty:** The right of Tribes to make their own laws and be ruled by them (*Williams v. Lee*, 1959). (Chapter 14)

**Trust responsibility:** The fiduciary and moral obligation of the federal government, based on treaties, agreements, case law, and statutes, to protect Tribal treaty rights, lands, and assets. (Chapter 14)

**Vaccination:** The act of introducing a killed or weakened organism into the body for the purpose of producing immunity to a specific disease. (Chapter 6)

**Vacuum preemption:** When a higher level government chooses not to enact any substantive regulations on a topic and forbids lower level governments from doing so, creating a regulatory vacuum. (Chapter 3)

**Vector-borne diseases:** Human illnesses caused by parasites, viruses, and bacteria that are transmitted by mosquitoes, sandflies, triatomine bugs, blackflies, ticks, tsetse flies, mites, snails, and lice. (Chapter 13)

**Wanton and willful misconduct:** Reckless disregard for others' safety and rights and knowing harm or injury may result. (Chapter 21)

**Zoning codes:** Local laws that designate areas for certain land uses, normally used for land planning; can designate areas for residential, industrial uses and can designate green space. (Chapter 13)

# INDEX

Printed in the United States
by Baker & Taylor Publisher Services